COLOR ATLAS OF
FARM ANIMAL DERMATOLOGY

CU00481454

COLOR ATLAS OF FARM ANIMAL DERMATOLOGY

DANNY W. SCOTT

Diplomate, American College of Veterinary Dermatology

Professor of Medicine

Department of Clinical Sciences and Department of Biomedical Sciences

College of Veterinary Medicine

Cornell University

Ithacca, New York

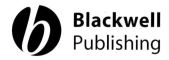

Blackwell Publishing Professional
2121 State Avenue, Ames, Iowa 50014, USA

Orders: 1-800-862-6657
Office: 1-515-292-0140
Fax: 1-515-292-3348
Web site: www.blackwellprofessional.com

Blackwell Publishing Ltd
9600 Garsington Road, Oxford OX4 2DQ, UK
Tel.: +44 (0)1865 776868

Blackwell Publishing Asia
550 Swanston Street, Carlton, Victoria 3053, Australia
Tel.: +61 (0)3 8359 1011

Authorization to photocopy items for internal or personal use, or the internal or personal use of specific
clients, is granted by Blackwell Publishing, provided that the base fee is paid directly to the Copyright
Clearance Center, 222 Rosewood Drive, Danvers, MA 01923. For those organizations that have been granted a
photocopy license by CCC, a separate system of payments has been arranged. The fee codes for users of the
Transactional Reporting Service are ISBN-13: 978-0-8138-0516-0/2007.

First edition, 2007

Library of Congress Cataloging-in-Publication Data

Scott, Danny W.
    Color atlas of farm animal dermatology / Danny W. Scott. — 1st ed.
       p.   ; cm.
    ISBN-13: 978-0-8138-0516-0 (alk. paper)
    ISBN-10: 0-8138-0516-3 (alk. paper)
    1. Livestock—Diseases—Atlases. 2. Skin—Diseases—Atlases. 3. Veterinary dermatology—Atlases. I. Title.
    [DNLM: 1. Skin Diseases—veterinary—Atlases. 2. Animals, Domestic—Atlases. 3. Skin Diseases—
    diagnosis—Atlases. SF 901 S425c 2006]

SF901.S37 2006
636.089′65—dc22

                                                                                           2006014702

The last digit is the print number: 9 8 7 6 5 4 3 2 1

This atlas is dedicated to my colleague and friend, Israel Yeruham, whose untimely death in 2005 left a huge void in the world of farm animal dermatology. Israel devoted much of his professional career to the recognition, reporting, and teaching of farm animal skin diseases. His work is liberally referenced in this atlas. Israel, thanx for all you did. I miss you. I look forward to seeing you again in the hereafter.

Danny Scott

CONTENTS

PREFACE AND ACKNOWLEDGEMENTS

For years veterinary students, practitioners, and Residents in Dermatology have asked me where to go to find concise information and color pictures of the skin diseases of farm ("food") animals: cattle, goats, sheep, and pigs. My answer was: "There ain't no such place."

To my knowledge, the only textbook ever devoted to the skin diseases of farm animals (it also included horses) was *Large Animal Dermatology*.[1] This book was published in 1988, and was mostly in black and white. My colleague and friend, Bill Miller, and I finally updated the equine portion in 2003.[2] Then people started asking me "When are you gonna write a new edition of *Large Animal Dermatology*?" My response was, and still is, "In my next lifetime." However, the idea of putting together an atlas of farm animal skin diseases—wherein color photographs and concise historical and physical information could be found in one place—appealed to me.

This, then, is my attempt to pull those aspects of the skin diseases of cattle, goats, sheep, and pigs together. A "short list" of reasonable differential diagnoses is provided. The essence of definitive diagnosis is presented. Therapy, prevention, and control are not addressed. The reader will have to dig into the references and current textbooks to pursue such information. The text is divided into four sections—bovine, caprine, ovine, and porcine—so that individuals interested in a particular species can dive right in. Because I did not have pictures of certain laboratory specimens from all four species, I have occasionally used the same photomicrograph of pus, the same louse, the same skin scraping, and so forth for multiple species. Oh, well. Ya know, at some level pus is pus and *Sarcoptes* is *Sarcoptes*.

Many of the diseases in this atlas are—from an American's viewpoint—foreign ("exotic"). I have had to draw upon the collections of many colleagues . . . and they have responded generously. If I have failed to acknowledge anyone for their contribution(s), please forgive me and let me know. I must single out two individuals for their many contributions. First, my colleague and friend Dr. Jean-Marie Gourreau (merci beaucoup, Jean-Marie, t'es ben super!). Second, my long-time friend and colleague, now deceased, Dr. Bill Rebhun (thanks for all those great years, Bill).

I would be remiss in my acknowledgements if I didn't specifically include two of my non-veterinary colleagues: Ray Kersey and Dede Anderson. Ray is a long-time friend and advisor from a former textbook and publisher. It was Ray that encouraged me to do this thing and to do it with Blackwell Publishing. Dede was my long-suffering editor on this project. We encountered and overcame big glitches, little glitches, and all kinda glitches in-between.

Lastly . . . but not leastly . . . thanx and so much more to my wife and soul-mate for the last 37 years, Kris: always there with the necessary encouragement, prodding, understanding, and love. Big smooch!

Hey vet students! Hey dermoids! You all are the best part of my career. Here's to you! Thanks!

Danny Scott
Ithaca, New York

1. Scott DW. 1988. Large Animal Dermatology. WB Saunders, Philadelphia, PA.

2. Scott DW, Miller WH. 2003. Equine Dermatology. Elsevier Science, St. Louis, MO.

REPORTABLE AND FOREIGN DISEASES

Many of the diseases presented in this atlas are infectious and pose serious threats to animal health and welfare. Some are transmissible to humans. Many are associated with huge economic losses and trade restrictions.

There are differences between countries and—in the United States—differences between states concerning which diseases are reportable. The following listing includes diseases that are officially reportable in New York state, and infectious diseases that currently do not occur in the United States (the appropriate authorities should be contacted when these are encountered).

Cattle
Anthrax
Besnoitiosis
Bluetongue
Bovine ephemeral fever
Bovine spongiform encephalopathy
Dermatophilosis
Foot-and-mouth disease
Hyalomma toxicosis
Lumpy skin disease
Malignant catarrhal fever (African)
Pseudorabies
Psoroptic mange
Rift Valley fever
Rinderpest
Sarcoptic mange
Screwworm
Theileriosis
Trypanosomiasis
Vesicular stomatitis

Goats
Anthrax
Bluetongue
Capripoxvirus infection

Foot-and-mouth disease
Peste des petits ruminants
Pseudorabies
Psoroptic mange
Rinderpest
Scrapie
Screwworm
Vesicular stomatitis

Sheep
Anthrax
Bluetongue
Capripoxvirus infection
Chorioptic mange
Foot-and-mouth disease
Peste des petits ruminants
Pseudorabies
Psoroptic mange
Rinderpest
Sarcoptic mange
Scrapie
Screwworm
Vesicular stomatitis

Swine
African swine fever
Anthrax
Classical swine fever
Erysipelas
Foot-and-mouth disease
Porcine respiratory and reproductive syndrome
Sarcoptic mange
Screwworm
Swine vesicular disease
Vesicular exanthema
Vesicular stomatitis

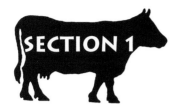

BOVINE

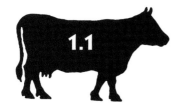

BACTERIAL SKIN DISEASES

IMPETIGO

Features

Impetigo (Latin: an attack; scabby eruption) is a superficial pustular dermatitis that does not involve hair follicles. It is common, cosmopolitan, and caused by *Staphylococcus aureus*, and predisposing factors include trauma, moisture, and the stress of parturition. Dairy breeds and lactating females are predisposed.

Lesions are most commonly seen on the udder (especially the base of the teats and the intramammary sulcus), teats, ventral abdomen, medial thighs, vulva, perineum, and ventral tail (Figs. 1.1-1 and 1.1-2). Superficial vesicles rapidly become pustular, rupture, and leave annular erosions and yellow-brown crusts.

Lesions are neither pruritic nor painful, and affected animals are otherwise healthy. Up to 48% of a herd may be affected. Staphylococcal mastitis is a possible, but uncommon complication.

Severe trauma (e.g., milking machine, laceration, crush) can lead to deeper staphylococcal infection—staphylococcal mammillitis. In such cases, ulceration, crusting, and variable degrees of necrosis are seen—usually affecting a solitary teat (Fig. 1.1-3).

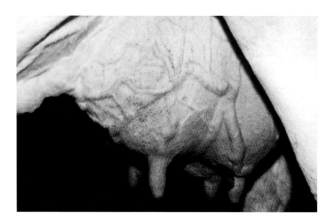

Figure 1.1-2 Impetigo. Pustules and erosions on the udder.

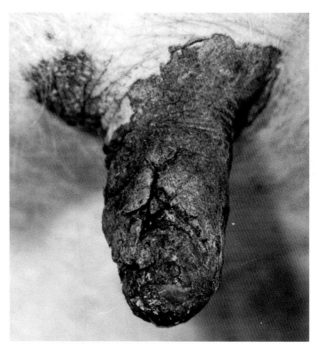

Figure 1.1-3 Staphylococcal Mammillitis. Ulceration, crusting, and necrosis due to milking machine trauma.

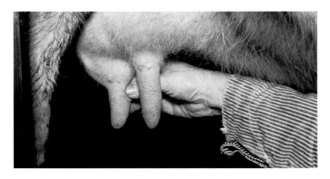

Figure 1.1-1 Impetigo. Superficial pustules on the base of the teats.

3

Occasional reports—often anecdotal—have indicated that humans can develop pustular dermatitis due to *S. aureus* infection on hands and arms that contact bovine impetigo lesions.

Differential Diagnosis

Other bacterial infections, dermatophilosis, dermatophytosis, stephanofilariasis, and viral infections.

Diagnosis

1. Microscopy (direct smears)—Suppurative inflammation with degenerate neutrophils, nuclear streaming, and phagocytosed cocci (Gram-positive, about 1 μm diameter, often in doublets or clusters) (see Figs. 1.1-8 and 1.1-9).
2. Culture (aerobic).
3. Dermatohistopathology—Subcorneal pustular dermatitis with degenerate neutrophils and intracellular cocci.

FOLLICULITIS AND FURUNCULOSIS

Features

Folliculitis (hair follicle inflammation) and furunculosis (hair follicle rupture) are uncommon, cosmopolitan, and caused by *Staphylococcus aureus* or less commonly *S. hyicus*, and predisposing factors include trauma and moisture. There are no apparent breed, sex, or age predilections.

Lesions can be seen anywhere, most commonly over the rump, tail, perineum, distal limbs, neck, and face (Figs. 1.1-4 to 1.1-7). Tufted papules become crusted, then alopecic. Intact pustules are often not seen. Furuncles are characterized by nodules, draining tracts, and ulcers. Lesions are rarely pruritic, but furuncles may be painful. Affected animals are usually otherwise healthy. Pending the inciting cause(s), single or multiple animals may be affected.

Differential Diagnosis

Dermatophilosis, dermatophytosis, demodicosis, stephanofilariasis, and sterile eosinophilic folliculitis and furunculosis.

Diagnosis

1. Microscopy (direct smears)—Suppurative inflammation with degenerate neutrophils, nuclear streaming, and phagocytosed

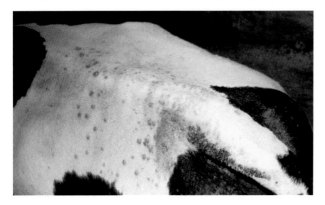

Figure 1.1-4 Staphylococcal Folliculitis. Multiple annular crusts over rump and tail.

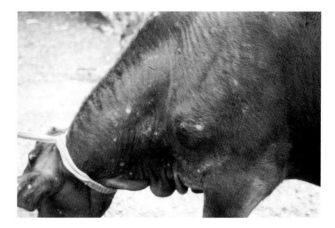

Figure 1.1-5 Staphylococcal Folliculitis and Furunculosis. Multiple tufted papules and annular areas of crusting, alopecia, and ulceration (courtesy J. Gourreau).

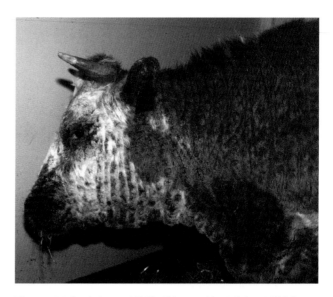

Figure 1.1-6 Staphylococcal Folliculitis caused by *S. hyicus*. Multiple annular crusts on face, neck, and shoulder (courtesy T. Clark).

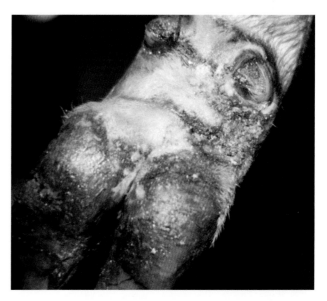

Figure 1.1-7 Staphylococcal Furunculosis. Plaque with draining tracts and ulceration on the caudolateral aspect of the pastern.

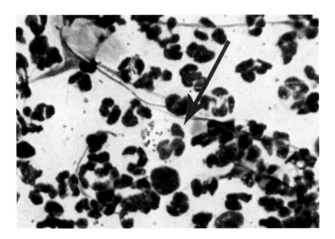

Figure 1.1-8 Staphylococcal Folliculitis. Direct smear (Diff-Quik stain). Suppurative inflammation with degenerate neutrophils, nuclear streaming, and phagocytosed cocci (arrow).

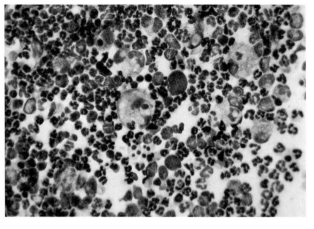

Figure 1.1-10 Staphylococcal Furunculosis. Direct smear (Diff-Quik stain). Pyogranulomatous inflammation with degenerate and nondegenerate neutrophils, macrophages, lymphocytes, and plasma cells.).

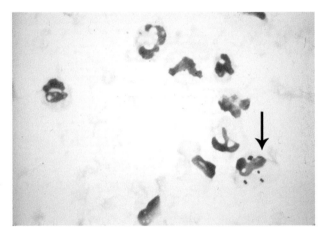

Figure 1.1-9 Staphylococcal Folliculitis. Direct smear (Gram stain). Degenerate neutrophils and phagocytosed Gram-positive cocci (arrow).

cocci (Gram-positive, about 1 μm diameter, often in doublets or clusters) with folliculitis (Figs. 1.1-8 and 1.1-9). Furunculosis is characterized by numerous macrophages, lymphocytes, eosinophils, and plasma cells in addition to the findings described for folliculitis (Fig. 1.1-10).
2. Culture (aerobic).
3. Dermatohistopathology—Suppurative luminal folliculitis with degenerate neutrophils and intracellular cocci; pyogranulomatous furunculosis.

ULCERATIVE LYMPHANGITIS

Features

Ulcerative lymphangitis is a rare bacterial infection of the cutaneous lymphatics. Cutaneous wounds may be contaminated by numerous bacteria, especially *Arcanobacterium pyogenes, Corynebacterium pseudotuberculosis, Staphylococcus aureus,* and ß-hemolytic streptococci. Mixed infections are not uncommon. There are no apparent breed, sex, or age predilections.

Lesions are typically unilateral and seen on the distal leg, shoulder, neck, or flank (Fig. 1.1-11). Firm to fluctuant nodules often ab-

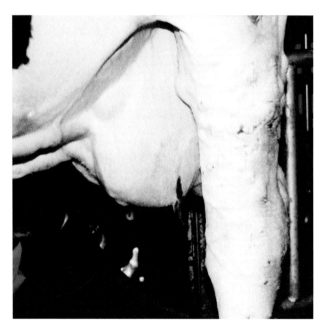

Figure 1.1-11 Mixed Bacterial Lymphangitis. Left pelvic limb is swollen and multiple papules, nodules, and draining tracts are present.

scess, ulcerate, and develop draining tracts. Affected lymphatics are often enlarged and palpable ("corded"). Lesions often take a linear distribution, and heat and pain are variable findings. Regional lymphadenopathy is very common. Affected animals are usually otherwise healthy. Typically only one animal in a herd is affected.

Differential Diagnosis

Opportunistic mycobacterial granuloma and farcy.

Diagnosis

1. Microscopy (direct smears)—Suppurative inflammation with degenerate neutrophils, nuclear streaming, phagocytosed bacteria (cocci and/or rods), and variable numbers of macrophages, lymphocytes, and plasma cells.

2. Culture (aerobic).
3. Dermatohistopathology—Nodular to diffuse suppurative or pyogranulomatous dermatitis and panniculitis with intracellular bacteria; lymphangitis often not seen.

CORYNEBACTERIUM PSEUDOTUBERCULOSIS GRANULOMA

Features

Corynebacterium pseudotuberculosis infection is an uncommon, perhaps geographically-restricted (Middle East) suppurative to pyogranulomatous disease. *Corynebacterium pseudotuberculosis* contaminates various wounds. Moisture and flies are important contributing factors. Older dairy cattle are predisposed.

Lesions may occur anywhere, especially the head, neck, shoulder, flank, and hind leg above the stifle (Figs. 1.1-12 and 1.1-13). Single or multiple subcutaneous abscesses rupture to drain a serosanguineous to blood-stained yellow pus. Ulcerated granulomas may have necrotic margins. Regional lymph nodes may be involved, but systemic signs are not usually seen.

Differential Diagnosis

Other bacterial infections, especially due to *Arcanobacterium pyogenes*, *Actinomyces bovis*, and *Actinobacillus lignieresii*.

Diagnosis

1. Microscopy (direct smears)—Pyogranulomatous inflammation. Intracellular Gram-positive pleomorphic bacteria (coccoid, club, rod forms) that may be arranged in single cells, palisades of parallel cells, or in annular clusters resembling "Chinese letters." Bacteria usually few in number and not seen.
2. Culture (aerobic).
3. Dermatohistopathology—Nodular to diffuse pyogranulomatous dermatitis and panniculitis. Intracellular Gram-positive bacteria not commonly seen.

DERMATOPHILOSIS

Features

Dermatophilosis ("streptothricosis," "rain rot," "rain scald") is a common, cosmopolitan skin disease. *Dermatophilus congolensis* proliferates under the influence of moisture (especially rain) and skin damage (especially ticks, insects, prickly vegetation, and ultraviolet light-damaged white skin). The disease is more common and more severe in tropical and subtropical climates and outdoor animals. In general, there are no breed, sex, or age predilections. However, endemic cattle are more resistant than exotic breeds.

Lesions may occur anywhere (Figs. 1.1-14 to 1.1-22). Common distributions include: dorsum and rump; brisket, axillae, groin; face and pinnae; distal legs; udder and teats or prepuce and scrotum; perineum and tail. Tufted papules and pustules coalesce and become exudative, which results in large ovoid to linear ("runoff" or "scald line") groups of hairs being matted together ("paint brush") in thick crusts. Erosions, ulcers, and thick, creamy, yel-

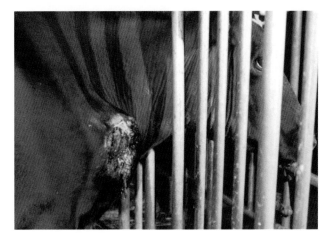

Figure 1.1-12 *Corynebacterium pseudotuberculosis* Granuloma. Large ulcerated nodule over shoulder. Note draining tracts.

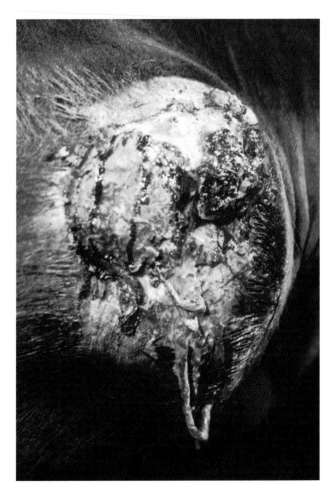

Figure 1.1-13 Close-up of Fig. 1.1-12. Note areas of necrosis, ulcerations, and draining tracts.

lowish to greenish pus underlie the crusts. Acute lesions are painful, but not pruritic. Chronic lesions consist of dry crusts, scale, and alopecia. Typically, multiple animals are affected.

In tropical climates, skin lesions can be generalized, and affected animals can become seriously ill, resulting in major economic losses. Generalized cases in endemic stock are invariably

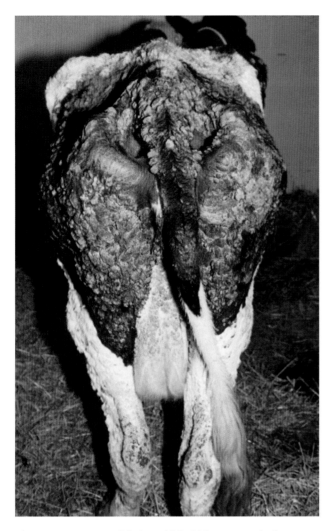

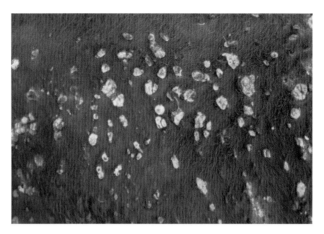

Figure 1.1-16 Dermatophilosis. Multiple annular to linear ("run-off," "scald line") crusts over trunk.

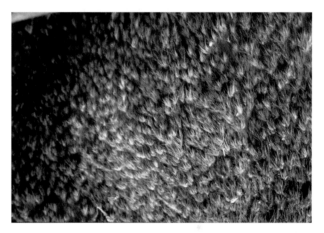

Figure 1.1-14 Dermatophilosis. Multiple thick crusts over back, rump, tail, and perineum.

Figure 1.1-17 Dermatophilosis. Multiple tufted ("paint brush") crusts over thorax.

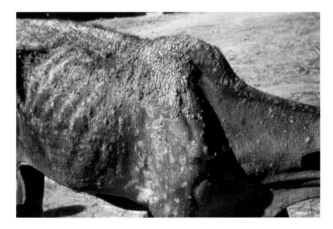

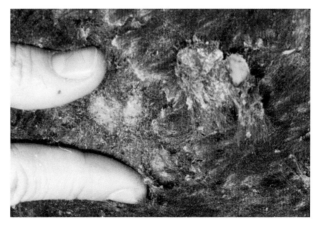

Figure 1.1-15 Dermatophilosis. Generalized crusts.

Figure 1.1-18 Dermatophilosis. Greenish pus coating ulcers and underside of avulsed crusts.

associated with concurrent diseases (e.g., poxvirus infection, trypanosomiasis, anaplasmosis, babesiosis).

Dermatophilosis is a zoonosis. Human skin infections are uncommon and characterized by pruritic or painful pustular lesions in contact areas (especially arms) (Fig. 1.1-23).

Differential Diagnosis

Staphylococcal folliculitis, dermatophytosis, demodicosis, stephanofilariasis, sterile eosinophilic folliculitis and furunculosis, and zinc-responsive dermatitis.

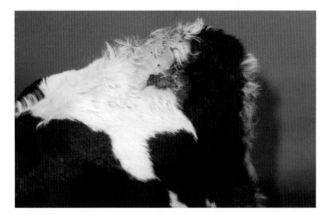

Figure 1.1-19 Dermatophilosis. Multiple crusts, ulcers, alopecia superimposed on erythematous, ultraviolet light-damaged white skin.

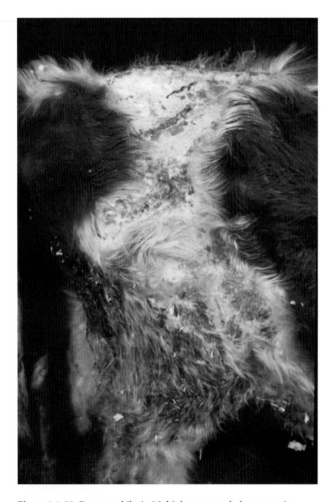

Figure 1.1-20 Dermatophilosis. Multiple crusts and ulcers superimposed on erythematous, ultraviolet light-damaged skin.

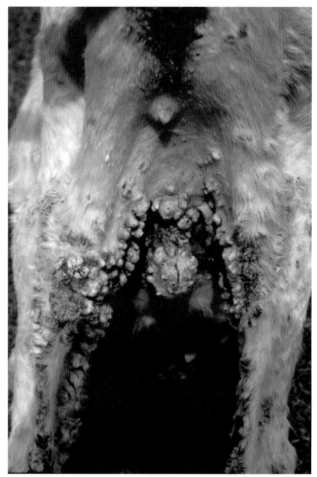

Figure 1.1-21 Dermatophilosis. Thick crusts on perineum, caudal thighs, groin, and scrotum associated with tick infestation.

3. Dermatohistopathology—Suppurative luminal folliculitis and epidermitis with palisading crusts containing Gram-positive cocci in branching filaments.

ACTINOMYCOSIS

Features

Actinomycosis (Greek *aktis*: rays and beams of light) is an uncommon, cosmopolitan suppurative to pyogranulomatous disease of the skin and bone. *Actinomyces bovis* and occasionally *A. israelii* contaminate various traumatic wounds. The disease is most commonly seen in 2- to 5-year-old cattle, with no apparent breed or sex predilections.

Lesions are most commonly seen on the mandible and maxilla ("lumpy jaw") (Figs. 1.1-25 to 1.1-28). Firm, variably painful, immovable bony swellings (osteomyelitis) extend to the overlying skin, resulting in nodules, abscesses, and draining tracts. The discharge is honey-like in color and consistency, and contains hard, yellowish-white granules ("sulfur granules"; 1 to 3 mm diameter) that are the size and consistency of sand (Fig. 1.1-29). Affected animals are usually healthy otherwise. Typically, a single animal is affected.

Diagnosis

1. Microscopy (direct smears)—Suppurative inflammation with degenerate neutrophils, nuclear streaming, and Gram-positive cocci (about 1.5 μm diameter) in 2 to 8 parallel rows forming branching filaments ("railroad tracks") (Fig. 1.1-24).
2. Culture (aerobic).

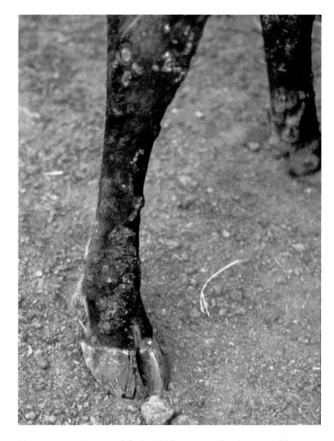

Figure 1.1-22 Dermatophilosis. Thick crusts on leg due to prickly vegetation damage.

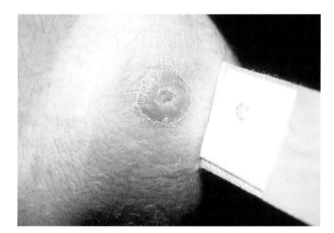

Figure 1.1-23 Dermatophilosis in a Human. Ruptured pustule and surrounding erythema on the elbow.

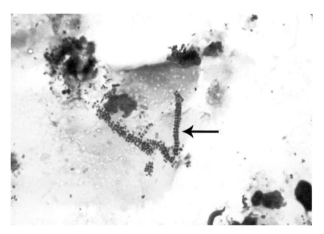

Figure 1.1-24 Dermatophilosis. Direct smear (Diff-Quik stain). Branching filaments composed of cocci ("railroad tracks").

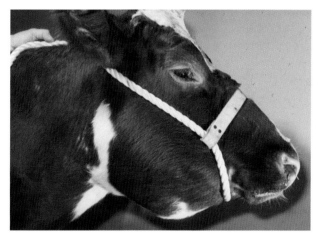

Figure 1.1-25 Actinomycosis. Firm, immovable swelling over mandible.

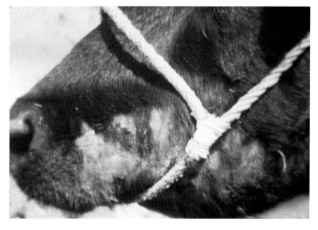

Figure 1.1-26 Actinomycosis. Firm, immovable swelling with alopecia and crusting over mandible (courtesy G. Bosquet, coll. J. Gourreau, AFSSA).

Differential Diagnosis

Other bacterial infections, especially due to *Actinobacillus lignieresii, Arcanobacterium pyogenes,* and *Corynebacterium pseudotuberculosis.*

Diagnosis

1. Microscopy (direct smears)—Suppurative to pyogranulomatous inflammation with degenerate neutrophils and nuclear streaming. Organisms may or may not be seen as Gram-positive, long filaments (less than 1 μm in diameter) and as shorter, V, Y, or T forms. Tissue granules contain Gram-positive long filaments (less than 1 μm diameter).

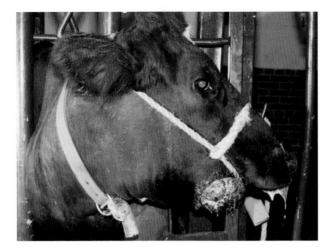

Figure 1.1-27 Actinomycosis. Firm, immovable, ulcerated nodule with draining tracts on mandible.

2. Culture (anaerobic).
3. Dermatohistopathology—Nodular to diffuse, suppurative to pyogranulomatous dermatitis and panniculitis. Tissue granules are coated with Splendore-Hoeppli material and contain Gram-positive filaments.

ACTINOBACILLOSIS

Features

Actinobacillosis is an uncommon, cosmopolitan suppurative to pyogranulomatous disease of the skin and lymph nodes. *Actinobacillus lignieresii* contaminates various traumatic wounds. There are no apparent breed, sex, or age predilections.

Lesions are most commonly seen on the face (cheek, lip, nostril, eyelid), head, and neck (Figs. 1.1-30 to 1.1-32). Lesions may be single or multiple; are usually unilateral but occasionally bilateral (bilateral facial swelling); and may be widespread on the back. Pyogranulomatous glossitis ("wooden tongue") is uncommon. Pyogranulomatous nodules and/or abscesses originate in regional lymph nodes and/or skin. Abscesses and draining tracts discharge a viscid to watery, mucoid white to greenish pus that is odorless and contains grayish-white to brownish-white granules ("sulfur granules"; less than 1 mm diameter). Lesions are neither hot nor painful. Affected animals are usually healthy otherwise. Typically, a single animal is affected.

Differential Diagnosis

Other bacterial infections, especially due to *Actinomyces bovis*, *Arcanobacterium pyogenes*, and *Corynebacterium pseudotuberculosis*.

Diagnosis

1. Microscopy (direct smears)—Suppurative to pyogranulomatous inflammation with degenerate neutrophils and nuclear streaming. Tissue granules contain Gram-negative coccobacilli or rods (about 0.4 μm × 1 μm).
2. Culture (aerobic).

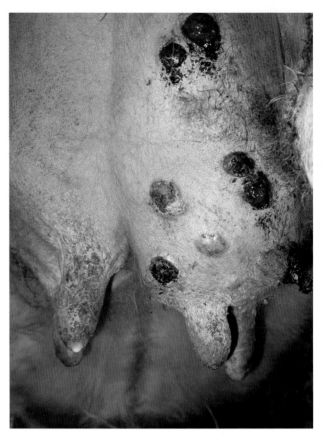

Figure 1.1-28 Actinomycosis. Firm, ulcerated nodules with draining tracts on udder (courtesy J. Nicol, coll. J. Gourreau, AFSSA).

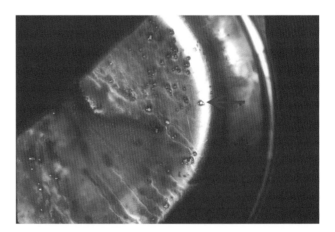

Figure 1.1-29 Actinomycosis. Seropurulent exudate containing "sulfur granules" (arrow) in a stainless steel bowl.

3. Dermatohistopathology—Nodular to diffuse suppurative to pyogranulomatous dermatitis and panniculitis. Tissue granules are coated with Splendore-Hoeppli material and contain Gram-negative coccobacilli.

CLOSTRIDIAL CELLULITIS

Features

Clostridial cellulitis is an uncommon cosmopolitan disease. *Clostridium* spp. contaminate a variety of wounds. These disor-

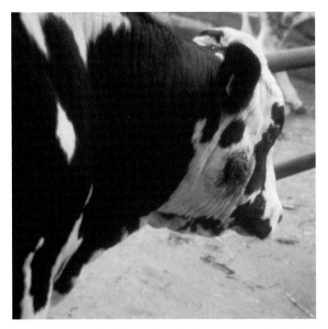

Figure 1.1-30 Actinobacillosis. Ulcerated subcutaneous mass below the ear (courtesy J. Gourreau).

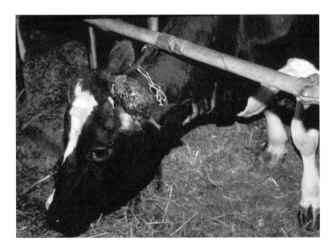

Figure 1.1-31 Actinobacillosis. Ulcerated, crusted mass subsequent to dehorning operation.

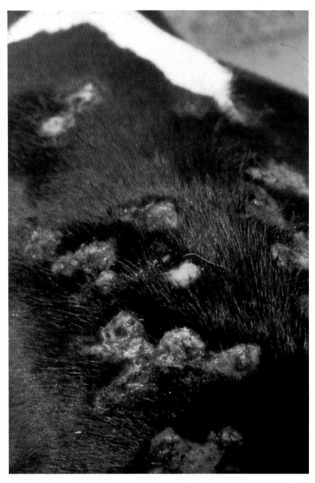

Figure 1.1-32 Actinobacillosis. Multiple ulcerated nodules over back.

ders are typically acute in onset and rapidly fatal (within 12 to 72 hours).

Malignant edema ("gas gangrene") is caused by *C. septicum, C. sordelli*, or *C. perfringens*. Lesions may occur anywhere, especially in the inguinal, axillary, abdominal, shoulder, neck, and head areas. Lesions are initially poorly circumscribed, painful, warm, pitting, deep swellings. Later, the swelling becomes cool and hypoesthetic or anesthetic, the skin becomes bluish to purplish, taut, necrotic, and sloughs. Crepitus (emphysema) may or may not be present. Affected animals are febrile, depressed, anorectic, and weak. Typically, a single animal is affected.

Blackleg is caused by *C. chauvoei*. Lesions commonly occur on a leg (Figs. 1.1-33 and 1.1-34), and are initially poorly-circumscribed, painful, warm, pitting, deep swellings. Later the swelling becomes cool and hypoesthetic or anesthetic, the skin becomes purplish to black, taut, cracked, necrotic, and sloughs.

Crepitus is often present. Affected animals are febrile, depressed, anorectic, and weak. Typically, a single animal is affected.

Differential Diagnosis

Other bacterial cellulitides, especially due to *Arcanobacterium pyogenes, Staphylococcus aureus, Fusobacterium necrophorum, Bacteroides* spp., and *Pasteurella septica*.

Diagnosis

1. Microscopy (direct smears)—Suppurative inflammation with numerous large (up to 5 μm length) Gram-positive straight or slightly curved rods.
2. Culture (anaerobic).
3. Necropsy—Skin lesions are characterized by suppurative and necrotizing cellulitis and numerous Gram-positive rods.

OPPORTUNISTIC MYCOBACTERIAL GRANULOMA

Features

Opportunistic ("atypical," "nontuberculous") mycobacterial granuloma ("skin tuberculosis") is an uncommon cosmopolitan disease. Infection occurs by wound contamination and *Mycobac-*

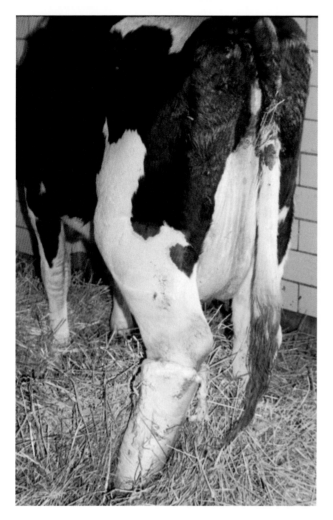

Figure 1.1-33 Clostridial Cellulitis. Swollen, painful left pelvic limb.

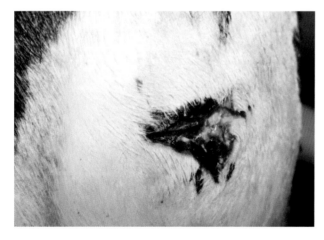

Figure 1.1-34 Clostridial Cellulitis. Area of necrosis, slough, and ulceration on pelvic limb.

terium kansasii has been isolated from some lesions. There are no apparent breed, sex, or age predilections.

Lesions are typically unilateral and affect the distal leg (Figs. 1.1-35 and 1.1-36) They may spread to the thigh, shoulder, or ab-

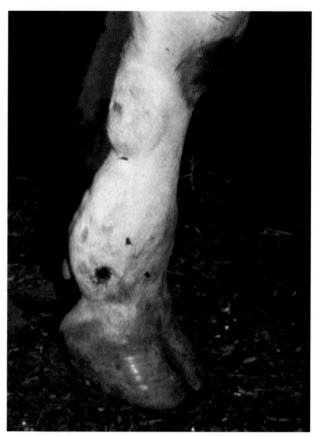

Figure 1.1-35 Opportunistic Mycobacterial Granuloma. Multiple papules and nodules, some having draining tracts on leg.

domen. Papules and nodules may be single or multiple, and often occur in chains with interlesional enlarged and palpable ("corded") lymphatics. Lesions may be hard or fluctuant, and may rupture and discharge a thick, cream to yellow to grayish pus. Pruritus and pain are absent. Regional lymph nodules are usually normal, and affected animals are healthy otherwise.

Differential Diagnosis

Ulcerative lymphangitis and farcy.

Diagnosis

1. Microscopy (direct smears)—Granulomatous inflammation with intracellular, Gram-positive and acid-fast slender rods (up to 4 μm long).
2. Culture (aerobic).
3. Dermatohistopathology—Nodular to diffuse granulomatous dermatitis and panniculitis with intracellular Gram-positive/acid-fast rods.

FARCY

Features

Farcy (Latin: full, stuffed) is a common geographically-restricted (Africa, Asia, South America) pyogranulomatous disease of skin

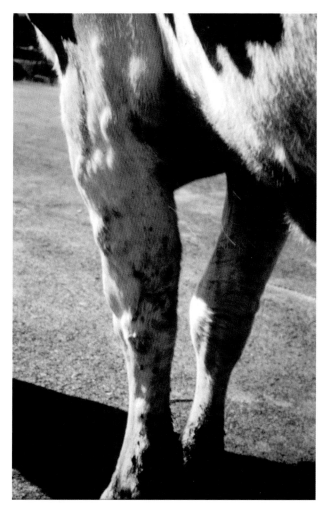

Figure 1.1-36 Opportunistic Mycobacterial Granuloma. Multiple papules and nodules on right pelvic limb.

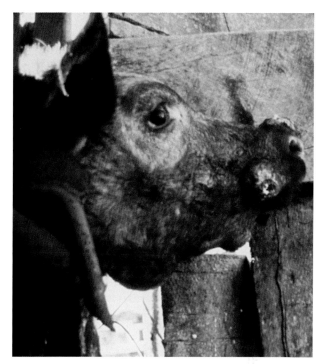

Figure 1.1-37 Farcy. Multiple papules and nodules, some of which are ulcerated, on face.

Diagnosis

1. Microscopy (direct smears)—Pyogranulomatous dermatitis with intracellular Gram-positive/acid-fast slender bacilli (up to 4 μm long) which are distinctly beaded and have a branching, filamentous appearance.
2. Culture (aerobic).
3. Dermatohistopathology—Nodular to diffuse pyogranulomatous dermatitis and panniculitis with intracellular Gram–positive/acid-fast bacilli.

and lymphatics. *Mycobacterium senegalense* contaminates a variety of wounds (especially tick damage). Farcy has previously been attributed to infections with *Nocardia farcinica* or *Mycobacterium farcinogenes*: but these reports are probably erroneous.

Skin lesions are most commonly seen on the head, neck, shoulder, and legs (Fig. 1.1-37). Firm, painless, slow-growing subcutaneous nodules may ulcerate and discharge a thick, stringy, odorless, grayish-white or yellowish material. Enlarged and palpable ("corded") lymphatics and regional lymphadenopathy are usually present. Farcy has a prolonged course with widespread organ involvement, emaciation, and death. Economic losses due to death, decreased productivity, hide damage, and carcass condemnation are considerable. Up to 32% of the animals in an endemic area may be affected.

Differential Diagnosis

Ulcerative lymphangitis and opportunistic mycobacterial granuloma.

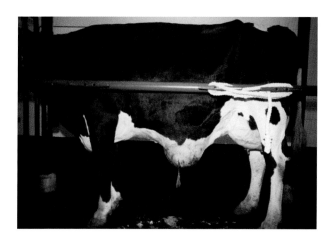

Figure 1.1-38 Subcutaneous Abscess (*Arcanobacterium pyogenes*) on ventral abdomen.

MISCELLANEOUS BACTERIAL DISEASES

Table 1.1-1 Miscellaneous Bacterial Diseases

Abscess (Figs. 1.1-38 and 1.1-39)	Common and cosmopolitan; anywhere (especially infected knee and hock hygromas); fluctuant, often painful, subcutaneous; numerous bacteria, especially *Arcanobacterium pyogenes*; culture
Cellulitis (Fig. 1.1-40)	Uncommon and cosmopolitan; leg (*Staphylococcus aureus* or *A. pyogenes*) or face, neck, brisket (*Fusobacterium necrophorum*, *Bacteroides* spp., *Pasteurella septica*); marked swelling and pain, variable exudation, draining tracts, necrosis; variable systemic signs; culture
Bacterial Pseudomycetoma ("botryomycosis")	Rare; udder; single or multiple crusted nodules and ulcers; *Pseudomonas aeruginosa*; culture and dermatohistopathology
Necrobacillosis (Figs. 1.1-41 to 1.1-43)	Uncommon and cosmopolitan; anywhere (especially axillae, groin, udder); moist, necrotic, ulcerative, foul-smelling; *Fusobacterium necrophorum*; variable systemic signs; culture
Nodular thelitis (Figs. 1.1-44 and 1.1-45)	Uncommon (Europe, Japan); teats, udder; painful papules, plaques, nodules, ulcers; occasional swollen teat with string of abscesses in lymphatics and yellowish, creamy pus; *Mycobacterium terrae* and *M. gordonae*; culture and dermatohistopathology
Nocardiosis	Uncommon (Africa); neck, chest, back, and occasionally rump, belly, scrotum, legs; thick, annular, exudative crusts; *Nocardia* spp.; culture and dermatohistopathology
Pasteurella granulomatis panniculitis ("Lechiguana")	Uncommon (Brazil); shoulder region; usually one large abscess; culture and dermatohistopathology
Anthrax (Greek: coal; black eschar)	Uncommon and cosmopolitan; neck, brisket, flanks, abdomen, perineum; massive edema; *Bacillus anthracis*; systemic signs; zoonosis (cutaneous, respiratory, intestinal); culture and necropsy
Septicemic slough (Figs. 1.1-46 and 1.1-47)	Rare and cosmopolitan; especially calves; distal legs, tail, pinnae; necrosis and slough; *Salmonella dublin* and *S. typhimurium*; systemic signs; zoonosis (intestinal); culture

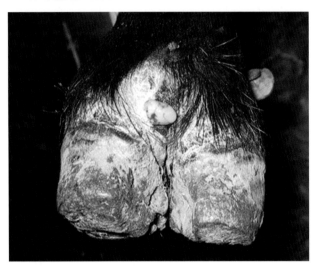

Figure 1.1-39 Subcutaneous Abscess. Abscess with purulent discharge on foot (courtesy G. Dauphin, coll. J. Gourreau, AFSSA).

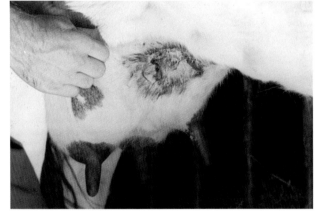

Figure 1.1-41 Necrobacillosis. Exudative, necrotic ulcer of udder.

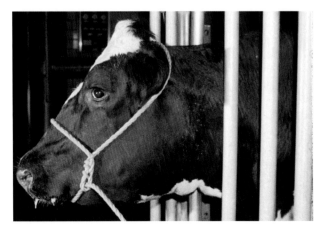

Figure 1.1-40 Cellulitis (Mixed Bacterial). Painful swelling involving side of face and neck.

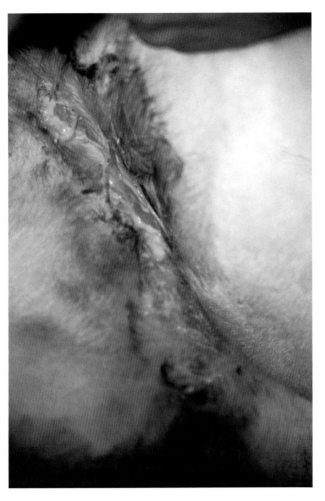

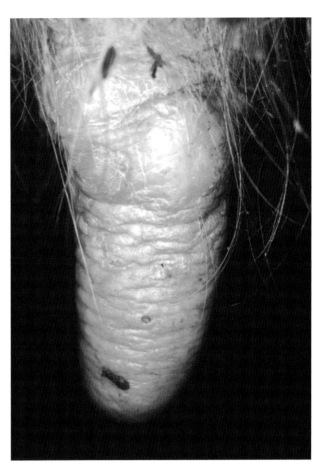

Figure 1.1-44 Nodular Thelitis. Nodule at mid-teat (courtesy G. Coussi, coll. J. Gourreau, AFSSA).

Figure 1.1-42 Necrobacillosis. Exudative, necrotic ulcer on intramammary sulcus.

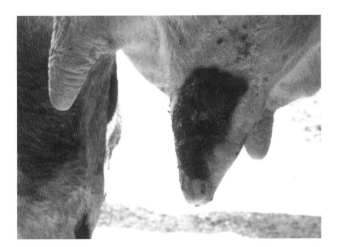

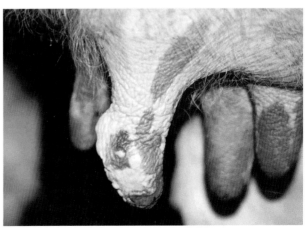

Figure 1.1-43 Necrobacillosis. Necrotic ulcer on teat (courtesy J. Gourreau).

Figure 1.1-45 Nodular Thelitis. Nodules and linear plaque (courtesy C. Husson, coll. J. Gourreau, AFSSA).

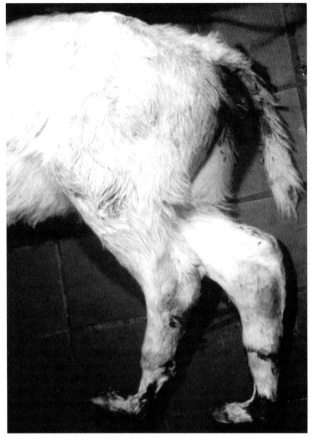

Figure 1.1-46 Septicemic Slough. Necrosis and slough of distal pelvic limbs in a calf with salmonellosis.

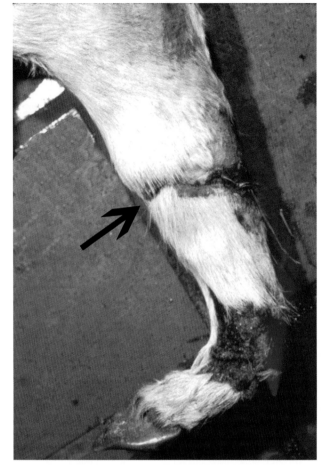

Figure 1.1-47 Close-up of Fig. 1.1-46. Note line (arrow) demarcating viable proximal from necrotic and sloughing distal limb.

REFERENCES

Fecteau G, et al. 1992. Ulcerative Lymphangitis and Periostitis in a Cow. *Agri-Practice* 13: 27.

Grinberg A, et al. 2004. Epidemiological and Molecular Evidence of a Monophyletic Infection with *Staphylococcus aureus* causing a Purulent Dermatitis in a Dairy Farmer and Multiple Cases of Mastitis in his Cows. *Epidemiol Infect* 132: 507.

Hamid ME, et al. 1991. Bovine Farcy: A Clinicopathological Study of the Disease and Its Aetiological Agent. *J Comp Path* 105: 287.

Hazarika RA, et al. 1991. Cutaneous Infection Associated with *Staphylococcus hyicus* in Cattle. *Res Vet Sci* 50: 374.

Howard JL, and Smith RA. 1999. Current Veterinary Therapy. Food Animal Practice. Ed 4. WB Saunders, Philadelphia, PA.

Jackson P. 1993. Differential Diagnosis of Common Bovine Skin Disorders part 1. *In Practice* 15: 119.

Marchot P, et al. 1989. Note sur Une Première Observation de Gangrène Sèche des Extrémités chez des Bovins, due à *Salmonella typhimurium*, au Ghana. *Rev Elev Méd Vét Pays Trop* 42: 510.

Milne MH, et al. 2001. Clinical Recognition and Treatment of Bovine Cutaneous Actinobacillosis. *Vet Rec* 148: 273.

Oyekunde MA, and Ojo MO. 1988. Preliminary Observations on Bovine Cutaneous Nocardiosis and Dermatophilosis in the Subhumid Climate of Southern Nigeria. *Rev Elev Méd Vét Pays Trop* 41: 347.

Radostits OM, et al. 2000. Veterinary Medicine. A Textbook of the Diseases of Cattle, Sheep, Pigs, Goats and Horses. Ed 9. WB Saunders, Philadelphia, PA.

Rebhun WC, et al. 1988. Atypical Actinobacillosis Granulomas in Cattle. *Cornell Vet* 78: 125.

Riet-Correa F, et al. 1992. Bovine Focal Proliferative Fibrogranulomatous Panniculitis (Lechiguana) Associated with *Pasteurella granulomatis*. *Vet Pathol* 29: 93.

Scott DW. 1988. Large Animal Dermatology. WB Saunders, Philadelphia, PA.

Scott DW, and Gourreau JM. 1991. La Folliculite et la Furonculose Staphylococciques des Bovins. *Point Vét* 23: 79.

Thorel MF, et al. 1990. Bovine Nodular Thelitis: A Clinicopathological Study of 20 Cases. *Vet Dermatol* 1.165.

Yeruham I, et al. 1991. Human Dermatophilosis (*Dermatophilus congolensis*) in Dairymen in Israel. *Israel J Vet Med* 46: 114.

Yeruham I, et al. 1996. Contagious Impetigo in a Dairy Cattle Herd. *Vet Dermatol* 7: 739.

Yeruham I, et al. 1997. *Corynebacterium pseudotuberculosis* infection in Israeli Cattle: Clinical and Epidemiological Studies. *Vet Rec* 140: 423.

Yeruham I, et al. 2004. A Herd Level Analysis of a *Corynebacterium pseudotuberculosis* Outbreak in a Dairy Cattle Herd. *Vet Dermatol* 15: 315.

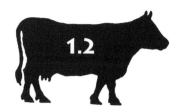

FUNGAL SKIN DISEASES

Dermatophytosis
Miscellaneous Fungal Diseases
    Aspergillosis
    Malassezia Otitis Externa
    Phaeohyphomycosis
    Pythiosis

DERMATOPHYTOSIS

Features

Dermatophytosis ("ringworm") is a common cosmopolitan disease. It is most commonly caused by *Trichophyton verrucosum*, and less frequently by *T. mentagrophytes, T. equinum, Microsporum gypseum, M. canis,* and *M. nanum.* In temperate climates the disease is most common in fall and winter, especially in confined animals. There are no apparent breed or sex predilections, and young animals (less than one year old) are most commonly affected.

Lesions can occur anywhere, but are most common on the face, head, pinnae, neck, rump, tail, and perineum (Figs. 1.2-1 to 1.2-3). Tufted papules enlarge into thick, grayish to whitish crusts. Lesions may be painful. Less commonly, annular areas of alopecia and scaling are seen. Pruritus is rare, and affected animals are otherwise healthy. From 10% to 100% of a herd may be affected.

Bovine dermatophytosis is a zoonosis. *T. verrucosum* infection in humans causes typical ringworm lesions or kerions in contact areas, especially hands (Fig. 1.2-4), arms, neck, face, and scalp.

Differential Diagnosis

Staphylococcal folliculitis, dermatophilosis, demodicosis, stephanofilariasis, sterile eosinophilic folliculitis and furunculosis, and zinc-responsive dermatitis.

Diagnosis

1. Microscopy (trichography)—Plucked hairs placed in mineral oil or potassium hydroxide contain hyphae and arthroconidia (spores) (Figs. 1.2-5 and 1.2-6).
2. Culture.
3. Dermatohistopathology—Suppurative luminal folliculitis and pyogranulomatous furunculosis with fungal hyphae and arthroconidia in and on hairs.

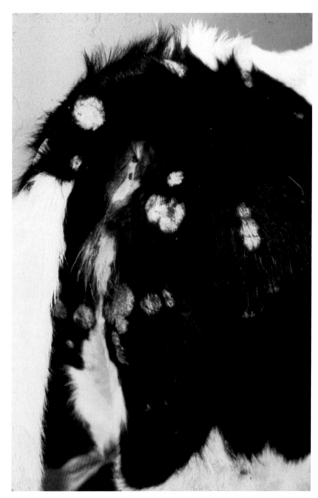

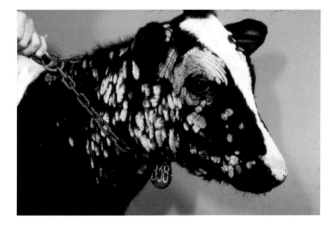

Figure 1.2-1 Dermatophytosis. Annular, thick, grayish-white crusts on face and neck.

Figure 1.2-2 Dermatophytosis. Annular, thick, grayish-white crusts on rump, tail, and perineum.

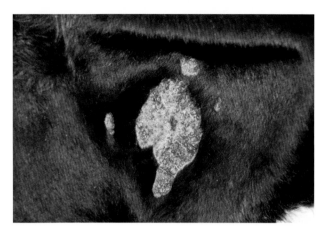

Figure 1.2-3 Dermatophytosis. Thick, grayish-white crusts in flank.

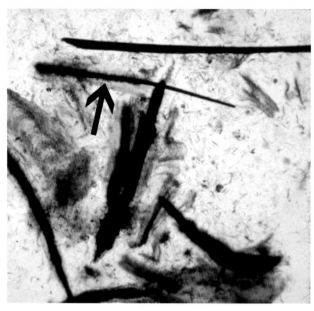

Figure 1.2-5 Dermatophytosis. Plucked hairs in mineral oil. Note thickened, irregular appearance of infected hair (arrow).

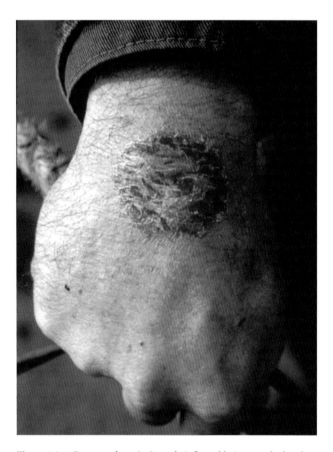

Figure 1.2-4 Dermatophytosis. Severely inflamed lesions on the hand caused by *Trichophyton verrucosum*.

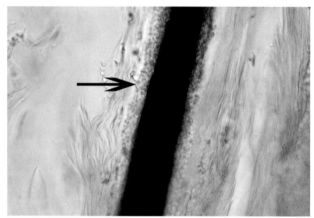

Figure 1.2-6 Dermatophytosis. Numerous arthroconidia (arrow) on surface of infected hair.

MISCELLANEOUS FUNGAL DISEASES

Table 1.2-1 Miscellaneous Fungal Diseases

Aspergillosis (Fig. 1.2-7)	Fungal placentitis results in skin lesions on aborted fetuses; lesions can be widespread or localized; annular, grayish, felt-like plaques; or yellow-white, dry plaques; especially *Aspergillus fumigatus*; culture and dermato-histopathology
Malassezia otitis externa	Common and perhaps geographically-restricted (South America); ceruminous to suppurative otitis externa; predominantly *Malassezia sympodialis* in summer, and *M. globosa* in winter; cytology and culture
Phaeohyphomycosis (Fig. 1.2-8)	Very rare and cosmopolitan; multiple ulcerated, oozing nodules over rump and thighs (*Dreschlera rostrata*); multiple nodules on pinnae, tail, vulva, and thighs (*D. spicifera*); culture and dermatohistopathology
Pythiosis	Rare; South America and southeastern United States; prolonged exposure to water; *Pythium insidiosum*; nodules, ulcers, draining tracts; especially distal legs; dermatohistopathology, immunohistochemistry, culture

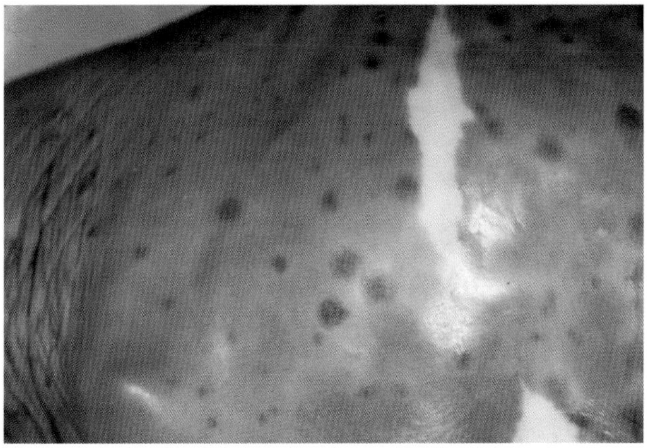

Figure 1.2-7 Aspergillosis. Aborted fetus. Multiple annular, brownish-black, felt-like lesions on skin.

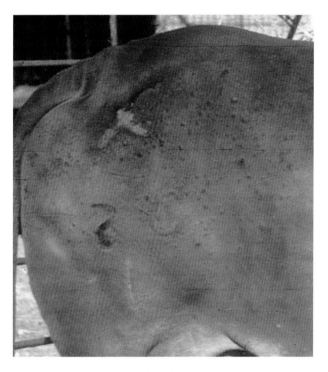

Figure 1.2-8 Phaeohyphomycosis. Multiple granulomatous nodules on hip and flank due to *Exserohilum* sp. (courtesy H. Whitford, coll. J. Gourreau, AFSSA).

REFERENCES

Duarte ER, et al. 1999. Prevalence of *Malassezia* spp. in the Ears of Asymptomatic Cattle and Cattle with Otitis in Brazil. *Med Mycol* 37: 159.

Duarte ER, et al. 2003. Factors Associated with the Prevalence of *Malassezia* species in the External Ears of Cattle from the State of Minas Gerais, Brazil. *Med Mycol* 41: 137.

Howard JL, and Smith RA. 1999. Current Veterinary Therapy. Food Animal Practice. Ed 4. WB Saunders, Philadelphia, PA.

Jackson P. 1993. Differential Diagnosis of Common Bovine Skin Disorders Part 1. *In Practice* 15: 100.

Pérez RC, et al. 2005. Epizootic Cutaneous Pythiosis in Beef Calves. *Vet Microbiol* 109: 121.

Radostits OM, et al. 2000. Veterinary Medicine. A Textbook of the Diseases of Cattle, Sheep, Pigs, Goats, and Horses. Ed. 9. WB Saunders, Philadelphia, PA.

Santurio JM, et al. 1998. Cutaneous Pythiosis insidiosi in Calves from the Pantanal Region of Brazil. *Mycopathologia* 141:123.

Scott DW. 1988. Large Animal Dermatology. WB Saunders, Philadelphia, PA.

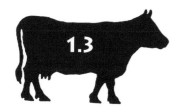

PARASITIC SKIN DISEASES

1.3

CHORIOPTIC MANGE

Features

Chorioptic mange ("foot mange," "tail mange") is uncommon in most parts of the world. It is caused by the mite *Chorioptes bovis*. There are no apparent breed, age, or sex predilections. The disease is especially common in stabled dairy cattle. Mite populations are usually much larger during cold weather. Thus, clinical signs are usually seen, or are more severe, in winter. Transmission occurs by direct and indirect contact.

Lesions are most commonly seen on the rump, tail, perineum, caudomedial thigh, caudal udder, and scrotum, and occasionally the distal hind legs and teats (Figs. 1.3-1 through 1.3-6). Erythema and papules progress to scaling, oozing, crusts, and alopecia. Pruritus varies from mild to intense. Stanchioned cattle exhibit restlessness, treading, violent swishing of the tail, and rubbing of the tail and perineum against stationary objects. Typically, multiple animals are affected. Severe infestations can cause weight loss, hide damage, and reduced milk and meat yields. Humans are not affected.

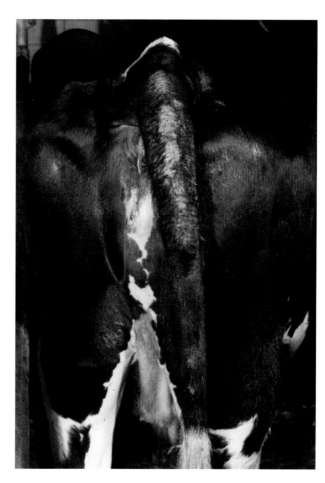

Figure 1.3-1 Chorioptic Mange. Crust and alopecia on proximal tail.

Differential Diagnosis

Sarcoptic mange, psoroptic mange, psorergatic mange, and pediculosis.

Diagnosis

1. Microscopy (Skin Scrapings in Mineral Oil)—Psoroptid mites, 0.3 to 0.5 mm in length (Figs. 1.3-7 and 1.3-8).
2. Dermatohistopathology—Hyperplastic eosinophilic perivascular-to-interstitial dermatitis with eosinophilic epidermal microabscesses and parakeratotic hyperkeratosis (mites rarely seen).

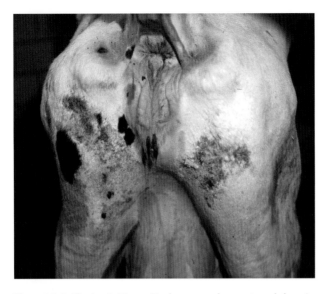

Figure 1.3-2 Chorioptic Mange. Erythema, papules, crusts, and alopecia on caudal thighs.

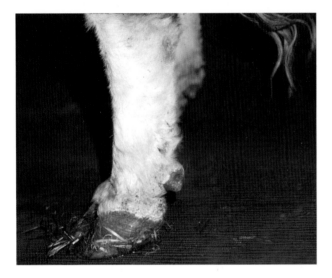

Figure 1.3-3 Chorioptic Mange. Erythema, alopecia, and excoriations on distal leg.

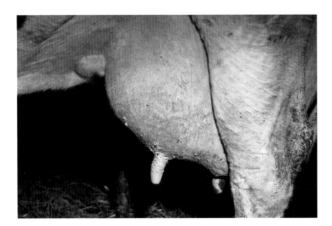

Figure 1.3-4 Chorioptic Mange. Erythema, crusts, and alopecia on udder and lateral hock.

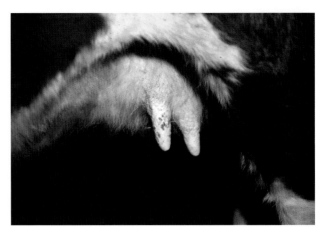

Figure 1.3-5 Chorioptic Mange. Crusts on teats.

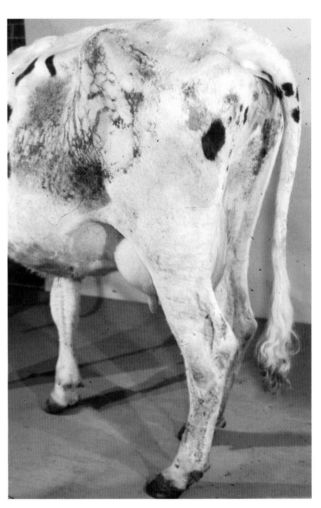

Figure 1.3-6 Chorioptic Mange. Erythema, alopecia, and excoriations on rump, tail, hindlegs, perineum, and flank.

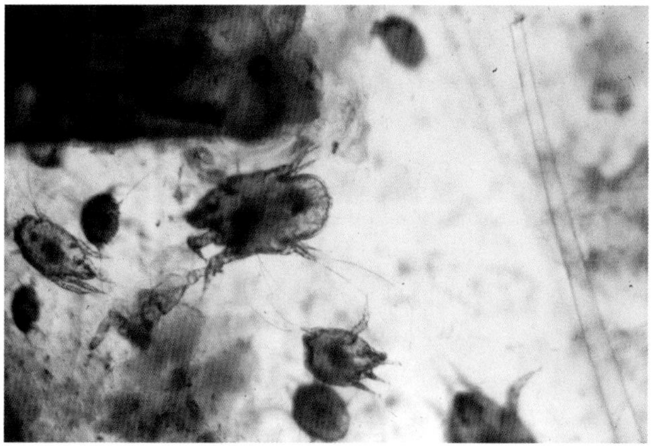

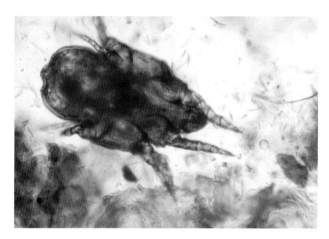

Figure 1.3-7 Chorioptic Mange. Multiple mites in a skin scraping.

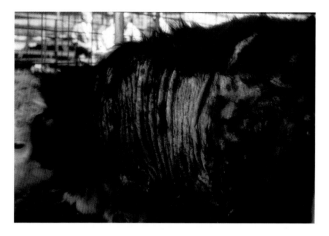

Figure 1.3-9 Psoroptic Mange. Alopecia, erythema, crusts, and lichenification over lateral trunk (courtesy U.S. Department of Agriculture).

Figure 1.3-8 Chorioptic Mange. Adult mite in a skin scraping.

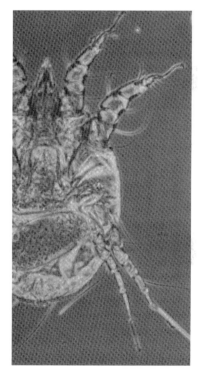

Figure 1.3-10 Psoroptic Mange. Adult *Psoroptes* mite (courtesy J. Georgi).

PSOROPTIC MANGE

Features

Psoroptic mange ("body mange") is common to uncommon in most parts of the world. It is caused by the mite *Psoroptes ovis (bovis)*. There are no apparent breed, age, or sex predilections. However, in the United States, psoroptic mange is mostly seen in range (beef) cattle in the western, southwestern, and central states. Transmission occurs by direct and indirect transmission. Mite populations are usually larger during cold weather. Thus, clinical signs are usually more severe in winter.

Lesions typically begin on the shoulders and rump (Fig. 1.3-9). Papules, pustules, exudation, crusts, alopecia, and excoriations are seen and pruritus is intense. Skin becomes lichenified and thickened with chronicity. Generalized skin involvement and secondary bacterial infections are common. Intense, unremitting pruritus results in annoyance, irritability, decreased food intake, decreased weight gains or weight loss, decreased milk production, hide damage, difficulty in estrus detection, and myiasis. Animals with 40% or more of their body involved may die. Typically, multiple animals are affected. Humans are not affected.

Differential Diagnosis

Sarcoptic mange, chorioptic mange, psorergatic mange, and pediculosis.

Diagnosis

1. Microscopy (Skin Scrapings in Mineral Oil)—Psoroptid mites, 0.4 to 0.8 mm in length (Fig. 1.3-10). Skin scrapings should be taken from the margin of lesions.
2. Dermatohistopathology—Hyperplastic eosinophilic perivascular-to-interstitial dermatitis with epidermal microabscesses and parakeratotic hyperkeratosis (mites uncommonly seen).

SARCOPTIC MANGE

Features

Sarcoptic mange (scabies, "head mange") is uncommon to rare in most parts of the world. It is caused by the mite *Sarcoptes scabiei var bovis*. There are no apparent breed, age, or sex predilections. Transmission occurs by direct and indirect contact.

Lesions are most commonly seen on the face, pinnae, neck, shoulders, and rump (Figs. 1.3-11 through 1.3-15). Erythema and papules progress to scaling, oozing, crusts, and alopecia. Pruritus is intense. Excoriation, lichenification, and hyperkeratosis are prominent in chronic cases. Peripheral lymphadenopathy is usually moderate to marked. Typically, multiple animals are affected. Decreased feed intake, weight loss, decreased milk production, hide damage, difficulty in estrus detection, secondary bacterial (usually staphylococcal) pyoderma, and myiasis can occur due to the intense pruritus and irritation.

Sarcoptic mange is a potential zoonosis. Affected humans develop pruritic erythematous papules with crusts and excoriations on the arms, chest, abdomen, and legs (Fig. 1.3-16).

Differential Diagnosis

Psoroptic mange, chorioptic mange, psorergatic mange, and pediculosis.

Diagnosis

1. Microscopy (Skin Scrapings in Mineral Oil)—Sarcoptid mites, 0.25 to 0.6 mm in length (Figs. 1.3-17 and 18). Ova (eggs) and scyballa (fecal pellets) may also be found (Fig. 1.3-19). Mites are often difficult to find, especially in chronic cases.
2. Dermatohistopathology—Hyperplastic eosinophilic perivascular-to-interstitial dermis with eosinophilic epidermal microabscesses and parakeratotic hyperkeratosis (mites rarely seen).

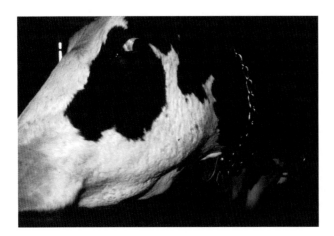

Figure 1.3-11 Sarcoptic Mange. Erythema, papules, crusts, and alopecia on face and muzzle.

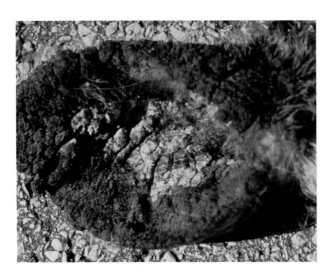

Figure 1.3-12 Sarcoptic Mange. Severe crusting of pinna (courtesy J. King).

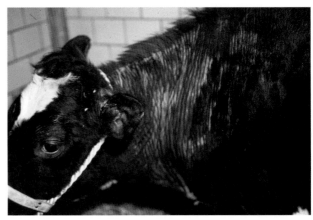

Figure 1.3-13 Sarcoptic Mange. Alopecia, crusts, and lichenification over face, pinna, neck, and shoulder.

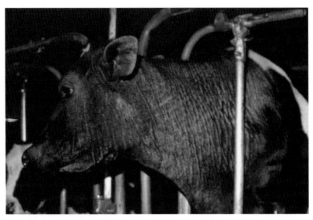

Figure 1.3-14 Sarcoptic Mange. Alopecia, lichenification, and crusts on face, pinna, neck, and shoulder.

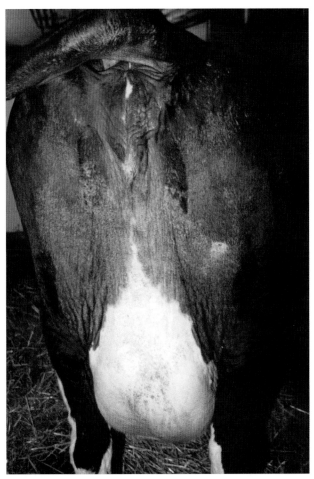

Figure 1.3-15 Sarcoptic Mange. Alopecia, erythema, and crusts on perineum, caudal thighs, and udder.

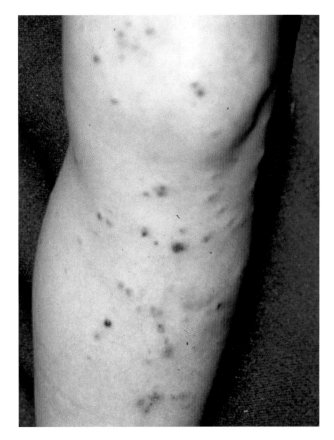

Figure 1.3-16 Sarcoptic Mange. Erythematous and crusted papules on the leg of a human with animal-origin scabies.

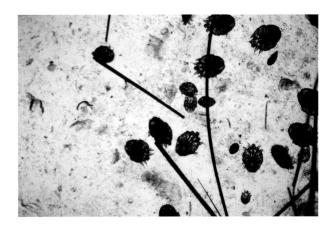

Figure 1.3-17 Sarcoptic Mange. Multiple mites in a skin scraping.

DEMODECTIC MANGE

Features

Demodectic mange (demodicosis, "follicular mange") is an uncommon, cosmopolitan dermatosis caused by the mite *Demodex bovis*. This mite is a normal resident of hair follicles, transmitted from the dam to nursing neonates during the first few days of life. It is assumed that all animals experiencing disease due to the excessive replication of this normal resident mite are in some way immunocompromised (e.g., concurrent disease, poor nutrition, debilitation, stress, genetic predilection). There are no apparent breed, age, or sex predilections. Demodectic mange is not a contagious disease. Although cattle harbor other demodicid mites (*D. ghanensis, D. tauri*), it is not clear if these mites are associated with skin disease.

Lesions consist of multiple (from 10 to hundreds) dermal papules and nodules, 0.5 to 2 cm in diameter (Figs. 1.3-20 and 1.3-21). The overlying hair coat and skin surface are normal, and the lesions are neither painful nor pruritic. There is often a seasonal (spring and summer) increase in the number of lesions. Occasionally, draining tracts, ulcers, abscesses, crusts, and alopecia may be seen when follicular rupture and/or secondary bacterial (usually staphylococcal) infection have occurred. Lesions are most commonly seen over the neck, shoulders, brisket, and forelegs, and occasionally on the back, flanks, head, and hind legs.

Differential Diagnosis

Insect bites, adverse cutaneous drug reaction, and lymphoma.

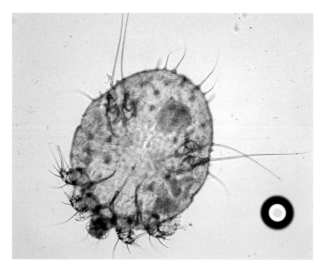

Figure 1.3-18 Sarcoptic Mange. Adult mite in a skin scraping.

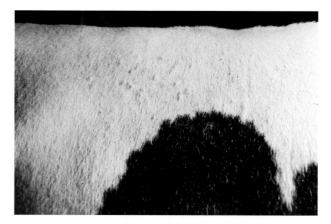

Figure 1.3-20 Demodectic Mange. Multiple papules over withers.

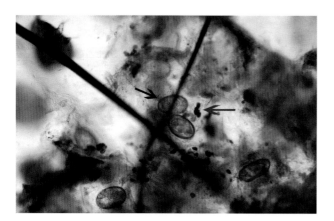

Figure 1.3-19 Sarcoptic Mange. Multiple eggs (black arrow) and fecal pellets (red arrow) in a skin scraping.

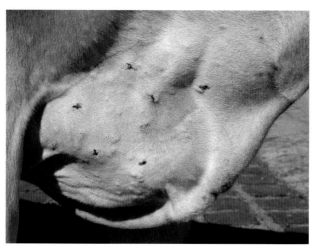

Figure 1.3-21 Demodectic Mange. Multiple papules on brisket (courtesy J. Gourreau).

Diagnosis

1. History and physical examination.
2. Microscopy (Incision and Manual Evacuation of Caseous Exudate from a Lesion Placed in Mineral Oil)—Multiple demodicid mites (0.2 to 0.3 mm in length) (Fig. 1.3-22).

PEDICULOSIS

Features

Pediculosis (lice) is a common, cosmopolitan infestation caused by various lice. In the United States, recognized cattle lice include *Damalinia (Bovicola) bovis* (biting louse, order Mallophaga) and *Haematopinus eurysternus*, *Linognathus vituli*, and *Solenopotes capillatus* (sucking lice, order Anoplura). There are no apparent breed, age, or sex predilections. Louse populations are usually much larger during cold weather. Thus, clinical signs are usually seen, or are more severe in winter. Transmission occurs by direct and indirect contact.

    D. bovis is most commonly seen over the neck, withers, and tail head (Fig. 1.3-23). Sucking lice are commonly found on the poll,

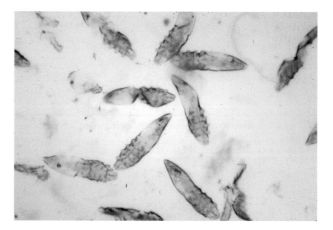

Figure 1.3-22 Demodectic Mange. Numerous mites from an incised and squeezed lesion.

pinnae, muzzle, periocular region, neck, brisket, withers, tail, axillae, and groin (Figs. 1.3-24 through 1.3-26). Some animals will show no clinical signs. Most animals will have variable combinations of scaling, crusting, erythema, excoriation, and hair loss.

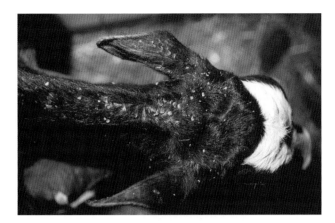

Figure 1.3-23 Pediculosis. Crusts and scales on pinnae, head, and dorsal neck.

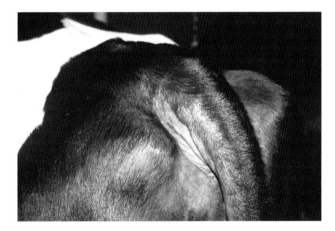

Figure 1.3-24 Pediculosis. Alopecia and scale on rump and tail (courtesy M. Sloet).

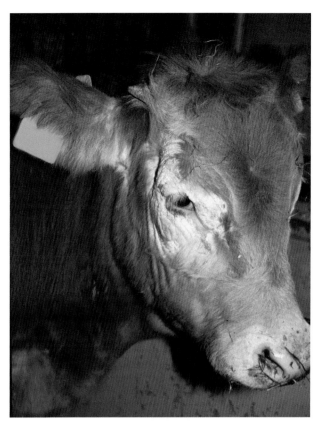

Figure 1.3-25 Pediculosis. Alopecia, scales, and crusts on base of pinna, muzzle, and periocular area (courtesy M. Sloet).

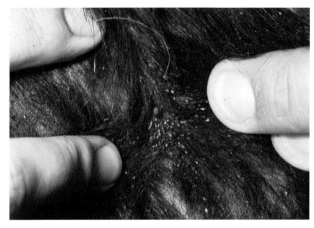

Figure 1.3-26 Pediculosis. Multiple lice over thorax (courtesy M. Sloet).

Pruritus is variable, but often moderate to marked, with affected animals constantly rubbing, licking, and scratching. Lick marks created by the tongue that resemble marks left by a wet paintbrush are classic on animals with lice (Fig. 1.3-27). Stanchioned cattle are very restless because their restraint limits their ability to lick or scratch. They tend to "rattle" the stanchions and rub vigorously back and forth or up and down in the stanchion, causing areas of hair loss on the neck and shoulders. Calves may develop hairballs. Louse infestations can be heavy in debilitated animals. Large populations of lice can cause anemia, especially in calves. Heavy infestations can cause unthriftiness, decreased growth, and damage to hides. Typically, multiple animals are affected. Humans are not affected.

Differential Diagnosis

Sarcoptic mange, chorioptic mange, psoroptic mange, and psorergatic mange.

Diagnosis

1. History and Physical Examination—Sucking lice are bluish-gray in color. Biting lice are pale to brownish in color.

2. Microscopy (Lice and Hairs Placed in Mineral Oil)—Adult lice are large (3 to 6 mm in length) (Figs. 1.3-28 and 1.3-29). Ova (nits) are 1 to 2 mm in length and may be found attached to hair shafts (Fig. 1.3-30).

STEPHANOFILARIASIS

Features

Stephanofilariasis is an uncommon disorder in many parts of the world. Many species of the genus *Stephanofilaria* are associated

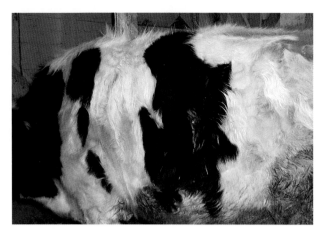

Figure 1.3-27 Pediculosis. Lick marks on the lateral aspect of the body (courtesy M. Smith).

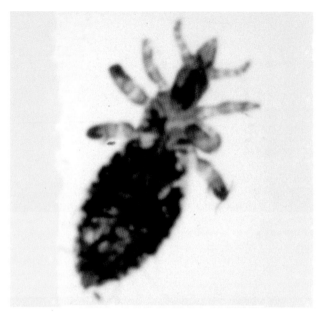

Figure 1.3-29 Pediculosis. Sucking louse (courtesy M. Sloet).

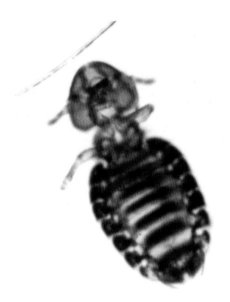

Figure 1.3-28 Pediculosis. Biting louse (courtesy M. Sloet).

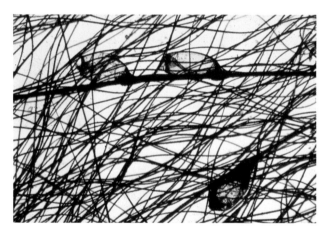

Figure 1.3-30 Pediculosis. Nits on hair shaft.

with skin disease in cattle (see Table 1.3-1). Stephanofilariasis is a nonseasonal disease, although it is often worse in warm weather, presumably the result of the activity of fly intermediate hosts (*Haematobia, Musca*). There are no apparent age or sex predilections. Range (beef) cattle are more commonly affected than dairy cattle.

In North America—especially in the west and southwest—stephanofilariasis is caused by *Stephanofilaria stilesi. Haematobia (Lyperosia) irritans* is the intermediate host. Lesions consist of papules, crusts, ulcers, alopecia, hyperkeratosis, and thickening of the skin. Pruritus is variable. The ventral chest and abdomen, flanks, udder, and teats are most commonly affected (Figs. 1.3-31 through 1.3-34). Lesions are occasionally seen over the face and neck. Teat lesions may predispose to mastitis. Typically, multiple animals are affected.

Differential Diagnosis

Contact dermatitis, chorioptic mange, trombiculosis, and *Pelodera* dermatitis.

Diagnosis

1. History and physical examination.
2. Dermatohistopathology—Adult nematodes in cyst-like structures at the base of hair follicles and microfilariae in surrounding dermis.

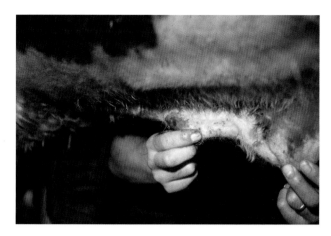

Figure 1.3-31 Stephanofilariasis. Alopecia, erythema, crusts, and excoriations on ventral midline.

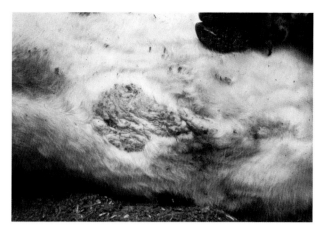

Figure 1.3-33 Stephanofilariasis. Annular areas of alopecia, erythema, and lichenification on ventrum (courtesy A. Stannard).

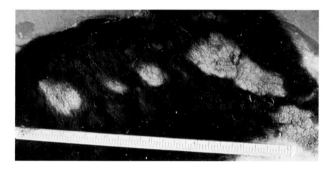

Figure 1.3-32 Stephanofilariasis. Annular areas of alopecia and crusting on ventral abdomen.

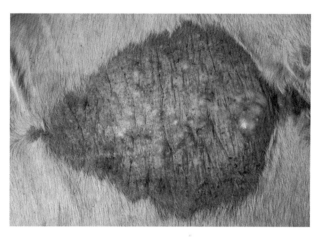

Figure 1.3-34 Stephanofilariasis. Alopecia, erythema, crusts, and lichenification on ventrum (courtesy A. Stannard).

MISCELLANEOUS PARASITIC DISEASES

Table 1.3-1 Miscellaneous Parasitic Diseases

Psorergatic mange	Uncommon; North America and Africa; *Psorergates (Psorobia) bos*, 0.1 to 0.2 mm in length; no breed, age, or sex predilections; varies from no clinical signs to severe alopecia, scaling, and pruritus over dorsum (head, neck, shoulders, back, rump); may require several skin scrapings
Trombiculosis ("chiggers," "harvest mite") (Figs. 1.3-35 and 1.3-36)	Rare and cosmopolitan; late summer and fall; infested woods and fields; legs, face, pinnae, axillae, groin; papulocrustous dermatitis and variable pruritus; trombiculid larvae (0.2 to 0.4 mm in length, red to orange in color); e.g., *Trombicula (Eutrombicula) alfreddugesi*, *T (Neotrombicula) autumnalis*, *T. sarcina*
Dermanyssus gallinae dermatitis ("poultry mite")	Rare and cosmopolitan; proximity to poultry roosts; especially late summer; especially legs and ventrum; pruritic, papulocrustous dermatitis; *D. gallinae* (0.6 to 1 mm in length)
Raillietia auris infestation ("ear mites")	Uncommon; Africa, Australia, and South America; *R. caprae* (*R. manfredi*), 0.5 to 0.8 mm in length; usually no clinical signs, but occasionally suppurative otitis externa, and can lead to suppurative otitis media, head tilt, facial paralysis, anorexia, emaciation, and deafness
Ticks (Fig. 1.3-37)	Common and cosmopolitan, most in spring and summer; especially ears, face, neck, axillae, groin, and legs; minimal lesions or papules and nodules centered around attached ticks; variable pain and pruritus; e.g., *Amblyomma americanum*, *A. cajenense*, *Otobius megnini*, *Ixodes scapularis*, *I. cookei*, *I. pacificus*, *Rhipicephalus sanguineous*, *Dermacentor andersonii*, and *D. variabilis* in the United States
Fleas	Uncommon and cosmopolitan; *Ctenocephalides felis* ("cat flea"), brown in color, 2 to 4 mm in length; especially summer and fall; variable degrees of pruritus and papulocrustous dermatitis; especially trunk and legs; heavy infestations in calves and debilitated animals may cause anemia and even death

(continued)

Table 1.3-1 Miscellaneous Parasitic Diseases (*continued*)

Biting flies	Uncommon to common and cosmopolitan; *Haematobia* irritans ("horn fly"), *Stomoxys calcitrans* ("stable fly"), *Simulium* spp. ("black fly"), and *Tabanus* spp. ("horse fly"); spring, summer, and fall; painful/pruritic papules, wheals, and plaques with central crusts and bleeding; especially legs, head, pinnae, abdomen, shoulders, and back
Louse flies ("forest flies") (Fig. 1.3-38)	Uncommon; *Hippobosca equina* (cosmopolitan), *H. maculata* (Africa and South America), and *H. rufipes* (Africa); 4 to 7 mm in length; especially summer; tend to cluster and suck blood in perineum and groin; source of irritation and fly-worry
Hypodermiasis ("cattle grubs") (Figs. 1.3-39 through 1.3-41)	Common in many parts of the Northern Hemisphere; younger cattle more frequently and more severely affected; *Hypoderma bovis* and *H. lineatum*; swarms of adult flies ("heel flies," "gad flies") cause annoyance and fright, often resulting in poor weight gain; larval-associated subcutaneous nodules and cysts ("warbles") over back in spring; lesions develop central pore in which larvae may be seen (about 25 mm in length); carcass and hide depreciation; occasional esophageal, spinal cord, toxic, or anaphylactic complications associated with larvae
Hydrotaea irritans flies ("head fly")	Common; Europe and Australia; especially summer; swarming flies initiate head shaking, rubbing, and scratching; excoriations progress to nonhealing ulcers and black crusts ("brown head," "black cap"); possible secondary bacterial infections and myiasis
Dermatobia hominis infestation	Uncommon; Central and South America; painful subcutaneous nodules with a central pore containing third-stage larvae (about 20 mm in length)
Calliphorine myiasis ("maggots," "flystrike")	Common and cosmopolitan; especially *Lucilia* spp., *Calliphora* spp., and *Phormia* spp.; especially late spring, summer, and early fall; any wounded/damaged skin; foul-smelling ulcers with scalloped margins and a "honeycombed" appearance, teeming with larvae ("maggots"); usually painful and pruritic
Screw-worm myiasis	Uncommon; Central and South America (*Callitroga hominivorax* and *C. macellaria*); Africa and Asia (*Chrysomyia bezziana* and *C. megacephala*); especially late spring, summer, and early fall; any wounded/damaged skin (e.g., branding, castration, dehorning); foul-smelling ulcers with scalloped margins and a "honeycombed" appearance, teeming with larvae; painful and pruritic; humans are also susceptible (e.g., skin, genitalia, ears, sinuses)
Parafilariasis (Figs. 1.3-42 and 1.3-43)	Uncommon; Africa, India, and Europe; *Parafilaria bovicola* (adults, 30 to 70 mm in length, in subcutaneous nodules); various *Musca* spp. serve as vectors or intermediate hosts; especially spring and summer; one to several subcutaneous nodules that discharge a bloody exudate; especially neck, shoulder, and trunk, and occasionally udder and teats; variable pain and pruritus; exudate contains larvae (about 0.2 mm in length)
Onchocerciasis	Common; *Onchocerca gutturosa* produces asymptomatic firm subcutaneous nodules over shoulder, hip, and stifle (North America, Europe, Africa, Australia; *Simulium* spp. and *Culicoides* spp. are intermediate hosts); *O. gibsoni* produces asymptomatic firm subcutaneous nodules over brisket, hip, and stifle (Africa, Asia, and Australia; *Culicoides* spp. are intermediate hosts); *O. ochengi* produces asymptomatic firm dermal and subcutaneous papules and nodules over scrotum, udder, flanks, and head (Africa; *Simulium* spp. are intermediate hosts); a number of *Onchocerca* spp. microfilariae may be associated with teat lesions (papules, plaques, ulcers); dermatohistopathology
Strongyloidosis	Uncommon and cosmopolitan; no breed, age, and sex predilections; *Strongyloides papillosus*; pruritic dermatitis of feet, legs, and ventrum; fecal flotation
Pelodera dermatitis ("rhabditic dermatitis") (Figs. 1.3-44 and 1.3-45)	Rare and mostly North America; no breed, age, or sex predilections; *Pelodera (Rhabditis) strongyloides* filthy environment; variably pruritic dermatitis of feet, legs, ventrum, udder, and teats; skin scrapings (0.4 to 0.8 mm in length nematode larvae)
Rhabditic otitis externa	Uncommon; Africa; *Rhabditis bovis* from contaminated soil; no breed, age, or sex predilections; painful, putrid otitis externa with brownish to yellowish purulent discharge; 0.3 to 0.6 mm in length larvae in otic discharge
Hookworm dermatitis	Rare and cosmopolitan; no breed, age, or sex predilections; *Bunostomum phlebotomum*; pruritic dermatitis of feet, legs, and ventrum; fecal flotation
Stephanofilariasis (Fig. 1.3-46)	Uncommon; *Stephanofilaria dedoesi* produces a papulocrustous dermatitis ("cascado") over the face, neck, and brisket (Indonesia); *S. kaeli* produces a papulocrustous dermatitis ("filarial" or "Krian sore") over the pinnae and distal limbs (Malaysia); *S. assamensis* produces a papulocrustous dermatitis ("hump sore") over the shoulders, neck, pinnae, and distal limbs (India and Russia): *S. okinawaensis* produces a papulocrustous dermatitis over the muzzle and teats (Japan); dermatohistopathology

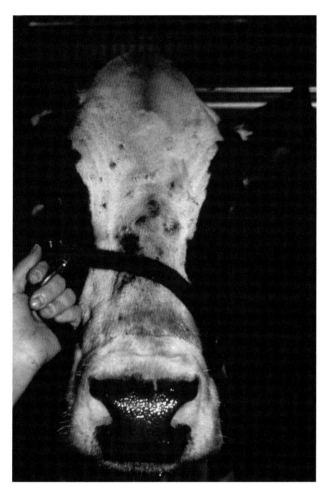

Figure 1.3-35 Trombiculosis. Erythema and crusts on face.

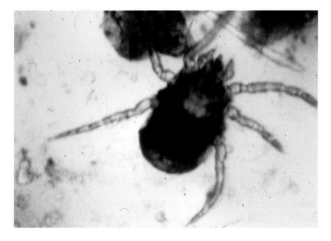

Figure 1.3-36 Trombiculosis. *E. alfreddugesi* in skin scraping.

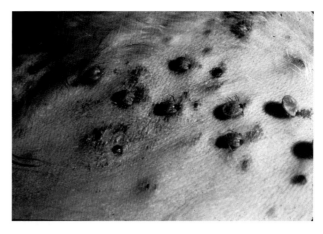

Figure 1.3-37 Ticks. Multiple engorged ticks and areas of erythema and hemorrhage (sites of previous tick attachment) (courtesy J. MacDonald).

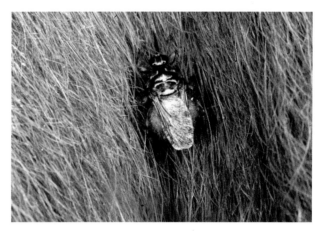

Figure 1.3-38 Louse Flies. *Hippobosca equina* on perineum (courtesy J. Gourreau).

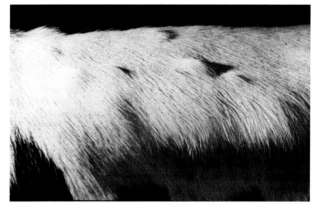

Figure 1.3-39 Hypodermiasis. Multiple subcutaneous nodules over back.

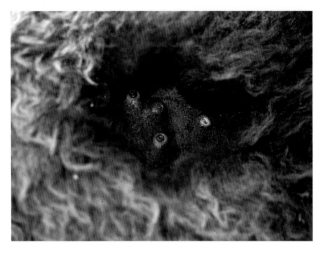

Figure 1.3-40 Hypodermiasis. Multiple nodules with pores and visible larvae (area has been clipped).

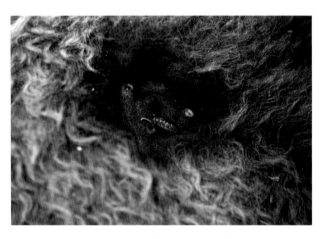

Figure 1.3-41 Hypodermiasis. Multiple nodules with pores. One larva has been extracted (area has been clipped).

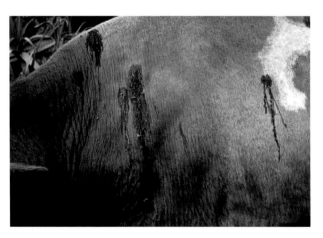

Figure 1.3-42 Parafilariasis. Multiple bleeding sores over lateral neck, shoulder, and thorax (courtesy P. Bland).

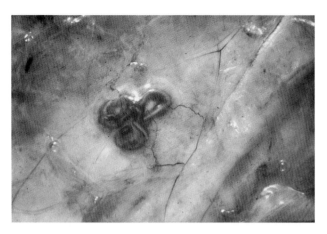

Figure 1.3-43 Parafilariasis. Adult nematode in subcutis (courtesy P. Bland).

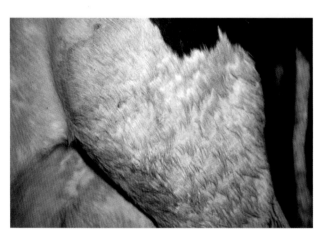

Figure 1.3-44 *Pelodera* Dermatitis. Annular areas of alopecia and erythema on lateral thigh.

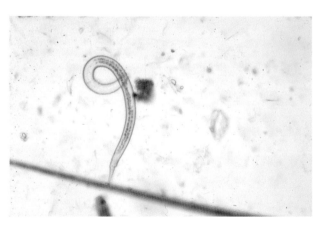

Figure 1.3-45 *Pelodera* Dermatitis. *P. strongyloides* in a skin scraping.

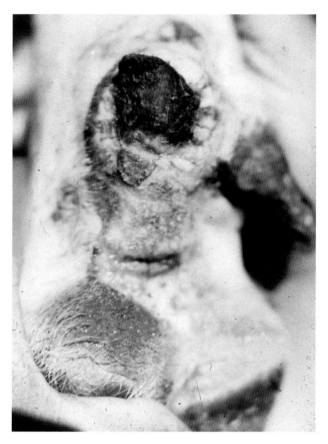

Figure 1.3-46 Stephanofilariasis. Erythema, crusts, and alopecia on pastern due to *S. assamensis* (courtesy A. Chatterjee).

REFERENCES

Alexander JL. 2006. Screwworms. *J Am Vet Med Assoc* 228: 357.

Barth D, et al. 1997. Efficacy of Eprinomectin Against Mange Mites in Cattle. *Am J Vet Res* 58: 1257.

Beytut E, et al. 2005. Teat Onchocercosis in Cows with Reference to Prevalence Species Involved and Pathology. *Res Vet Sci* 78: 45.

Bukva V. 1986. *Demodex tauri* sp. n. (Acari:Demodicidae), a New Parasite of Cattle. *Folia Parasitol* 33: 363.

Bussiéras J, et al. 1987. Nouvelles Observations sur les Plaies d'Eté des Bovins de l'Est de la France. *Rec Méd Vét* 163: 853.

Jubb TF, et al. 1993. Suppurative Otitis in Cattle Associated with Ear Mites (*Raillietia auris*). *Aust Vet J* 70: 354.

Lima WS, et al. 2004. Evaluation of the Prophylactic Efficacy of Fipronil 1% Pour-On (Topline®) on Post-Castration Scrotal Myiasis Caused by *Cochliomyia hominivorax* in Cattle. *Vet Parasitol* 125: 373.

Losson B, et al. 1988. Haematological and Immunological Responses of Unrestrained Cattle to *Psoroptes ovis*, the Sheep Scab Mite. *Res Vet Sci* 44: 197.

Losson BJ, et al. 1998. Field Efficacy of Injectable Doramectin Against *Chorioptes bovis* in Naturally Infected Cattle. *Vet Rec* 142: 18.

Matthes HF. 1994. Investigations of Pathogenesis of Cattle Demodicosis: Sites of Predilection, Habitat, and Dynamics of Demodectic Nodules. *Vet Parasitol* 53: 283.

Otter A, et al. 2003. Anaemia and Mortality in Calves Infested with the Long-Nosed Sucking Louse (*Linognathus vituli*). *Vet Rec* 153: 176.

Radostits OM, et al. 2000. Veterinary Medicine. A Textbook of the Diseases of Cattle, Sheep, Pigs, Goats, and Horses. Ed. 9. WB Saunders, Philadelphia, PA.

Rooney KA, et al. 1999. Efficacy of a Pour-On Formulation of Doramectin Against Lice, Mites, and Grubs of Cattle. *Am J Vet Res* 60: 402.

Scott DW. 1988. Large Animal Dermatology. WB Saunders, Philadelphia, PA.

Scott DW, and Gourreau JM. 1993. La Dermatite à *Pelodera strongyloides* et l'Otite Externe à *Rhabditis bovis* chez les Bovins. *Méd Vét Québec* 23: 112.

Stromberg PC, and Guillot FS. 1987. Bone Marrow Response in Cattle with Chronic Dermatitis Caused by *Psoroptes ovis*. *Vet Pathol* 24: 365.

Stromberg PC, and Guillot FS. 1987. Hematology in the Regressive Phase of Bovine Psoroptic Scabies. *Vet Pathol* 24: 371.

Stromberg PC, and Guillot FS. 1989. Pathogenesis of Psoroptic Scabies in Hereford Heifer Calves. *Am J Vet Res* 50: 594.

Yeruham I, Perl S. 2005. Dermatitis in a Dairy Herd Caused by *Pelodera strongyloides* (Nematoda: Rhabditidae). *J Vet Med B* 52: 197.

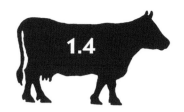

VIRAL AND PROTOZOAL SKIN DISEASES

Pseudocowpox
Bovine Papular Stomatitis
Herpes Mammillitis
Malignant Catarrhal Fever
Bovine Viral Diarrhea
Infectious Bovine Rhinotracheitis
Vesicular Stomatitis
Foot-and-Mouth Disease
Lumpy Skin Disease
Besnoitiosis
Miscellaneous Viral and Protozoal Diseases
   Bluetongue
   Bovine Ephemeral Fever
   Bovine Spongiform Encephalopathy
   Cowpox
   Herpes Mammary Pustular Dermatitis
   Jembrana Disease
   Pseudolumpy Skin Disease
   Pseudorabies
   Rift Valley Fever
   Rinderpest
   Sarcocystosis
   Theileriosis
   Trypanosomiasis

PSEUDOCOWPOX

Features

Pseudocowpox is a common cosmopolitan infectious disease caused by *Parapoxvirus bovis-2*. It is the most common infectious cause of teat lesions. Transmission occurs via contamination of skin abrasions. There are no apparent breed or age predilections, and milking cows and heifers are most commonly affected.

Initial signs include focal areas of erythema and edema, and pain of affected teats. Vesicles are not commonly seen. Orange papules evolve into dark red crusts. These lesions undergo progressive peripheral enlargement and become umbilicated (Figs. 1.4-1 through 1.4-3). When the central crust falls off, the classical "ring" or "horseshoe" lesion—pathognomonic for pseudocowpox—is formed. The udder is often affected. The medial thighs, perineum, and scrotum are occasionally involved (Figs. 1.4-4 and 1.4-5). Typically, 5% to 10% of the animals in a herd are affected at any given time.

Pseudocowpox is a zoonosis. In humans, the condition is often called "milker's nodule" or "farmyard pox." Transmission can be direct, indirect, and even human-to-human. Lesions are often solitary, and occur most commonly on the fingers, arm, face, and

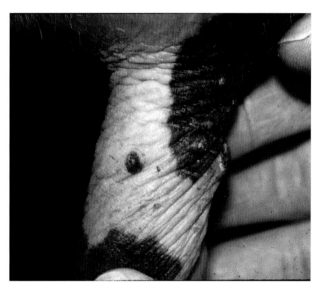

Figure 1.4-1 Pseudocowpox. Umbilicated, crusted papules on teat.

leg (Fig. 1.4-6). Erythematous papules evolve into nodules with a red center, a white middle ring, and a red periphery. The lesions initially have a red, oozing surface, which then develop a dry crust through which black dots may be seen. Lastly, the lesions develop a papillomatous surface, a thick crust, then regress. There is variable pain and pruritus.

Differential Diagnosis

Staphylococcal dermatitis, insect bites, traumatized viral papillomas, and herpes mammillitis (Table 1.4-1).

Diagnosis

1. Histopathology and Electron Microscopy—Eosinophilic intracytoplasmic inclusion bodies in epidermal keratinocytes.
2. Virus isolation.

BOVINE PAPULAR STOMATITIS

Features

Bovine papular stomatitis is a common, cosmopolitan infectious disease caused by *Parapoxvirus bovis -1*. Transmission occurs via contamination of skin abrasions. There are no breed or sex predilections, and the disease is seen more commonly in animals less than 1 year of age.

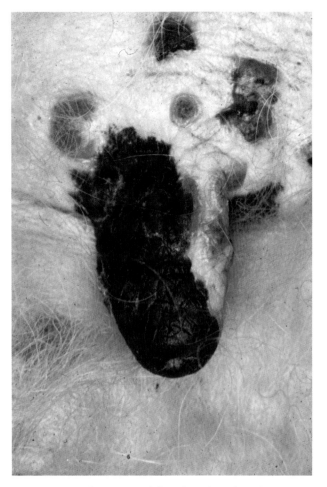

Figure 1.4-2 Pseudocowpox. Umbilicated papules and annular to crescentic red crusts on teat.

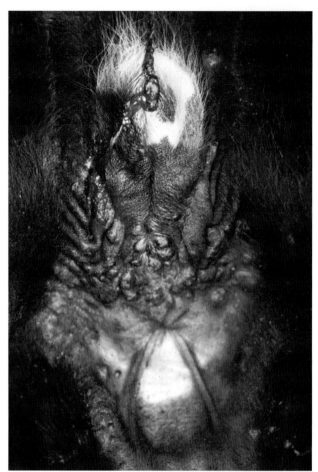

Figure 1.4-4 Pseudocowpox. Multiple crusted papules between anus and vulva.

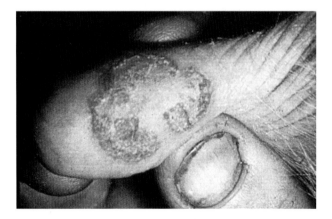

Figure 1.4-3 Pseudocowpox. Horseshoe-shaped red crust on teat.

Initial lesions are erythematous macules and papules which may become papillomatous, or may undergo central necrosis and become crusted. Mature lesions vary in color from red, to brownish, to yellowish-orange. These lesions are most common on the muzzle, nostrils, and lips (Figs. 1.4-7 and 1.4-8). Lesions in the oral cavity may be papular or flat and plaque-like. Occasionally, lesions can be widespread and involve the abdomen, prepuce,

scrotum, teats (Fig. 1.4-9), udder, hind legs, and sides. A chronic form of bovine papular stomatitis in calves is characterized by a proliferative and necrotic stomatitis, a generalized necrotic and exudative dermatitis, and marked hyperkeratosis around the mouth, anus, and ventral tail.

A necrotic dermatitis of the tail of feedlot cattle ("rat-tail syndrome") has been associated with bovine papular stomatitis. Affected cattle lose the tail switch, leaving an eroded to ulcerated area.

Bovine papular stomatitis is a zoonosis. In humans, the condition is often called, "milker's nodule" or "farmyard pox". Transmission can be direct, indirect, and even human-to-human. Lesions are often solitary, and occur most commonly on the fingers, arm, face, and leg (Fig. 1.4-10). Erythematous papules evolve into nodules with a red center, a white middle ring, and a red periphery. The lesions initially have a red, oozing surface, which then develops a dry crust through which black dots may be seen. Lastly, the lesions develop a papillomatous surface, a thick crust, then regress. There is variable pain and pruritus.

Differential Diagnosis

Bovine viral diarrhea, bluetongue, malignant catarrhal fever, rinderpest, vesicular stomatitis, and foot-and-mouth disease.

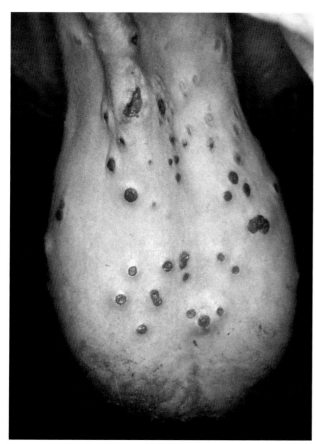

Figure 1.4-5 Pseudocowpox. Multiple crusted and umbilicated papules on scrotum (courtesy J. Gourreau).

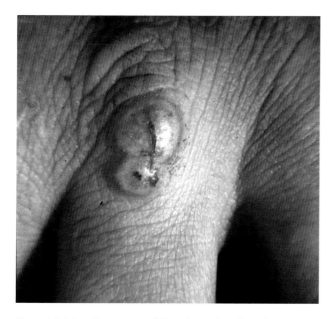

Figure 1.4-6 Pseudocowpox. Umbilicated pustule with erythematous halo ("milker's nodule") on dairyman's finger.

Table 1.4-1 Differential Diagnosis of Bovine Teat and Udder Lesions

Viral
Bluetongue
Bovine papular stomatitis
Bovine viral diarrhea
Cowpox
Foot-and-mouth disease
Herpes mammary pustular dermatitis
Herpes mammillitis
Infectious bovine rhinotracheitis
Lumpy skin disease
Malignant catarrhal fever
Pseudocowpox
Pseudolumpy skin disease
Rinderpest
Vaccinia
Vesicular stomatitis
Viral papillomatosis
Bacterial
Bacterial pseudomycetoma
Dermatophilosis
Impetigo
Necrobacillosis
Nodular thelitis
Fungal
Dermatophytosis
Parasitic
Chorioptic mange
Insect bites
Onchocerciasis
Pelodera dermatitis
Sarcoptic mange
Stephanofilariasis
Trombiculosis
Protozoal
Besnoitiosis
Miscellaneous
Black pox
Burns
Chapping
Contact dermatitis
Dermatitis, pyrexia, and hemorrhage syndrome
Frostbite
Intertrigo
Neoplasms
Photodermatitis
Trauma

Diagnosis

1. Histopathology and Electron Microscopy—Eosinophilic intracytoplasmic inclusion bodies in epidermal keratinocytes.
2. Viral isolation.

HERPES MAMMILLITIS

Features

Herpes mammillitis is a cosmopolitan infectious disease caused by *bovine herpesvirus–2*. Transmission occurs via contact and in-

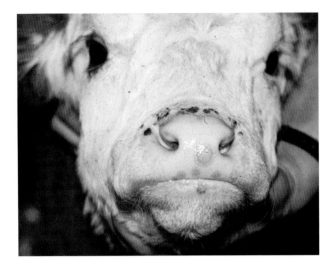

Figure 1.4-7 Bovine Papular Stomatitis. Multiple erythematous flat-topped papules and plaques on muzzle.

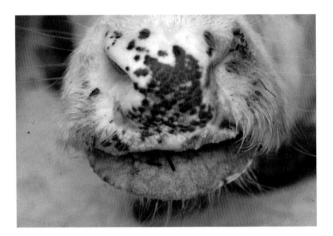

Figure 1.4-8 Bovine Papular Stomatitis. Orange papillomatous lesions on lips.

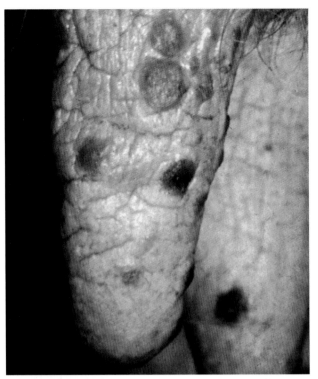

Figure 1.4-9 Bovine Papular Stomatitis. Crusted and umbilicated papules on teats (courtesy A. Mayr, coll. J. Gourreau, AFSSA).

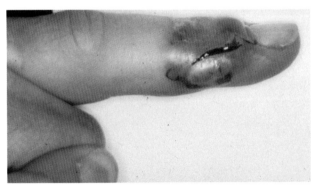

Figure 1.4-10 Bovine Papular Stomatitis. Bruised, pustular lesion on finger (lesion has been lanced).

sect vectors. Disease occurs in lactating cattle, and heifers tend to be more severely affected. Disease is most common in summer and fall.

Most cattle show no signs of systemic illness. Lesions may be confined to one teat, or involve all teats. Disease is typically sudden in onset, with swollen, tender teats. Irregularly shaped vesicles may be seen (Fig. 1.4-11), but usually sloughing and ulceration are the lesions noted. Serum oozing and thick dark red to brown crusting follow (Fig. 1.4-12). Severity of lesions varies from: (1) lines of erythema, often in circles, which enclose dry skin or papules with occasional ulceration to, (2) annular red to blue plaques which evolve into ulcers, 0.5 to 2 cm in diameter, to (3) large areas of bluish discoloration, necrosis, slough, ulceration, and serum exudation. These lesions are painful, and cows often kick at milking machines or their operators. Lesions may extend to the udder (Fig. 1.4-13), perineum, and vulva. Occasionally, lesions occur on the muzzle and in the oral cavity of nursing calves.

Morbidity varies from 18 to 96%, but mortality is rare. However, economic losses can be severe as a result of decreased milk production and an increased incidence of mastitis.

Differential Diagnosis

Trauma, photodermatitis, bluetongue, malignant catarrhal fever, foot-and-mouth disease, vesicular stomatitis, cowpox, and pseudocowpox.

Diagnosis

1. Virus isolation.

MALIGNANT CATARRHAL FEVER

Features

Malignant catarrhal fever ("malignant head catarrh," "bovine malignant catarrh," "snotsiekte") is a cosmopolitan, highly fatal pan-

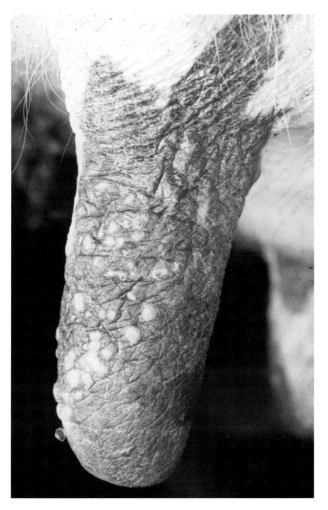

Figure 1.4-11 Herpes Mammillitis. Irregularly shaped vesicles on teat.

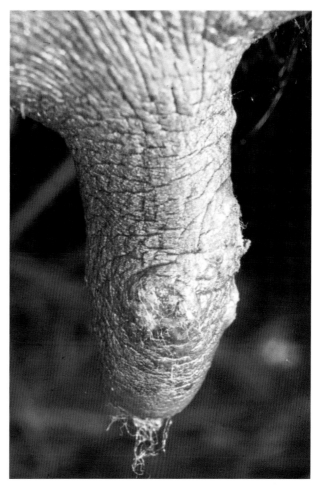

Figure 1.4-12 Herpes Mammillitis. Crusted ulcers on teat.

systemic infectious disease. There are two forms of the disease: (1) wildebeest-associated (alcelaphine herpesvirus 1) in Africa, and (2) sheep-associated (*ovine herpesvirus-2*) worldwide. Details of transmission are incomplete. There are no apparent breed, age, or sex predilections.

Initial clinical signs include fever, nasal discharge, anorexia, and severe depression. Bilateral photophobia, excessive lacrimation, and conjunctivitis develop into severe panophthalmitis and corneal opacity. The muzzle is crusted and burnt in appearance (Fig. 1.4-14) and may become necrotic, cracked, and slough. Similar lesions occasionally occur on the udder, teats, (Fig. 1.4-15), vulva, and scrotum. There is a copious nasal discharge which is frequently fetid. The mucosa of the nasal septum becomes fiery red, then purple, and may necrose. The oral mucosa is hyperemic, and the hard palate and tongue develop punched-out ulcers.

Erythematous-to-purplish macules and papules ooze, crust and may become superficially necrotic and slough. These lesions are most easily seen in the axillae, groin, perineum, coronets (Fig. 1.4-16). In haired skin—especially ears, the trunk, face, and neck—these lesions are covered by characteristically tufted hairs, which epilate leaving heavily crusted areas (Figs. 1.4-17 through 1.4-19). Occasionally the hooves may slough. Rarely, a general-

ized exudative and crusting dermatitis, resembling dermatophilosis, is seen in the absence of systemic signs.

Most animals have neurologic signs such as stupor, head jerking, and periods of extreme irritability and mania.

Differential Diagnosis

Bovine viral diarrhea, infectious bovine rhinotracheitis, rinderpest, and bluetongue.

Diagnosis

1. Necropsy examination.
2. Viral isolation.
3. Viral antigen detection.

BOVINE VIRAL DIARRHEA

Features

Bovine viral diarrhea is a cosmopolitan infectious disease caused by a *Pestivirus*. Transmission occurs via direct and indirect contact. There are no apparent breed, age, or sex predilections.

Acute infections are characterized by fever, diarrhea, cough, nasal and ocular discharges, and erosions and ulcers of the oral

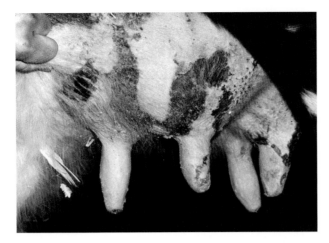

Figure 1.4-13 Herpes Mammillitis. Linear areas of necrosis, ulceration, and crust on udder.

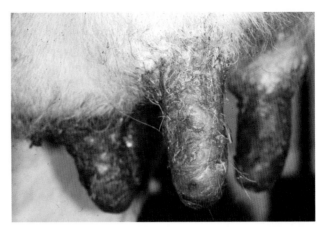

Figure 1.4-15 Malignant Catarrhal Fever. Erythema, necrosis, and crusting on teats.

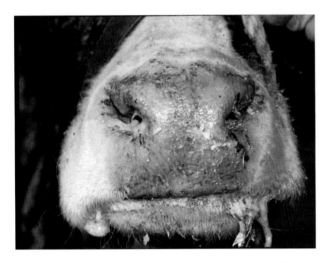

Figure 1.4-14 Malignant Catarrhal Fever. Erythema, necrosis, and ulcers on muzzle.

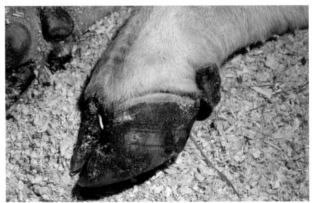

Figure 1.4-16 Malignant Catarrhal Fever. Coronitis.

cavity. Chronic infections ("mucosal disease") are characterized by diarrhea, nasal and ocular discharge, necrosis and ulceration of oral mucosa, erosion and ulceration and crusting of the muzzle (Fig. 1.4-20), lips, nostrils, coronet (Fig. 1.4-21), interdigital spaces (Fig. 1.4-22), teats (Fig. 1.4-23), vulva (Fig. 1.4-24), and prepuce. Scales, crusts, hyperkeratosis, and alopecia may occur on the neck, medial thighs, and perineum. A generalized crusting dermatitis may occur. *In utero* infections may cause generalized hypotrichosis that may spare the head, tail, and distal legs.

Differential Diagnosis

Malignant catarrhal fever, rinderpest, bovine papular stomatitis, infectious bovine rhinotracheitis, bluetongue, vesicular stomatitis, and foot-and-mouth disease.

Diagnosis

1. Virus isolation.
2. Viral antigen detection.

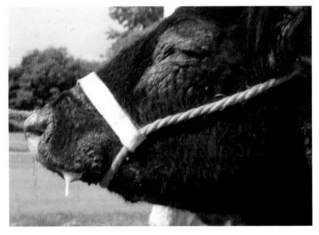

Figure 1.4-17 Malignant Catarrhal Fever. Tufted hairs and thick crusts on face.

INFECTIOUS BOVINE RHINOTRACHEITIS

Features

Infectious bovine rhinotracheitis (IBR) is a cosmopolitan infectious disease caused by bovine herpesvirus-1. Transmission oc-

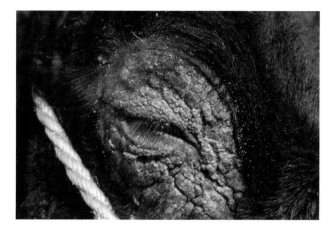

Figure 1.4-18 Malignant Catarrhal Fever. Thick crusts periocularly.

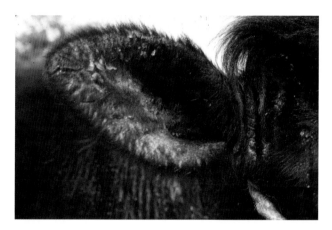

Figure 1.4-19 Malignant Catarrhal Fever. Erythema and crusting on pinna.

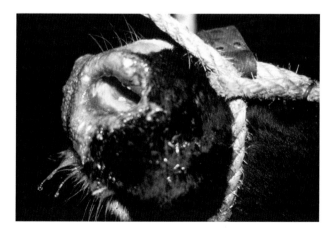

Figure 1.4-20 Bovine Viral Diarrhea. Erythema and ulceration of muzzle.

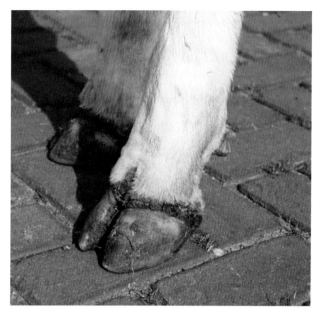

Figure 1.4-21 Bovine Viral Diarrhea. Coronitis (courtesy M. Sloet).

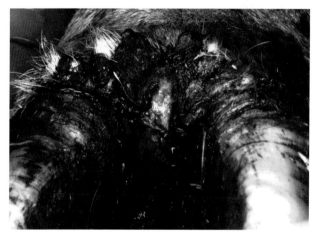

Figure 1.4-22 Bovine Viral Diarrhea. Interdigital ulceration and crusting (courtesy J. Gourreau).

Genital IBR (infectious pustular vulvovaginitis [IPV], infectious pustular balanoposthitis [IPB]) is characterized by pustules and necrotic white plaques on the vulva, vagina, prepuce, and penis. Lesions are often painful. Rarely, pustules, crusts, alopecia, and lichenification are seen on the perineum, udder (Fig. 1.4-26), and scrotum.

Differential Diagnosis

Pasteurellosis, pinkeye (*Moraxella bovis*), necrotic vaginitis from parturition injuries or sadism, irritation from caustic materials, granular vaginitis.

Diagnosis

1. Virus isolation.
2. Viral antigen detection.

curs via aerosol and venereal methods. There are no apparent breed, age, or sex predilections.

Respiratory IBR is characterized by fever, decreased appetite, dyspnea, and erythema and crusting of the muzzle ("red nose") (Fig. 1.4-25). The muzzle may become necrotic and ulcerated. Conjunctivitis and abortion occur frequently.

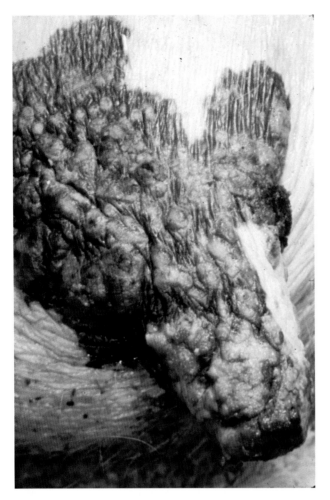

Figure 1.4-23 Bovine Viral Diarrhea. Ulcers and crusts on teat.

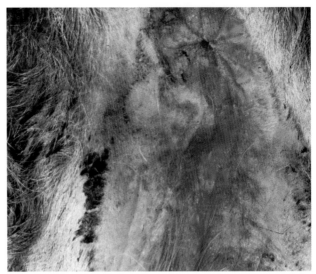

Figure 1.4-24 Bovine Viral Diarrhea. Erythema and ulceration of vulva (courtesy J. Gourreau).

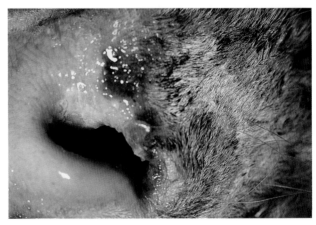

Figure 1.4-25 Infectious Bovine Rhinotracheitis. Erythema and crusts on muzzle (courtesy J. Gourreau).

VESICULAR STOMATITIS

Features

Vesicular stomatitis is an uncommon infectious disease caused by a *Vesiculovirus*. The disease is enzootic in North, Central, and South America, and is most common between late spring and early fall. Transmission occurs via aerosols and insect vectors. There are no apparent breed, age, or sex predilections.

Vesicles and bullae progress to painful erosions and ulcers. Lesions are often confined to one of three body regions: (1) the muzzle, lips, and oral cavity (Fig. 1.4-27), (2) the teats, udder, and prepuce (Fig. 1.4-28), and (3) the coronets and interdigital spaces (Fig. 1.4-29). Fever, depression, inappetence, and lameness are variable findings. Mastitis is a potential sequela of teat lesions, and hooves may rarely slough. Morbidity varies from 10 to 95%, but mortality is rare.

Vesicular stomatitis is a potential zoonosis. Humans develop influenza-like symptoms and occasionally mucocutaneous vesicles and erosions. Swine, sheep, goats, and horses are also affected.

Differential Diagnosis

Foot-and-mouth disease is clinically indistinguishable from vesicular stomatitis. Other differentials include bovine viral diarrhea, rinderpest, malignant catarrhal fever, bluetongue, and bovine papular stomatitis.

Diagnosis

1. Virus isolation.
2. Viral antigen detection.

FOOT-AND-MOUTH DISEASE

Features

Foot-and-mouth disease ("aphthous fever"—Greek: painful vesicles and ulcers in mouth) is a highly contagious infectious disease of cattle, sheep, goats, and swine caused by an *Aphthovirus* having 7 principal serotypes: A, O, C, South African Territories (SAT) 1, SAT 2, SAT 3, and Asia 1. It is the most dreaded of cattle diseases. The disease is endemic in Africa, Asia, and South America, and sporadic in Europe. Transmission oc-

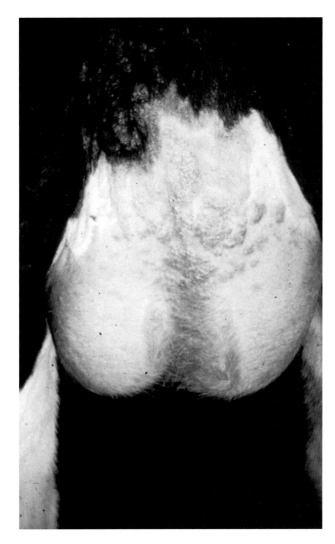

Figure 1.4-26 Infectious Bovine Rhinotracheitis. Erythema and crusts on udder.

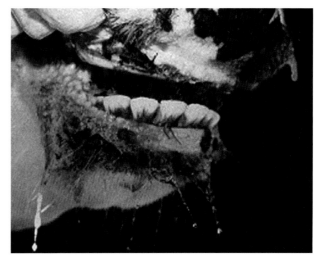

Figure 1.4-27 Vesicular Stomatitis. Ulcers on lips (courtesy J. Gourreau).

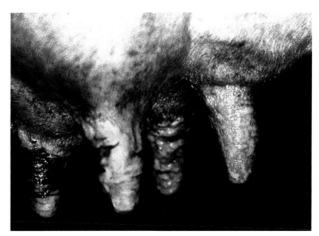

Figure 1.4-28 Vesicular Stomatitis. Ulcers and crusts on teats (courtesy J. Gourreau).

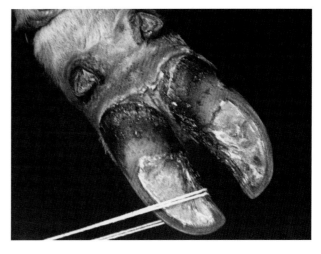

Figure 1.4-29 Vesicular Stomatitis. Ulceration of coronet and interdigital space (courtesy J. Gourreau).

curs via aerosol, contact, insect vectors, and fomites. There are no breed, age or sex predilections.

Fever, depression, and inappetence are usually the first signs of infection. As vesicle formations begin, hypersalivation and nasal discharge are evident, and cattle may exhibit lip smacking, a classic early sign. Lameness becomes obvious. Vesicles and bullae (up to 10 cm in diameter) develop into painful erosions and ulcers. Lesions are most commonly seen on the muzzle, nostrils, lips, oral mucosa, teats, coronets, and interdigital spaces and heels of the feet (Fig. 1.4-30 through 1.4-32). Pregnant animals may abort. In severe cases, the hooves may detach or severe laminitis may be followed by deformed hooves.

Morbidity varies from 50% to 100%, and mortality is usually low (less than 5%), although occasional outbreaks are characterized by over 50% mortality. Economic losses can be devastating: quarantine, slaughter, embargoes, and loss of trade. Foot-and-mouth disease is the number one foreign animal disease threat in the United States, and the most significant disease affecting free trade in animals and animal products internationally.

Humans may rarely develop vesicles on the hands and/or in the mouth (Fig. 1.4-33).

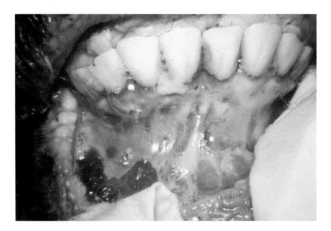

Figure 1.4-30 Foot-and-Mouth Disease. Ulcers on oral mucosa (courtesy L. Dhennin, coll. J. Gourreau, AFSSA).

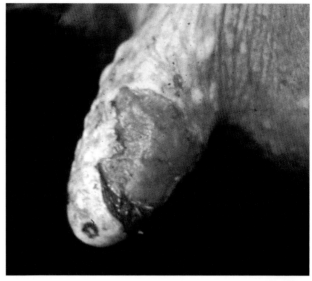

Figure 1.4-32 Foot-and-Mouth Disease. Ulceration of teat.

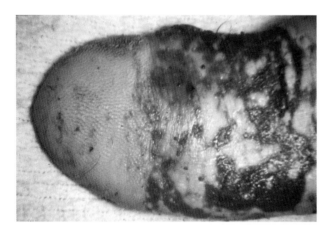

Figure 1.4-31 Foot-and-Mouth Disease. Ulcers on tongue (courtesy L. Dhennin, coll. J. Gourreau, AFSSA).

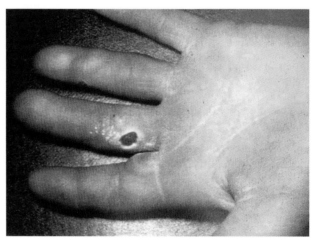

Figure 1.4-33 Foot-and-Mouth Disease. Ruptured vesicle on finger of a human (courtesy J. Gourreau).

Differential Diagnosis

Vesicular stomatitis is clinically indistinguishable from foot-and-mouth disease. Other differentials include bovine viral diarrhea, rinderpest, malignant catarrhal fever, bluetongue, and bovine papular stomatitis.

Diagnosis

1. Virus Isolation—Vesicular fluid, epithelial lesions, and heparinized blood.
2. Viral antigen detection.
3. Serology—Clotted blood.

LUMPY SKIN DISEASE

Features

Lumpy skin disease ("knopvelsiekte") is a chronic infectious disease caused by a *Capripoxvirus* ("Neethling Virus"). Transmission occurs via insect vectors (especially *Stomoxys calcitrans*). There are no apparent breed, age, or sex predilections. Severe, generalized lumpy skin disease-like lesions have occurred in dairy cattle

vaccinated with a sheeppox virus strain meant to prevent the naturally-occurring disease.

Initial clinical signs include fever, anorexia, ocular discharge, nasal discharge, hypersalivation, and lymphadenopathy. Firm papules and nodules (0.5 to 5 cm diameter) are initially recognized as erect tufts of hair. Lesions are often confined to the head, neck, legs, perineum, teats, udder, scrotum and tail, but may be generalized (Fig. 1.4-34). Some lesions ooze and ulcerate (Figs. 1.4-35 through 1.4-37), others only develop a dry crust. Larger lesions undergo necrosis, wherein a "moat" develops around them and separates them from surrounding normal skin. These so-called "sitfasts" then slough, leaving crateriform—often full skin thickness—ulcers which heal by scar (Fig. 1.4-38).

Edema is evident in the legs (sometimes swollen to 3 to 4 times normal size), dewlap, brisket, and genitalia. Severely swollen limbs may develop areas of necrosis, sloughing, and ulceration, leading to secondary bacterial infection and/or myiasis. Yellowish white papules and nodules that slough leaving erosions and ul-

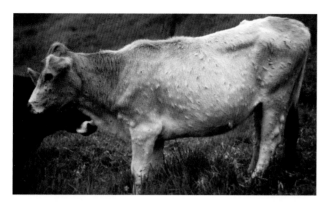

Figure 1.4-34 Lumpy Skin Disease. Generalized tufted papules and nodules (courtesy H. Meyer, coll. J. Gourreau, AFSSA).

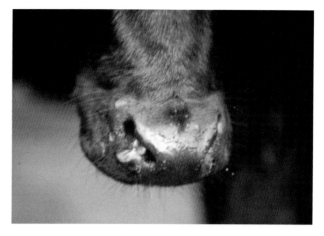

Figure 1.4-36 Lumpy Skin Disease. Small papules and ulcerated nodules on muzzle (courtesy H. Meyer, coll. J. Gourreau, AFSSA).

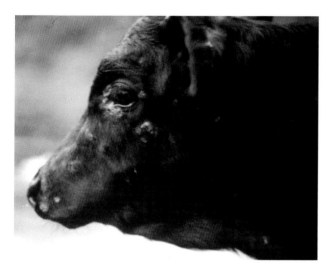

Figure 1.4-35 Lumpy Skin Disease. Ulcerated nodules on face (courtesy H. Meyer, coll. J. Gourreau, AFSSA).

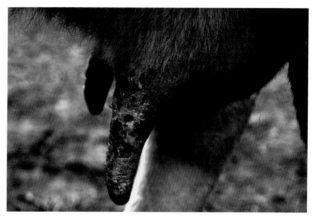

Figure 1.4-37 Lumpy Skin Disease. Ulcerated nodules on teat (courtesy J. Gourreau).

cers occur in the nasal and oral mucosae. Weight loss, reduced milk production, and abortion occur. Hide damage can be extensive, and teat lesions may lead to mastitis. Morbidity varies from 5 to 80%, but mortality rarely exceeds 3%.

Differential Diagnosis

Pseudolumpy skin disease.

Diagnosis

1. Necropsy examination.
2. Dermatohistopathology—Eosinophilic intracytoplasmic inclusion bodies in epidermal keratinocytes.
3. Virus isolation.

BESNOITIOSIS

Features

Besnoitiosis ("globidiosis") is an uncommon to common protozoal disease caused by *Besnoitia besnoiti*. Transmission occurs by

ingestion (vegetation contaminated with cat feces containing oocysts) or biting arthropods and insects (bradyzoites). The disease is most common in summer. Besnoitiosis occurs in Africa, Asia, and parts of Europe and South America. There are no apparent breed or sex predilections, and animals 2 to 4 years of age are most commonly affected.

Initial clinical signs include fever, depression, anorexia, photophobia, and reluctance to move. Hair is seen standing on end, especially on the perineum, pinnae, and face, and the underlying skin is hot and painful. Marked edema then develops, especially on the head, legs, udder (Fig. 1.4-39) and scrotum (Fig. 1.4-40). Edematous skin is hot, painful, and loses its elasticity. Peripheral lymphadenopathy is pronounced. Edema gradually recedes, but the skin becomes thick, folded and wrinkled ("elephantiasis"), alopecic, and hyperkeratotic (Fig. 1.4-41). The skin over limb joints becomes fissured and secondarily infected. Small, 1 mm diameter, shiny white parasitic cysts occur in the conjunctiva (Fig. 1.4-42), and are virtually pathognomonic.

Typically, multiple animals are affected. Economic losses are heavy because of emaciation, carcass condemnation, and death.

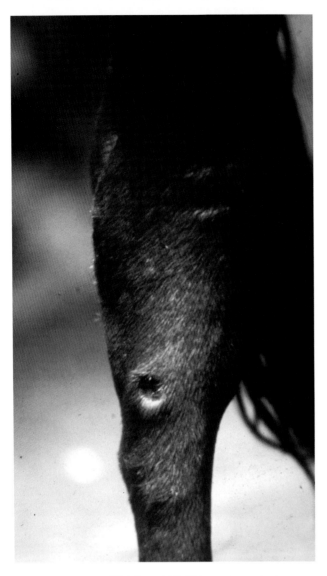

Figure 1.4-38 Lumpy Skin Disease. Full-thickness ulcer on leg (courtesy D. Thiaucourt, coll. J. Gourreau, AFSSA).

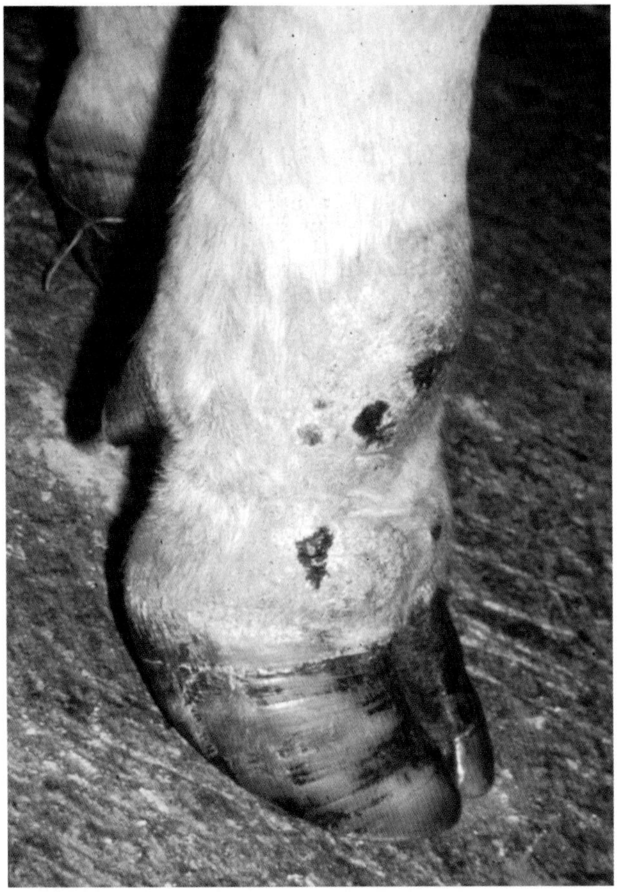

Figure 1.4-39 Besnoitiosis. Edema, erythema, crusting, and alopecia of distal leg (courtesy M. Franc, coll. J. Gourreau, AFSSA).

Diagnosis

1. Physical Examination—Parasitic cysts in conjunctiva.
2. Microscopy (Direct Smear of Scraped Conjunctival Cysts)—Numerous crescent- or banana-shaped bradyzoites (2 to 7 µm in length by 1 to 2 µm in width).
3. Dermatohistopathology—Parasitic cysts (up to 600 µm diameter) containing numerous crescentic or banana-shaped bradyzoites (2 to 7 µm long).

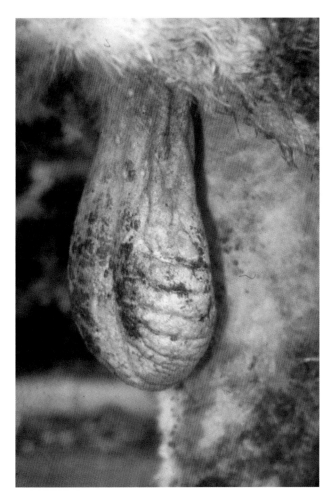

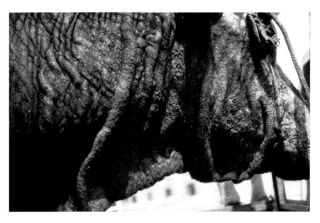

Figure 1.4-41 Besnoitiosis. Alopecia, crusting, thickening, and folding of skin over face and neck (courtesy P. Bland).

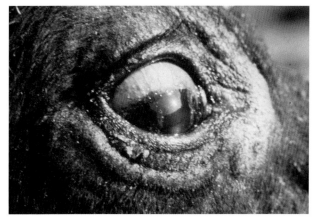

Figure 1.4-40 Besnoitiosis. Edema, thickening, and folding of scrotal skin (courtesy M. Franc, coll. J. Gourreau, AFSSA).

Figure 1.4-42 Besnoitiosis. Small, white parasitic cysts on sclera (courtesy M. Franc, coll. J. Gourreau, AFSSA).

MISCELLANEOUS VIRAL AND PROTOZOAL DISEASES

Table 1.4-2 Miscellaneous Viral and Protozoal Diseases

Bluetongue (*Orbivirus*) (Figs. 1.4-43 through 1.4-46)	Uncommon; cosmopolitan; *Culicoides* spp. vectors; erythema, edema, necrosis, ulcerations, and crusts; especially muzzle ("burnt muzzle"), oral cavity, coronets, udder, and teats; rarely hooves slough; fever, nasal discharge, hypersalivation, lameness; viral isolation, viral antigen detection, serology
Bovine ephemeral fever (*Ephemerovirus*)	Uncommon; Africa, Asia, and Australia; especially summer; mosquito vectors; edema (especially head) and subcutaneous emphysema (especially back); fever, lameness, anorexia, depression, hypersalivation, nasal and ocular discharge, abortion, decreased milk production; viral isolation, serology
Bovine spongiform encephalopathy ("mad cow disease")	Rare; widespread; prion protein; licking, wrinkling nose, head rubbing; neurological disorders; brain histopathology, various immunohistochemical and Western blot procedures
Cowpox (*Orthopoxvirus*)	Rare; Europe and the Middle East; field mice and vole reservoirs, and cats infected; an identical syndrome was produced by vaccinia virus; fever and tender teats are followed by the typical sequence of pox lesions on the teats and udder; the classic thick, red crust, 1 to 2 cm in diameter, is said to be pathognommic; in severe cases, lesions occur on the medial thighs, perineum, vulva, scrotum, and mouth of nursing calves; zoonosis (skin lesions in humans identical to those produced by pseudo-cowpox); virus isolation
Herpes mammary pustular dermatitis (Bovine herpesvirus-4)	Rare; United States; lactating cattle; vesicles and pustules on the lateral and ventral aspects of the udder; viral isolation
Jembrana disease (*Lentivirus*)	Uncommon; Indonesia; blood oozes from skin ("blood sweating"); fever, anorexia, oculo-nasal discharge, oral erosions, diarrhea, lymphadenopathy; serology
Pseudolumpy skin disease (*Bovine herpesvirus-2* ["Allerton virus"]) (Figs. 1.4-47 through 1.4-49)	Uncommon; cosmopolitan; sudden appearance of firm, round, raised papules and nodules that develop a characteristic flat surface and slightly depressed center; superficial sloughing and alopecia occurs—without scarring; lesions are usually widespread, especially on the head, neck, back, and perineum; nursing calves may develop ulcers of the muzzle and oral cavity; virus isolation
Pseudorabies (Aujeszky's disease, "mad itch") (Porcine herpesvirus-1) (Figs. 1.4-50 and 1.4-51)	Uncommon; cosmopolitan; bite, lick, scratch, rub, producing self-mutilation; especially flanks, hindquarters, anus, vulva, face, and neck; fever, depression, hypersalivation, anorexia, bellowing, convulsing; necropsy examination, viral isolation
Rift Valley fever (*Phlebovirus*)	Uncommon; Africa; mosquito vectors; coronitis and dry, thick skin on unpigmented areas of teats, udder, and scrotum; fever, stomatitis, diarrhea, lameness and abortion; humans —influenza-like disease, and occasional fatal encephalitis and hemorrhagic fever; viral isolation, serology
Rinderpest ("cattle plague") (*Morbillivirus*) (Figs. 1.4-52 and 1.4-53)	Uncommon; Africa and Asia; grey-white necrotic foci that slough and ulcerate in oral cavity and on lips and nasal, vulvar and prepucial mucosae with fetid smell; fever, depression, anorexia, nasal and ocular discharge, diarrhea; rarely, a skin form (pustules and crusts on neck, withers, medial thighs, and scrotum) with mild systemic signs; viral isolation, viral antigen detection
Sarcocystosis (Fig. 1.4-54)	Common; cosmopolitan; *Sarcocystis cruzi*; loss of tail switch ("rat tail"); may develop alopecia of pinnae, neck, rump, and distal limbs; fever, anorexia, hypersalivation, lameness, anemia, abortion; necropsy examination
Theileriosis	Uncommon; Africa and Mediterranean; tick vectors; *Theileria parva* ("East Coast Fever") may be associated with papules and nodules over neck and trunk; fever, lymphadenopathy, oculonasal discharge, dyspnea, wasting; *T. annulata* ("Mediterranean Coast Fever") may be associated with wheals or papules that begin on face, neck, and shoulders, and then generalize; pruritus may be intense; fever, lymphadenopathy, wasting; *T. lawrencei* associated with edema of eyelids, face, and throat; fever, lymphadenopathy, oculonasal discharge; histopathology of lymph nodes (schizonts), serology
Trypanosomiasis	Uncommon; Africa; *Trypanosoma congolense*; papules on neck, chest, and flanks; fever, apathy, anemia, lymphadenopathy, wasting; blood smears (trypanosomes), serology

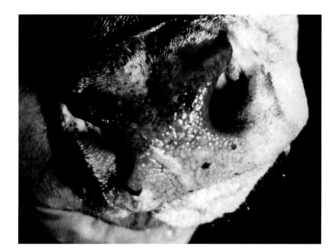

Figure 1.4-43 Bluetongue. Erythema and necrosis of muzzle (courtesy J. Gourreau).

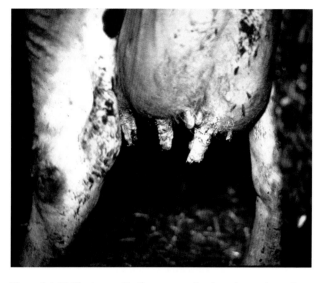

Figure 1.4-46 Bluetongue. Erythema, necrosis, ulceration, and crusting of teats.

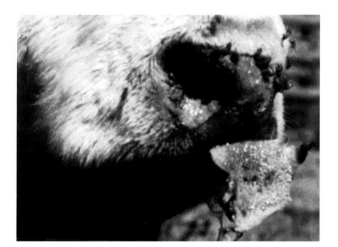

Figure 1.4-44 Bluetongue. Necrosis and sloughing of muzzle skin (courtesy A. Weaver, coll. J. Gourreau, AFSSA).

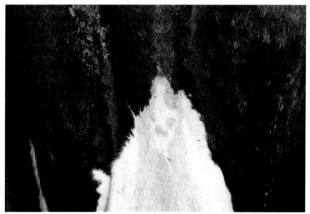

Figure 1.4-47 Pseudolumpy Skin Disease. Tufted crusts in perineal area.

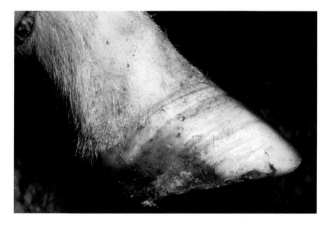

Figure 1.4-45 Bluetongue. Coronitis.

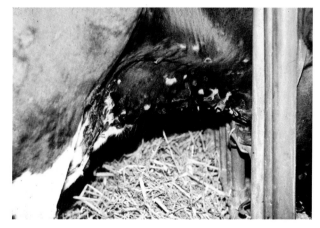

Figure 1.4-48 Pseudolumpy Skin Disease. Multiple areas of superficial necrosis and sloughing on neck and shoulder.

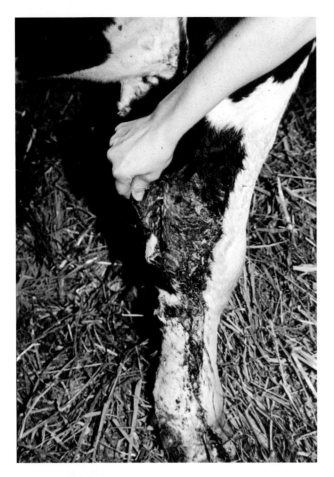

Figure 1.4-49 Pseudolumpy Skin Disease. Large area of necrosis, slough, and ulceration on leg.

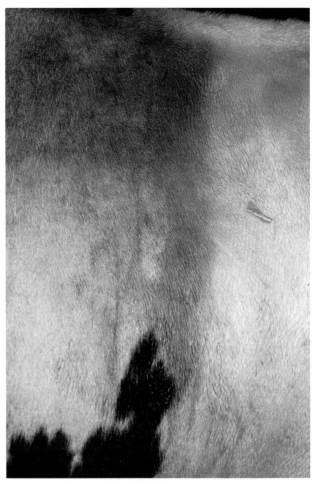

Figure 1.4-51 Pseudorabies. Linear area of erythema and excoriation produced by frenzied licking (courtesy M. Sloet).

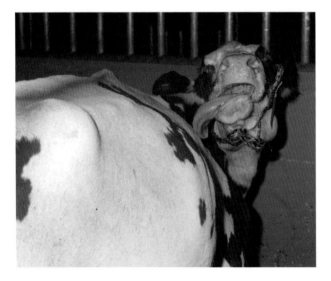

Figure 1.4-50 Pseudorabies. Frenzied, focal, unilateral licking (courtesy M. Sloet).

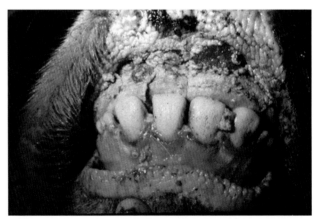

Figure 1.4-52 Rinderpest. Necrosis and ulceration of oral mucosa (courtesy J. Gourreau).

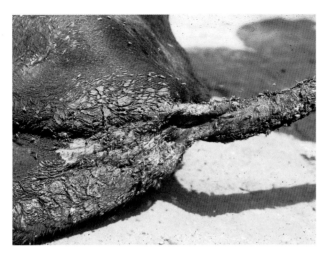

Figure 1.4-53 Rinderpest. Erythema and crusting of perineum and ventral tail (courtesy J. Gourreau).

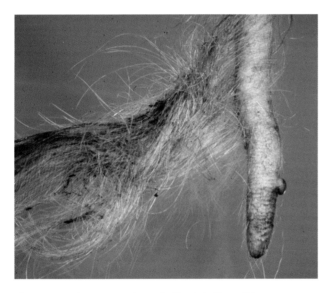

Figure 1.4-54 Sarcocystosis. Loss of tail switch ("rat tail").

REFERENCES

Ali AA, et al. 1990. Clinical and Pathological Studies on Lumpy Skin Disease in Egypt. *Vet Rec* 127: 549.

Andrews AH, et al. 2005. Bovine Medicine, Ed 2. Blackwell Scientific, Oxford, UK.

Büttner M, Rziha HJ. 2002. Parapoxviruses: From the Lesion to the Viral Genome. *J Vet Med B* 49: 7.

Cortes H, et al. 2005. Besnoitiosis in Bulls in Portugal. *Vet Rec* 157: 262.

David D, et al. 2005. Two Cases of the Cutaneous Form of Sheep–Associated Malignant Catarrhal Fever in Cattle. *Vet Rec* 156: 118.

Davies FG. 1991. Lumpy Skin Disease, an African *Capripoxvirus* Disease of Cattle. *Br Vet J* 147: 489.

d'Offay JM, et al. 2003. Use of a Polymerase Chain Reaction Assay to Detect Bovine Herpesvirus Type 2 DNA in Skin Lesions from Cattle, Suspected to have Pseudolumpy Skin Disease. *J Am Vet Med Assoc* 222: 1404.

Franc M, et al. 1987. La Besnoitiose Bovine. *Point Vét* 19: 445.

Gavier-Widén D, et al. 2005. Diagnosis of Transmissible Spongiform Encephalopathies in Animals: A Review. *J Vet Diagn Invest* 17: 509.

Gourreau JM, et al. 1988. La Thélite Ulcérative Herpétique des Bovins. *Point Vét* 20: 507.

Grootenhuis JG, et al. 1990. Susceptibility of African Buffalo and Boran Cattle to *Trypanosoma congolense* Transmitted by *Glossina morsitans centrales*. *Vet Parasitol* 35: 219.

Guo WZ, et al. 1988. Comparison of an Enzyme-Linked Immunosorbent Assay and a Complement-Fixation Test for the Detection of IgG to Bovine Herpesvirus type IV (Bovine Cytomegalovirus). *Am J Vet Res* 49: 667.

Kahrs RF. 2001. Viral Diseases of Cattle. Ed 2. Iowa State University Press, Ames, IA.

Miller JM, et al. 1988. Effects of a Bovine Herpesvirus–1 Isolate on Reproductive Function in Heifers: Classifications of a Type–2 (Infectious Pustular Vulvovaginitis) Virus by Restriction Endonuclease Analysis of Viral DNA. *Am J Vet Res* 49: 1653.

Odéon AC, et al. 2003. Bovine Viral Diarrhea Virus Genomic Associations and Generalized Dermatitis Outbreaks in Argentina. *Vet Microbiol* 96: 133.

Radostits OM, et al. 2000. Veterinary Medicine. A Textbook of the Diseases of Cattle, Sheep, Pigs, Goats and Horses. Ed 9. WB Saunders, Philadelphia, PA.

Scott DW. 1988. Large Animal Dermatology. WB Saunders, Philadelphia, PA.

Stachurski F, et al. 1988. La Fièvre Catarrhale Maligne des Bovins (Coryza Gangreneux). *Point Vét* 20: 715.

Yeruham I, et al. 1994. Adverse Reactions in Cattle to a Capripox Vaccine. *Vet Rec* 135: 330.

Yeruham I, et al. 1994. Clinical and Pathological Description of a Chronic Form of Bovine Papular Stomatitis. *J Comp Pathol* 111: 279.

Yeruham I, et al. 1996. Occurrence of Cowpox-like Lesions in Cattle in Israel. *Rev Elev Méd Vet Pays Trop* 49: 299.

Yeruham I, et al. 2005. Bovine Ephemeral Fever in a Dairy Cattle Herd in the Jordan Valley. *Vet Rec* 156: 284.

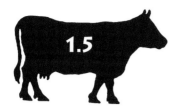

IMMUNOLOGICAL SKIN DISEASES

Urticaria
Cutaneous Adverse Drug Reaction
Alopecia Areata
Miscellaneous Immunological Diseases
    Bovine Exfoliative Erythroderma
    Erythema Multiforme
    Food Hypersensitivity
    Insect Hypersensitivity
    Toxic Epidermal Necrolysis
    Vasculitis

URTICARIA

Features

Urticaria ("hives") is a rarely reported, cosmopolitan, variably pruritic, edematous skin disorder. It may be immunologic or nonimmunologic in nature. Incriminated causes include insects, arthropods, infections, systemic medications (penicillin, streptomycin, oxytetracycline, chloramphenicol, neomycin, sulfonamides, diethylstilbestrol, carboxymethylcellulose, hydroxypropylmethylcellulose), biologicals (various vaccines and toxoids, especially leptospirosis, *Brucella abortus* strain 19, foot and mouth disease, shipping fever, salmonellosis, rinderpest, rabies, contagious pleuropneumonia, horse serum), physical trauma (dermatographism), hypodermiasis, feed stuffs (pasture plants, moldy hay or straw, potato, walnut leaves), and plants (stinging nettle). Milk allergy is a unique autoallergic disease. It is seen most commonly in Jerseys and Guernseys—wherein cows become sensitized to the casein in their own milk. Except for milk allergy, bovine urticaria has no apparent age, breed, or sex predilections.

Urticarial reactions are characterized by the sudden onset of more-or-less bilaterally symmetric wheals, which may or may not be erythematous or pruritic. Lesions are typically flat-topped, steep-walled, covered by normal appearing skin and haircoat, of normal body temperature, and pit with digital pressure. Lesions may be annular, angular, arciform, or serpiginous (Figs. 1.5-1 and 1.5-2). Individual lesions are typically evanescent, disappearing within 24 to 72 hours as new ones appear. They commonly occur on the face, neck, and trunk.

Milk allergy is associated with milk retention, unusual engorgement of the udder, and occasionally variable degrees of respiratory distress.

Differential Diagnosis

Erythema multiforme, vasculitis, and early cutaneous lymphoma.

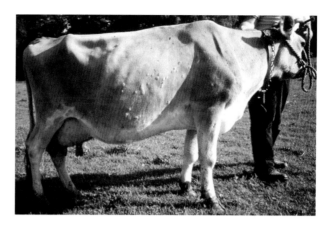

Figure 1.5-1 Milk Allergy. Multiple wheals over shoulder, lateral thorax and abdomen.

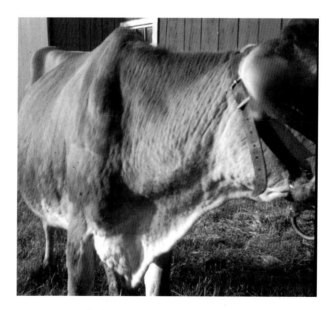

Figure 1.5-2 Milk Allergy. Multiple wheals over neck and shoulder.

Diagnosis

1. History and physical examination (the three differentials typically produce persistent lesions that do not pit with digital pressure).
2. Dermatohistopathology—Pure superficial to deep, perivascular to interstitial, eosinophilic dermatitis.

CUTANEOUS ADVERSE DRUG REACTION

Features

Cutaneous adverse drug reactions (drug eruption, drug allergy, dermatitis medicamentosa) are rarely reported, cosmopolitan, variably pruritic, and pleomorphic cutaneous or mucocutaneous reactions to a drug. Agents responsible for skin eruptions may be administered orally, topically, or by injection. Any drug may cause a skin eruption, and cutaneous adverse drug reactions can mimic virtually any dermatosis. There are no apparent age, breed or sex predilections.

Numerous agents have been reported to cause urticarial reactions (see Urticaria) (Figs. 1.5-3 and 1.5-4). Inactivated foot-and-mouth disease vaccines can produce skin reactions in 0.1% to 14.6% of the animals vaccinated. Reactions only occur in previously vaccinated animals, appear one to two weeks post-vaccination, and persist for three to five weeks. Skin reactions may be urticarial and/or vasculitic (necrotic, exudative) (Figs. 1.5-5 and 1.5-6) and are associated with weight loss, decreased milk production (average of 21.5%/day), and lymphadenopathy. Other cutaneous reaction patterns potentially produced by drugs include erythema multiforme and toxic epidermal necrolysis (see Table 1.5-1).

Differential Diagnosis

Urticaria, vasculitis, and early cutaneous lymphoma.

Diagnosis

Helpful criteria include:

1. Reactions occur in a minority of patients receiving the drug.
2. Observed manifestations do not resemble known pharmacologic actions for the drug.
3. Previous experience that the suspect drug is known for causing this type of skin reaction.
4. Lack of alternative etiologies.
5. Appropriate timing—Reactions generally occur within the first 1 to 3 weeks of the initiation of therapy, or within hours to days if there has been previous exposure.

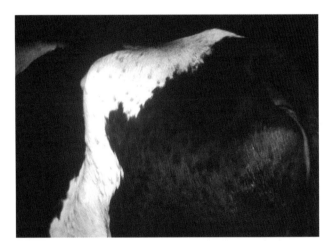

Figure 1.5-4 Cutaneous Adverse Drug Reaction. Multiple wheals over rump and flank associated with rabies vaccination (courtesy J. Segaud, Coll. J. Gourreau, AFSSA).

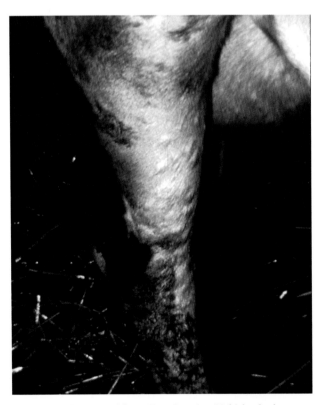

Figure 1.5-3 Cutaneous Adverse Drug Reaction. Multiple wheals on hind leg and udder associated with rabies vaccination (courtesy J. Segaud, Coll. J. Gourreau, AFSSA).

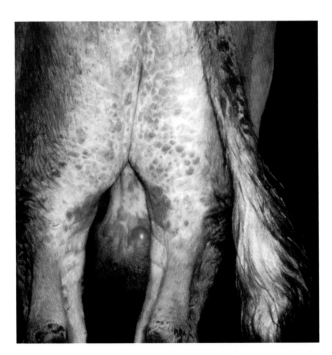

Figure 1.5-5 Cutaneous Adverse Drug Reaction. Multiple purpuric papules and plaques on perineum and udder associated with foot-and-mouth disease vaccination (courtesy A. Mayr, coll. J. Gourreau, AFSSA).

6. Dechallenge—Resolution begins to occur within 1 to 2 weeks after drug is discontinued.

7. Rechallenge—Reaction reproduced by readministration of drug (definitive, but not usually recommended nor approved).

ALOPECIA AREATA

Features

Alopecia areata is a rare cosmopolitan autoimmune dermatosis. Anagen hair follicle antigens are the targets of cell-mediated and humoral autoimmune responses. There are no apparent age, sex, or breed predilections.

Lesions, may be solitary or multiple, and consist of annular–to-oval areas of alopecia (Figs. 1.5-7 to 1.5-11). The exposed skin

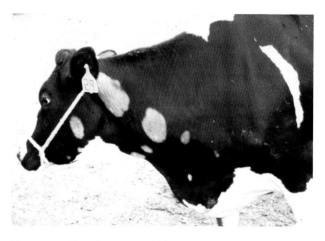

Figure 1.5-8 Alopecia Areata. Multiple annular to oval areas of alopecia over face and neck.

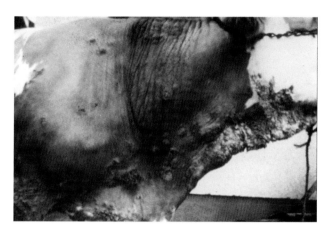

Figure 1.5-6 Cutaneous Adverse Drug Reaction. Papules and plaques with necrotic centers over neck and shoulder associated with foot-and-mouth disease vaccination (courtesy A. Mayr, coll. J. Gourreau, AFSSA).

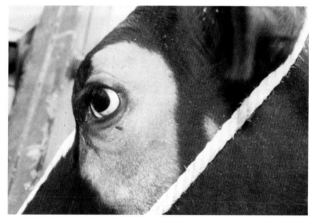

Figure 1.5-9 Alopecia Areata. Periocular alopecia with regrowth of fine, white hairs.

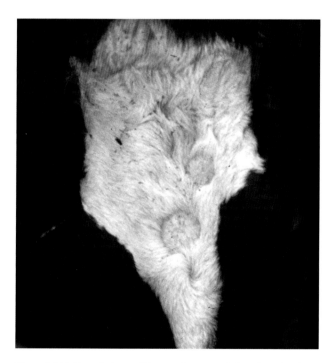

Figure 1.5-7 Alopecia Areata. Two annular areas of alopecia on head (orange color due to topical iodophor applications).

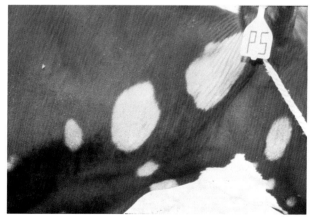

Figure 1.5-10 Alopecia Areata. Multiple annular to oval areas of alopecia over cheek, neck, and shoulder.

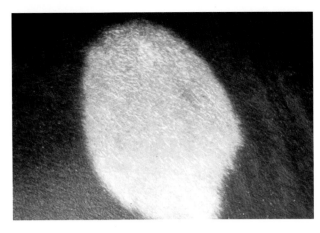

Figure 1.5-11 Alopecia Areata. Annular area of alopecia with regrowth of fine, white hairs.

appears normal. Lesions most commonly occur on the face, neck, brisket, and shoulder. Pruritus and pain are absent, and affected animals are otherwise healthy. Spontaneous regrowth of hair often features hairs that are lighter in color and smaller in size than normal. Only a single animal in a herd is affected.

Differential Diagnosis

Follicular dysplasia.

Diagnosis

1. The normal-appearing skin rules out infectious (bacteria, fungi) and parasitic causes of annular alopecic lesions.
2. Dermatohistopathology—Lymphocytic bulbitis.

MISCELLANEOUS IMMUNOLOGICAL DISEASES

Table 1.5-1 Miscellaneous Immunological Diseases

Bovine exfoliative erythroderma	Very rare; colostrum-associated; erythema and vesicles on muzzle from birth to 4 days old, becoming generalized erythema, scale, and alopecia between 4 and 50 days old; spontaneous recovery by 4 months old; dermatohistopathology
Erythema multiforme	Very rare; host-specific cell-mediated hypersensitivity against various antigens (infections, drugs, neoplasia); more-or-less symmetrical urticarial or vesicular lesions; especially neck and dorsum; dermatohistopathology
Food hypersensitivity	Very rare and anecdotal; generalized pruritus with or without papules, plaques, wheals; attributed to wheat, maize, soybeans, rice, bran, clover hay, milk-replacer; elimination diet and rechallenge
Insect hypersensitivity (Fig. 1.5-12)	Rare; presumed hypersensitivity to salivary allergens of *Culicoides* spp.; seasonal (spring to fall); severe pruritic dermatitis of face, forehead, pinnae, and neck
Toxic epidermal necrolysis	Very rare; host-specific cell-mediated response associated with various antigens (drugs, infections); localized areas of necrosis and ulceration, especially abdomen, hind legs, and rump; reported cases neither compatible clinically (no oral mucosal or mucocutaneous involvement, no systemic illness) nor convincing histopathologically
Vasculitis (Figs. 1.5-13 to 1.5-17)	Very rare; immune-complex vascular disease (infections, drugs); more-or-less symmetrical urticarial or necroulcerative lesions (infarcts); lesions often punctate and/or linear; especially pinnae, tail tip, legs, udder, teats; dermatohistopathology

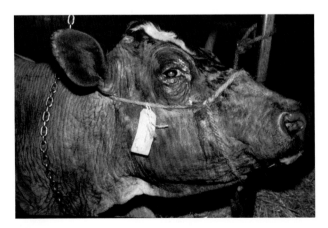

Figure 1.5-12 Presumptive Insect Hypersensitivity. Pruritic, lichenified, crusted, alopecic dermatitis of face, neck, and pinnae.

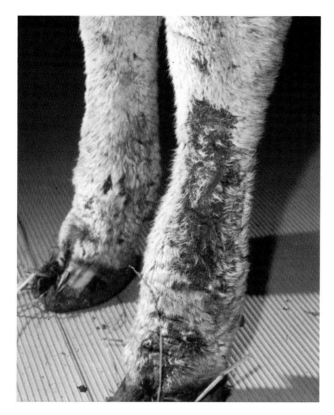

Figure 1.5-13 Idiopathic Vasculitis. Edema and linear areas of necrosis and ulceration of front legs.

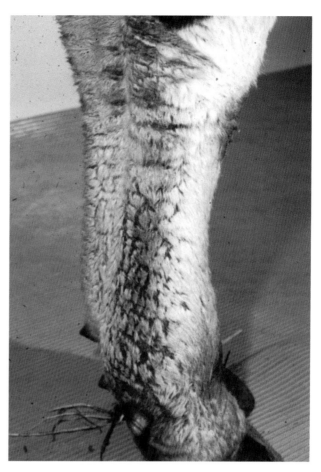

Figure 1.5-14 Idiopathic Vasculitis. Edema and linear areas of necrosis and ulceration of hind legs.

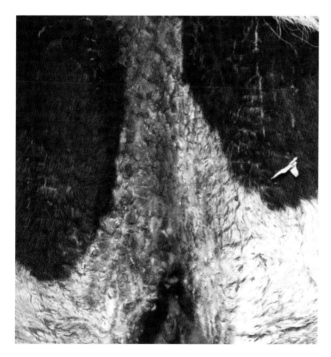

Figure 1.5-15 Idiopathic Vasculitis. Ulceration and necrosis of perineum.

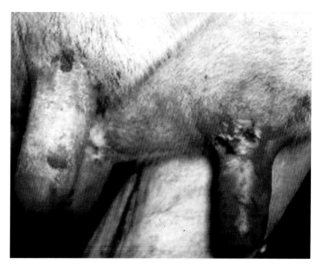

Figure 1.5-16 Drug-associated Vasculitis. Multiple annular areas of necrosis and ulceration (infarcts) on teats and udder. Animal was receiving multiple drugs.

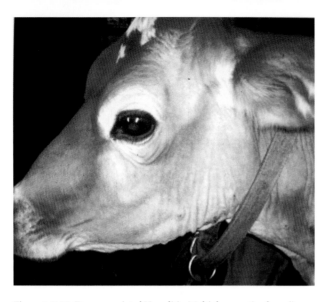

Figure 1.5-17 Drug-associated Vasculitis. Multiple necrotic ulcers (infarcts) on mandibular area. Animal was receiving multiple drugs.

REFERENCES

Fleddérus A, et al. 1988. Conjunctivitis, Rednose and Skin Hypersensitivity as Signs of Food Allergy in Veal Calves. *Vet Rec* 122: 633.

Paradis M, et al. 1988. Alopecia Areata (Pelade) in a Cow. *Can Vet J* 29: 727.

Scott DW. 1988. Large Animal Dermatology. WB Saunders, Philadelphia, PA.

Scott DW. 1991. Analyse de la Modalité de Réaction Histopathologique dans le Diagnostic des Dermatoses Inflammatoires chez les Bovins. *Point Vét* 23: 163.

Scott DW, Guard CL. 1988. Alopecia Areata in a Cow. *Agri-Pract* 9: 16.

Vomand KC, Sumano H. 1990. Adverse Drug Reactions in Cattle. *J Am Vet Med Assoc* 197: 899.

Yeruham I, et al. 1993. Field Observations in Israel on Hypersensitivity in Cattle, Sheep and Donkeys caused by *Culicoides*. *Aust Vet J* 70: 348.

Yeruham I, et al. 1999. Case Report: Idiopathic Toxic Epidermal Necrolysis in a One-Week Old Calf. *Berl Munch Tierärztl Wschr* 112: 172.

Yeruham I, et al. 1999. Nine Cases of Idiopathic Toxic Epidermal Necrolysis in Cattle in Israel. *J Vet Med B* 46: 493.

Yeruham I, et al. 2001. Adverse Reactions to FMD Vaccine. *Vet Dermatol* 12: 197.

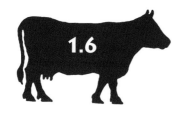

CONGENITAL AND HEREDITARY SKIN DISEASES

1.6

HYPOTRICHOSIS

Features

Hypotrichosis implies *clinically* a less than normal amount of hair that is hereditary and often congenital, and *histopathologically* a hypoplasia of hair follicles. These conditions are rare, cosmopolitan, and characterized by symmetrical hair loss and skin that is initially normal in appearance. Exposed skin is susceptible to sunburn, infections, and contact dermatitis. Affected animals are often intolerant to cold. In some instances, dental abnormalities are also present, wherein the condition is often referred to as a "congenital ectodermal dysplasia." Some forms of hypotrichosis are viable, others are lethal. The reported hypotrichoses in cattle are presented in Table 1.6-1 (Figs. 1.6-1 through 1.6-5).

Table 1.6-1 Hypotrichoses of Cattle	
Lethal hypotrichosis	Holstein-Friesians; autosomal recessive; sparse hair only on muzzle, eyelids, pinnae, tail, and pasterns; death within a few hours after birth
Hypotrichosis and partial anodontia	Simmental/Holstein cross, Charolais and Maine-Anjou-Normandy; sex-linked recessive in males; hairless and toothless at birth, and after several weeks a fine, downy haircoat and partial dentition; macroglossia and defective horns; death by 6 months old
Hypotrichosis and incisor anodontia (Fig. 1.6-1)	Holstein-Friesians; autosomal dominant; congenital patchy hypotrichosis on face, neck, pinnae, thorax, dorsum, tail, and medial thighs; Friesian crosses; x-linked incomplete dominant in males; congenital generalized hypotrichosis; viable
Ectodermal dysplasia	Black and white and red and white German Holsteins; x-linked recessive; hypotrichosis over head, neck, pinnae, back and tail; eyelashes and vibrissae few and short; dysplastic teeth
Streaked hypotrichosis	Holstein-Friesians; sex-linked dominant in females; congenital hypotrichosis in vertical streaks over hips and sometimes sides and legs; viable
Tardive hypotrichosis	Friesians; sex-linked recessive in females; hair loss on face, neck, and legs beginning at 6 weeks to 6 months old; viable
Hypotrichosis with prognathia inferior	Friesians; females; hair present only on topline
Dominant hypotrichosis (Fig. 1.6-2)	Herefords and Polled Herefords; autosomal dominant; widespread hair loss at birth; hairs thin, soft, curly, and easily broken and epilated; viable
Inherited epidermal dysplasia ("baldy calf syndrome") (Figs. 1.6-3 and 1.6-4)	Holstein-Friesians; autosomal recessive; normal at birth, except for absent horn buds and elongated, narrow, pointed hooves; at 1–2 months old, begin to lose condition and develop generalized thin haircoat and areas of scale, crust, and thickened/ wrinkled skin over the neck, flanks, shoulders, axillae, stifles, hocks, elbows, and periocular region; tips of pinnae curl medially; ulcers and crusts appear on the cranial surface of the carpi and lateral surface of the stifles and hocks; slow, painful, stilted gait, death by 8 months old
Congenital goiter and hypothyroidism	Many breeds associated with maternal dietary iodine deficiency; Friesians and Afrikanders with presumed hereditary thyroid dysplasia or defective thyroglobulin synthesis; born weak and die in hours or weeks; haircoat varies from short and fuzzy to completely absent; the skin is often thickened and puffy (myxedema)
Congenital hypotrichosis due to BVD (Fig. 1.6-5)	BVD (bovine viral diarrhea) infection of pregnant cow produces *in utero* infection of fetus; born with generalized hypotrichosis that may be less severe on the head, tail, and distal limbs

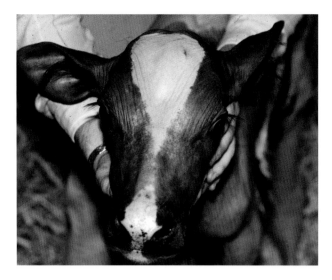

Figure 1.6-1 Hypotrichosis and Incisor Anodontia. Hypotrichosis of face and pinnae.

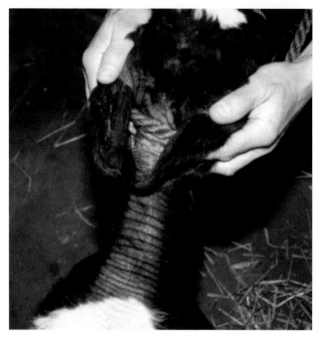

Figure 1.6-3 Inherited Epidermal Dysplasia ("Baldy Calf"). Hypotrichosis of head and neck, and medial curling of tips of pinnae.

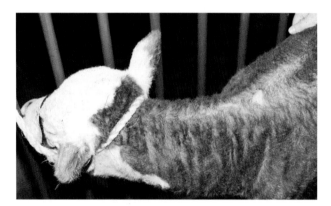

Figure 1.6-2 Dominant Hypotrichosis. Hypotrichosis of head, pinnae, and neck.

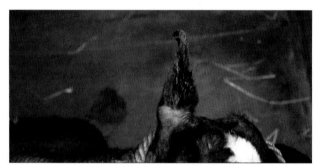

Figure 1.6-4 Same calf as in Figure 1.6-3. Medial curling of tip of pinna.

Differential Diagnosis

Follicular Dysplasias

Diagnosis

1. History and physical examination.
2. Dermatohistopathology.
   a. Hypoplastic hair follicles in most forms.
   b. Follicular hypoplasia, megalotrichohyalin granules, and vacuolization of the inner root sheath in dominant hypotrichosis.
   c. Hypoplasia of all adnexae in inherited epidermal dysplasia.
   d. Hypoplastic hair follicles and no nasiolabial glands in ectodermal dysplasia.

FOLLICULAR DYSPLASIA

Features

Follicular dysplasia implies *clinically* variable degrees of hair loss, and *histopathologically* dysplasia of hair follicles and hair shafts. These conditions are rare, cosmopolitan, and characterized by symmetrical hair loss and skin that is initially normal in appearance. The hair loss may be color-related. Exposed skin is susceptible to sunburn, infections, and contact dermatitis. All reported conditions are viable. The reported follicular dysplasias in cattle are as follows:

1. Semi-hairlessness—Herefords, Polled Herefords, and Ayrshires; autosomal recessive; thin coat of short, fine, curly hairs at birth; later a sparse coat of coarse, wiry hairs which is thickest on the legs.
2. Viable Hypotrichosis—Guernseys, Jerseys, Holsteins, and Ayrshires; autosomal recessive; hair only on legs, tail, eyelids, and pinnae at birth.
3. Color-related Follicular Dysplasia—Black and white or tan ("buckskin") and white Holsteins; normal or mildly affected at birth, then hair loss and scaling only in black- or tan-coated areas (Figs. 1.6-6 through 1.6-10).
4. Follicular Dysplasia of Black Cattle—Black Angus and black Brangus-cross; generalized hair loss begins at 3 to 5 years old.

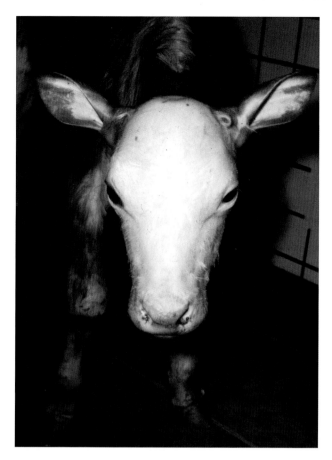

Figure 1.6-5 Congenital Hypotrichosis Due to Bovine Viral Diarrhea. Hypotrichosis of face and pinnae.

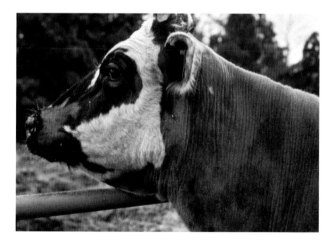

Figure 1.6-6 Black Hair Follicular Dysplasia. Hypotrichosis of only the black-haired areas of face and neck (courtesy J. Gourreau).

Differential Diagnosis

Hypotrichoses.

Diagnosis

1. History and physical examination.
2. Dermatohistopathology—Dysplasia of hair follicles and hair shafts.

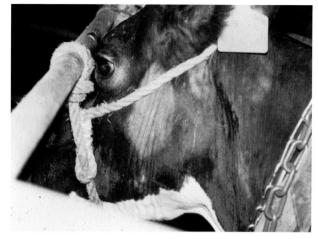

Figure 1.6-7 Black Hair Follicular Dysplasia. Patchy hypotrichosis of the face and neck.

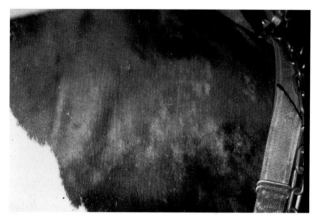

Figure 1.6-8 Same cow as Figure 1.6-7. Patchy hypotrichosis on only black-haired areas of thorax.

CUTANEOUS ASTHENIA

Features

Cutaneous asthenia (dermatosparaxis, cutis hyperelastica, Ehlers-Danlos syndrome) is a group of inherited, congenital collagen dysplasias characterized by loose, hyperextensible, abnormally fragile skin that is easily torn by minor trauma. These disorders are rare and cosmopolitan. In most cattle, cutaneous asthenia is inherited as an autosomal recessive trait, and is associated with a deficiency in procollagen peptidase (aminopropeptidase, type I procollagen N-proteinase) activity. Cutaneous asthenia has been reported in a number of breeds, including Belgian, Charolais, Hereford, Holstein-Friesian, Simmental, and crossbreeds.

From birth, affected cattle show variable degrees of cutaneous fragility and hyperextensibility, as well as joint laxity. The skin is often thin and easily torn, resulting in gaping ("fish mouth") wounds that heal with thin, papyraceous ("cigarette paper-like") scars (Fig. 1.6-11 and Fig. 1.6-12). Wound healing may be delayed. In about one-third of the animals, cutaneous edema develops shortly after birth, especially involving the eyelids, dewlap, and distal limbs.

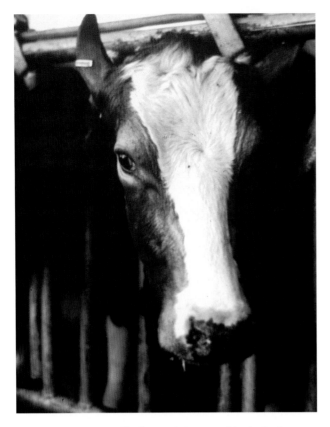

Figure 1.6-9 Tan Hair Follicular Dysplasia. Hypotrichosis of only tan-coated areas of face (courtesy A. Evans).

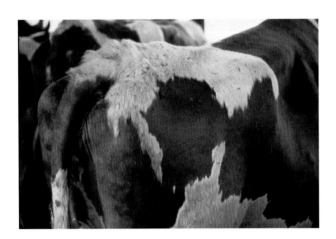

Figure 1.6-10 Tan Hair Follicular Dysplasia. Hypotrichosis of only tan-coated areas of rump (courtesy A. Evans).

Diagnosis

1. History and physical examination.
2. Dermatohistopathology—Collagen dysplasia, with small, fragmented, disorganized, loosely packed fibers.
3. Electron Microscopy—Abnormal structure and packing of collagen fibrils.

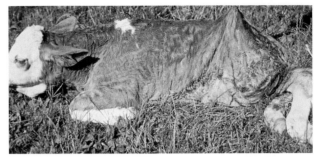

Figure 1.6-11 Cutaneous Asthenia. Loose, hyperextensible skin (courtesy K. Doll, coll. J. Gourreau, AFSSA).

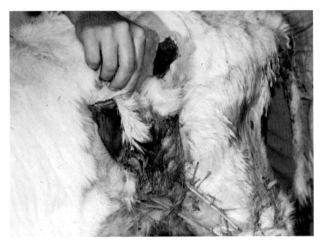

Figure 1.6-12 Cutaneous Asthenia. Large skin tears in flank.

EPIDERMOLYSIS BULLOSA

Features

Epidermolysis bullosa is a group of hereditary mechanobullous diseases whose common primary feature is the formation of vesicles and bullae following trivial trauma. It is rare and cosmopolitan. In older veterinary literature, epidermolysis bullosa was misdiagnosed as "aplasia cutis," "epitheliogenesis imperfecta" or "familial acantholysis." The condition has been reported in several breeds, including Holstein-Friesian, Ayrshire, Jersey, Shorthorn, Angus, Brangus, Dutch Black Pied, Swedish Red Pied, German Yellow Pied, Blonde d'Aguitaine, Charolais, Simmental, Red Breed of West Flanders. There is no apparent sex predilection.

Most reported cases of bovine epidermolysis bullosa resemble *junctional epidermolysis bullosa*, and are thought to be of autosomal recessive inheritance. In Simmentals and their crosses, the condition resembles *epidermolysis bullosa simplex*, and is autosomal dominant with incomplete penetrance. *Dystrophic epidermolysis bullosa* was reported in the Red Breed of West Flanders and thought to be an autosomal recessive trait.

Vesiculobullous lesions and well-circumscribed ulcers are present at birth or within a few days after. Lesions are especially common in the oral cavity, and on the distal limbs, pinnae, muzzle, and pressure points (Figs. 1.6-13 through 1.6-15). One or

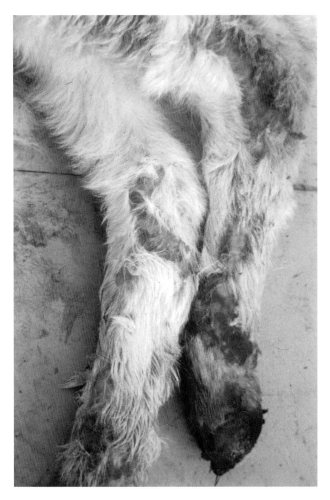

Figure 1.6-13 Epidermolysis Bullosa. Multiple ulcers on hind legs and sloughing of hoof (courtesy J. Gourreau).

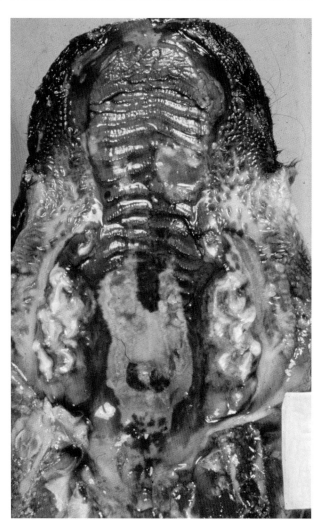

Figure 1.6-14 Epidermolysis Bullosa. Multiple ulcers on lips, gingiva, and hard and soft palates (courtesy M. Alley).

more hooves may be dysplastic or slough. Most animals die shortly after birth. Simmentals with less severe disease may improve clinically as they get older.

Diagnosis

1. History and physical examination.
2. Dermatohistopathology and electron microscopy.
   a. Subepidermal vesicular dermatitis with cleavage through the stratum basale of the epidermis (epidermolysis bullosa simplex).
   b. Subepidermal vesicular dermatitis with cleavage through the lamina lucida of the basement membrane (junctional epidermolysis bullosa).
   c. Subepidermal vesicular dermatitis with cleavage through the superficial dermis (dystrophic epidermolysis bullosa).

HEREDITARY ZINC DEFICIENCY

Features

Hereditary zinc deficiency (hereditary parakeratosis, lethal trait A46, Adema disease, hereditary thymic hypoplasia) is characterized by skin disease and profound immunodeficiency, and a wast-

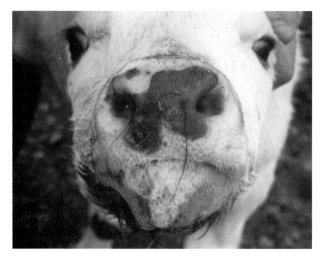

Figure 1.6-15 Epidermolysis Bullosa. Ulceration of muzzle (courtesy P. Dudal, coll. J. Gourreau, AFSSA).

ing syndrome resulting from intestinal malabsorption of zinc (analogous to acrodermatitis enteropathica in humans). It is an autosomal recessive trait reported in Friesians, Danish Black Pieds, Shorthorns, Holsteins, and Angus. There is no apparent sex predilection. The condition is rare and cosmopolitan.

Affected animals are normal at birth, but develop diarrhea (often dark green and watery with a sweet metallic odor) by 3 to 8 weeks of age. Lethargy, depression, and a poor appetite are accompanied by increased lacrimation and a clear nasal discharge. Erythema, scaling, crusting, and alopecia begin on the face (Fig. 1.6-16) and spread to the neck, flanks, perineum, ventrum, distal limbs, and mucocutaneous areas. Affected skin often fissures and oozes, especially around the joints of the limbs (Fig. 1.6-17). Dark-coated areas often fade, especially periocularly ("spectacles"). Untreated animals die by 6 months of age.

Diagnosis

1. History and physical examinations.
2. Decreased concentrations of serum alkaline phosphatase.
3. Decreased concentrations of serum zinc.
4. Dermatohistopathology—Marked diffuse parakeratotic hyperkeratosis.
5. Necropsy—hypoplasia of thymus and lymph nodes.

ICHTHYOSIS

Features

Ichthyosis (Greek: fishy condition) consists of a heterogeneous group of hereditary disorders of keratinization. It is rare and cosmopolitan. There is no apparent sex predilection.

A *severe form* ("ichthyosis fetalis") has been reported in Norwegian Red Polls, Friesians, and Brown Swiss. It is inherited as a simple autosomal recessive trait. Affected calves either are dead at birth or die within a few hours or days. The entire skin is alopecic, covered with thick scales and hyperkeratosis, and divided into plates by fissures (Figs. 1.6-18 and 1.6-19). The skin

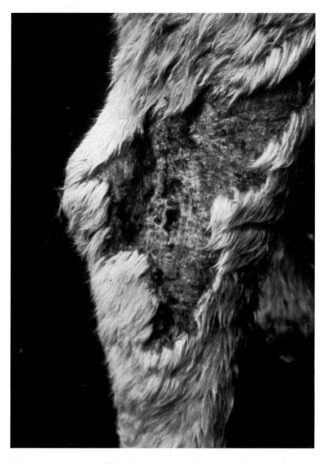

Figure 1.6-17 Same calf as Figure 1.6-16. Alopecia, erythema, and crusts on lateral aspect of hock (courtesy J. Baird).

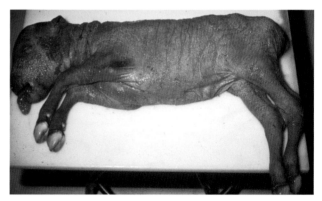

Figure 1.6-18 Ichthyosis. Generalized alopecia and hyperkeratosis in a newborn calf (courtesy J. King).

around the lips (eclabium), eyelids (ectropion), and other body orifices tends to be everted (Fig. 1.6-20).

A *milder form* ("ichthyosis congenita") has been reported in German Pinzgauers, Jerseys, Holsteins, and Chianinas. It is inherited as a simple autosomal recessive trait. Affected calves are born with, or develop over the course of several weeks, variable degrees of generalized hyperkeratosis and alopecia. This form may be associated with microtia and cataracts.

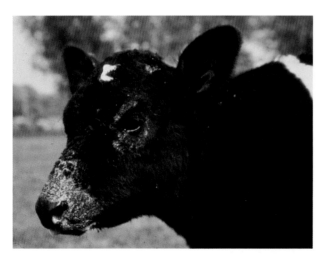

Figure 1.6-16 Hereditary Zinc Deficiency. Crusting and alopecia of muzzle, periocular area, and pinnae (courtesy J. Baird).

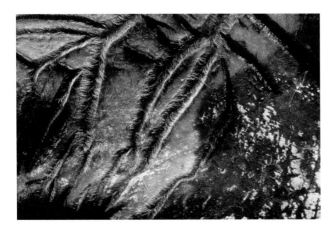

Figure 1.6-19 Ichthyosis. Alopecia, hyperkeratosis, and fissures of skin over thorax (courtesy J. King).

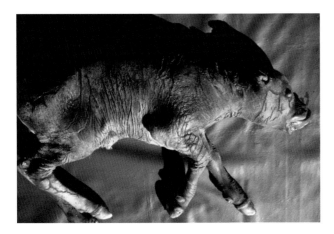

Figure 1.6-20 Ichthyosis. Generalized alopecia and hyperkeratosis, eclabium, and ectropion (courtesy J. King).

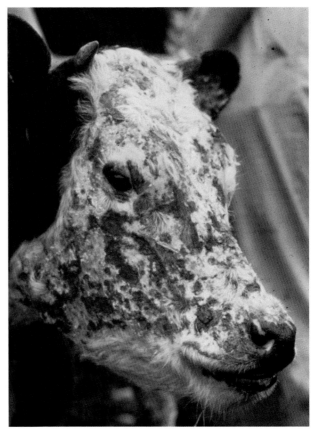

Figure 1.6-21 Erythropoietic Porphyria. Erythema, crusting, ulceration, and alopecia of only white-haired areas of face.

Diagnosis

1. History and physical examination.
2. Dermatohistopathology—Diffuse orthokeratotic hyperkeratosis.

PORPHYRIA

Features

Porphyria is characterized by the abnormal accumulation of various photodynamic porphyrins in the blood and body tissues as a result of aberrant porphyrin synthesis. Photodermatitis is the classical clinical sign of porphyria. These conditions are rare and cosmopolitan.

Erythropoietic porphyria (congenital porphyria, pink tooth, ochronosis, osteohemochromatosis, porphyrinuria) has been reported in many breeds. It is inherited as an autosomal recessive trait with no sex predilection. Decreased levels of uroporphyrinogen III cosynthetase result in increased levels of uroporphyrin I and coproporphyrin I in blood and tissues. Clinical signs include retarded growth, anemia, discolored teeth and urine, and photodermatitis (see "Photodermatitis" in Chapter 1.7) (Figs. 1.6-21

and 1.6-22). Teeth vary in color from light pink, pinkish-red, purplish-red, red-brown, to mahogany (Fig. 1.6-23). Urine is usually reddish-brown or turns red on exposure to sunlight.

Protoporphyria has been reported in Limousins and their crosses and Blonde d'Aquitaine. It is inherited as an autosomal recessive trait with no sex predilection. Decreased levels of heme synthetase (ferrochelatase) result in increased levels of protoporphyrin in blood and tissues. Clinical signs include photodermatitis and photophobia. Teeth and urine are normal in color.

Differential Diagnosis

Other causes of photodermatitis (see Chapter 1.7).

Diagnosis

1. History and physical examination.
2. Discolored teeth and urine with erythropoietic porphyria.
3. Wood's Light Examination—Teeth and urine fluoresce a bright orange or red with erythropoietic porphyria.
4. Hemogram—Macrocytic, normochromic anemia with eythropoietic porphyria.
5. Blood Porphyrin Levels—Increased uroporphyrin I and coproporphyrin I (erythropoietic porphyria) or protoporphyrin (protoporphyria).
6. Dermatohistopathology—Subepidermal vesicular dermatitis, festooning, and PAS-positive material in blood vessel walls.

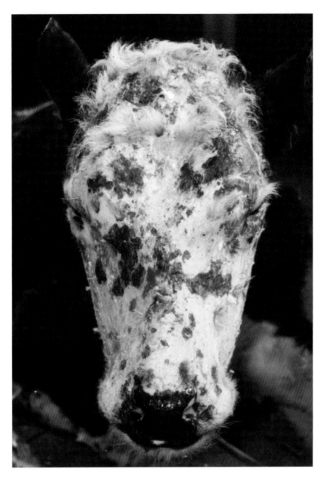

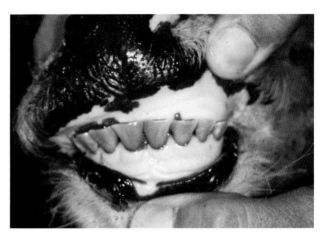

Figure 1.6-23 Erythropoietic Porphyria. Purplish teeth and pale oral mucous membranes.

Figure 1.6-22 Erythropoietic Porphyria. Alopecia, erythema, crusting, and ulceration of only white-haired areas of face.

MISCELLANEOUS DISEASES

Table 1.6-2 Miscellaneous Congenital/Hereditary Skin Diseases	
Chédiak-Higashi Syndrome	Herefords, Japanese Blacks and Grey Brangus; autosomal recessive; partial oculocutaneous albinism, photophobia hemorrhagic tendencies, and increased susceptibility to infection; abnormal granules in leukocytes
Congenital dyserythropoiesis and dyskeratosis	Polled Herefords; often small at birth and prominent forehead; hyperkeratotic muzzle attracts dirt and saliva, producing "dirty-faced appearance"; haircoat wiry, kinked and easily epilated; alopecia and hyperkeratosis initially over bridge of nose, lateral pinnal margins, and base of ears; progressive widespread hypotrichosis and keratinization abnormality; skin becomes markedly wrinkled over face and neck; anemia, exercise intolerance; failure to thrive; death by 6 months old; dermatohistopathology (diffuse orthokeratotic hyperkeratosis, apoptosis ("dyskeratosis") of epidermal and follicular keratinocytes)
Curly coat	Ayrshires (autosomal dominant), Swedish cattle (autosomal recessive), and Herefords, Polled Herefords (autosomal recessive); curly ("wooly") coat is a phenotypic marker for cardiomyopathy in Herefords and Polled Herefords
Dermal dysplasia	Holstein; at 2 years old develop loose folded skin on head, neck, and legs; poor wound healing; no hyperextensibility; dermatohistopathology (collagen dysplasia)
Hypertrichosis	European Friesians; autosomal dominant; excessive haircoat is associated with decreased productivity and polypnea during hot weather
Lymphedema	Ayrshires (autosomal recessive) and Herefords (autosomal dominant) with variable expressivity and incomplete penetration; variable degrees of edema of hind limbs and occasionally forelimbs, tails, prepuce, pinnae, and face; dermatohistopathology (hypoplasia and aplasia of lymph vessels)
Vitiligo	Holstein-Friesians, Japanese Blacks, Balis, Maduras; early onset, symmetrical depigmentation of skin and haircoat on muzzle, lips, and eyelids, may become widespread; dermatohistopathology (absence of melanocytes)

REFERENCES

Bassett H. 1987. A Congenital Bovine Epidermolysis Resembling Epidermolysis Bullosa Simplex of Man. *Vet Rec* 121: 8.

Braun U, et al. 1988. Hypotrichose und Oligodontie, Verbunden mit einer Xq-Deletion, bei einem Kalb der Schweizerischen Fleckviehrasse. *Tierärztl Prax* 16: 39.

Buchanan M, and Crawshaw WM. 1995. Bovine Congenital Erythropoietic Protoporphyria in a Pedigree Limousin Heifer. *Vet Rec* 136: 640.

Burton SA, et al. 1994. Congenital Dyserythropoiesis and Dyskeratosis in a Polled Hereford Calf. *Can Vet J* 35: 519.

Deprez P, et al. 1993. Een Geval van Epidermolysis Bullosa bij een Kalf. *Vlaams Diergeneeskd Tijdschr* 62: 155.

Drögemüller C, et al. 2002. Congenital Hypotrichosis with Anodontia in Cattle: A Genetic, Clinical and Histological Analysis. *Vet Dermatol* 13: 307.

Drögemüller C, et al. 2003. Kongenitale Hypotrichose und Oligodontie beim Rind. *Tierärztl Prax* 31: 66.

Gourreau JM, et al. 1986. L'Epitheliogenesis Imperfecta des Bovins. *Point Vét* 18: 361.

Hanna PE, and Ogilvie TH. 1989. Congenital Hypotrichosis in an Ayrshire Calf. *Can Vet J* 30: 249.

Healy PJ, et al. 1991. Protoporphyria in Limousin Cattle. *Aust Vet J* 69: 114.

Howard JL, and Smith RA. 1999. Current Veterinary Therapy. Food Animal Practice. Ed 4. WB Saunders, Philadelphia, PA.

Jubb TF, et al. 1990. Inherited Epidermal Dysplasia in Holstein-Friesian Calves. *Aust Vet J* 67: 16.

Kawaguchi T, et al. 1988. Dermal Dysplasia Characterized by Collagen Disorder—Related Skin Fragility in a Cow. *Am J Vet Res* 49: 965.

Machen M, et al. 1996. Bovine Hereditary Zinc Deficiency: Lethal Trait A46. *J Vet Diag Invest* 8: 219.

Mansell JL. 1999. Follicular Dysplasia in Two Cows. *Vet Dermatol* 10: 143.

Meyer W, et al. 1992. Integumental Structure in a Friesian Calf with Congenital Hypo- or Atrichosis Combined with Prognathia Inferior. *Vet Dermatol* 3: 413.

Miller WH, and Scott DW. 1990. Black-Hair Follicular Dysplasia in a Holstein Cow. *Cornell Vet* 80: 273.

Ogawa H, et al. 1997. Clinical, Morphologic, and Biochemical Characteristics of Chédiak-Higashi Syndrome in Fifty-Six Japanese Black Cattle. *Am J Vet Res* 58: 1221.

Ostrowski S, and Evans A. 1989. Coat-Color-Linked Hair Follicle Dysplasia in "Buckskin" Holstein Cows in Central California. *Agri-Pract* 10: 12.

Peixoto PV, et al. 1994. Ocorrência da Paraqueratose Hereditária (Linhagem Letal A-46) no Brasil. *Pesq Vet Bras* 14: 79.

Pence ME, and Liggett AD. 2002. Congenital Erythropoietic Protoporphyria in a Limousin Calf. *J Am Vet Med Assoc* 221: 277.

Radostits OM, et al. 2000. Veterinary Medicine. A Textbook of the Diseases of Cattle, Sheep, Pigs, Goats, and Horses. Ed. 9. WB Saunders, Philadelphia, PA.

Schelcher F, et al. 1991. Observations on Bovine Congenital Erythrocytic Protoporphyria in Blonde d'Aquitaine Breed. *Vet Rec* 129: 403.

Schild AL, et al. 1991. Hereditary Lymphedema in Hereford Cattle. *J Vet Diag Invest* 3: 47.

Scott DW. 1988. Large Animal Dermatology. WB Saunders, Philadelphia, PA.

Steffen DJ, et al. 1991. Congenital Anemia, Dyskeratosis, and Progressive Alopecia in Polled Hereford Calves. *Vet Pathol* 28: 234.

Steffen DJ, et al. 1992. Ultrastructural Findings in Congenital Anemia, Dyskeratosis, and Progressive Alopecia in Polled Hereford Calves. *Vet Pathol* 29: 203.

Stocker H, et al. 1995. Epidermolysis Bullosa bei einem Kalb. *Tierärztl Prax* 23: 123.

Tajima M, et al. 1999. Genetic Defect of Dermatan Sulfate Proteoglycan of Cattle Affected with a Variant Form of Ehlers-Danlos Syndrome. *J Vet Intern Med* 13: 202.

Troyer DL, et al. 1991. Gross, Microscopic and Ultrastructural Lesions of Protoporphyria in Limousin Calves. *Zentralb Veterinarmed A* 38: 300.

Vestweber JG, et al. 1994. Difficult Dermatologic Diagnosis. *J Am Vet Med Assoc* 204: 1567.

Vogt, DW et al. 1988. Hereditary Parakeratosis in Shorthorn Beef Calves. *Am J Vet Res* 49: 120.

Whittington RJ, and Cook RW. 1988. Cardiomyopathy and Woolly Haircoat Syndrome of Polled Hereford Cattle: Electrocardiographic Findings in Affected and Unaffected Calves. *Aust Vet J* 65: 341.

Wijeratne WVS, et al. 1988. A Genetic, Pathological and Virological Study of Congenital Hypotrichosis and Incisor Anodontia in Cattle. *Vet Rec* 122: 149.

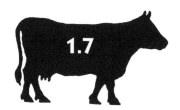

ENVIRONMENTAL SKIN DISEASES

Intertrigo
Hematoma
Teat Injuries
Burns
Frostbite
Primary Irritant Contact Dermatitis
Ergotism
Fescue Toxicosis
Hyalomma Toxicosis
Dermatitis, Pyrexia, and Hemorrhage Syndrome
Photodermatitis
Miscellaneous Diseases
   Amanita Toxicosis
   Arsenic Toxicosis
   Chlorinated Naphthalene Toxicosis
   Foreign Bodies
   Hairy Vetch Toxicosis
   Iodism
   Mercurialism
   Mimosine Toxicosis
   Oat Straw Toxicosis
   Polybrominated Biphenyl Toxicosis
   Selenium Toxicosis
   Snake Bite
   Stachybotryotoxicosis
   Subcutaneous Emphysema
   Vampire Bat Bite

INTERTRIGO

Features

Intertrigo (Latin: a rubbing between) ("udder-thigh dermatitis," "flexural seborrhea") is a superficial inflammatory dermatitis that occurs where skin is in apposition and is thus subject to the friction of movement, increased local heat, maceration from retained moisture, and irritation from accumulated debris. It is common in dairy cattle, especially in association with the udder edema of parturition.

Intertrigo is characterized by variable degrees of erythema, edema, and oozing at the junction of the lateral aspect of the udder and the medial thigh (Figs. 1.7-1 and 1.7-2). It is typically more-or-less symmetrical. The condition is usually nonpruritic and nonpainful, unless secondary bacterial infection (*Staphylococcus; Fusobacterium necrophorum*) occurs, whereupon severe dermatitis, crusting, necrosis, ulceration, and foul odor are present. Affected animals are typically otherwise healthy.

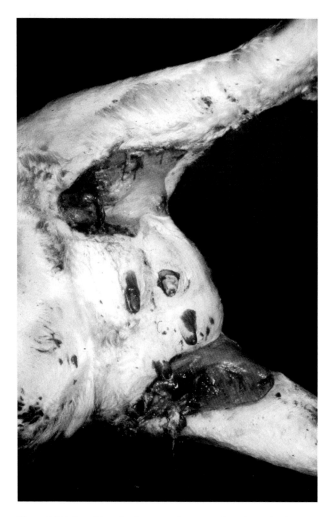

Figure 1.7-1 Intertrigo. Erythema, oozing, necrosis and crusting in inguinal areas (courtesy M. Sloet).

Differential Diagnosis

Various bacterial infections.

Diagnosis

1. History and physical examination.
2. Microscopy (direct smears)—No evidence of infection (uncomplicated cases).

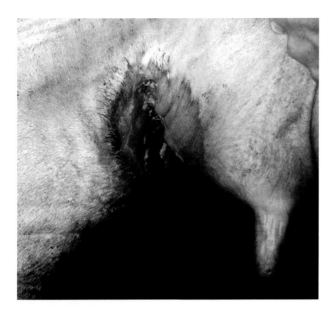

Figure 1.7-2 Intertrigo. Erythema, oozing, and crusting between udder and thigh (courtesy M. Sloet).

HEMATOMA

Features

A hematoma is a circumscribed area of hemorrhage into the tissue arising from vascular damage due to sudden, severe, blunt external trauma (e.g., a fall, a kick).

The lesions are usually acute in onset, subcutaneous, fluctuant, and may or may not be painful (Figs. 1.7-3 to 1.7-5). The lesions are usually not warm to the touch. Hematomas are seen most commonly over the stifle, ischial tuberosity, lateral thorax, and the point of the shoulder.

Differential Diagnosis

Abscess, neoplasm.

Diagnosis

1. History and physical examination.
2. Needle aspiration (blood).

TEAT INJURIES

Features

Teat injuries are common in dairy cattle, and include:

1. Treading injuries—Especially housed cattle; especially large teats that project laterally.
2. Lacerations—Barbed wire, sharp objects (Fig. 1.7-6).
3. Bite wounds—Especially dogs.
4. Fissures—Due to chapping when damp teats exposed to cold winds after milking; excessive sucking/biting by older calves (Fig. 1.7-7).
5. Milking machine injuries—Vacuum defects; ill-fitting teat cup liners (Figs. 1.7-8 and 1.7-9).

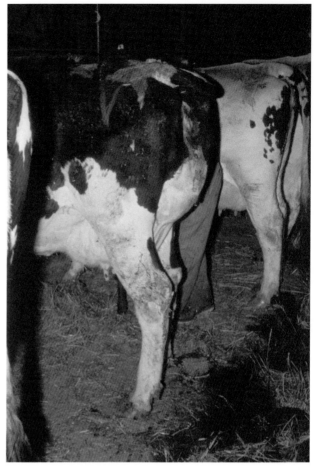

Figure 1.7-3 Hematoma. Large swelling on caudal udder and perineum.

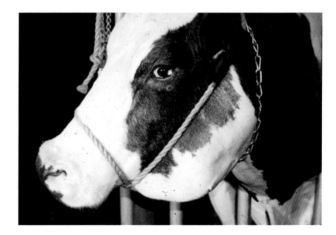

Figure 1.7-4 Hematoma. Large swelling on side of face.

6. Photodermatitis (see "Photodermatitis" later in chapter).
7. Frostbite (see "Frostbite" later in chapter).

Ischemic necrosis at the base of teats in dairy cattle has been associated with poor attention to husbandry; poor milking parlor design, layout, and installation; improper teat disinfection; improper cluster position.

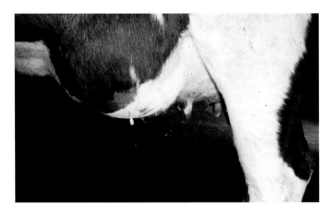

Figure 1.7-5 Hematoma. Large swelling on ventrolateral abdomen cranial to udder.

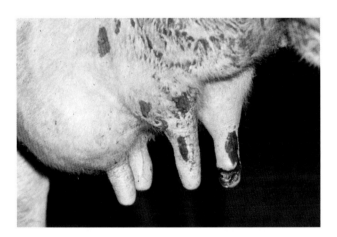

Figure 1.7-6 Laceration. Laceration on distal teat.

Diagnosis

1. History and physical examination.

BURNS

Features

Burns are occasionally seen and may be thermal (barn, forest, or brush fires; accidental spillage of hot solutions) (Figs. 1.7-10 and 1.7-11), electrical (electrocution; lightning strike), frictional (ropes; falls), chemical (improperly used topicals), or radiational (radiotherapy).

First degree burns involve the superficial epidermis and are characterized by erythema, edema, heat, and pain. *Second degree burns* affect the entire epidermis and are characterized by erythema, edema, heat, pain, and vesicles. *Third degree burns* affect the entire epidermis, dermis, and appendages, and are characterized by necrosis, ulceration, anesthesia, and scarring. Burns are most commonly seen over the dorsum and face or udder and teats.

Diagnosis

1. History and physical examination.

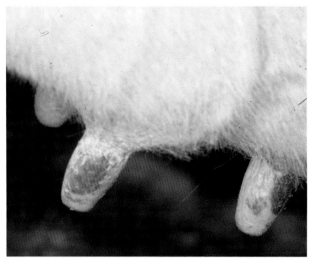

Figure 1.7-7 Chapping. Erythema and scaling on teats.

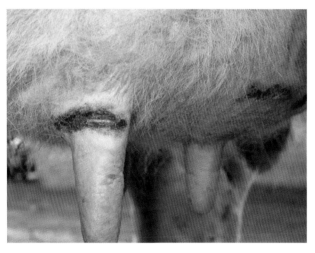

Figure 1.7-8 Pressure Necrosis. Ring of necrosis and ulceration at base of teat due to milking machine (courtesy J. Nicol, coll. J. Gourreau, AFSSA).

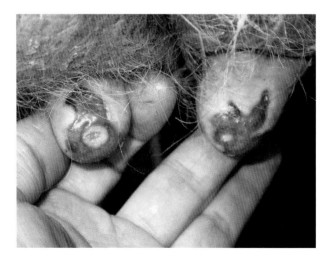

Figure 1.7-9 Traumatic Ulceration. Ulcers on teats due to milking machine (courtesy J. Nicol, coll. J. Gourreau, AFSSA).

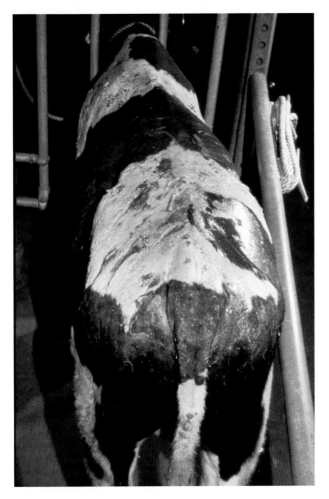

Figure 1.7-10 Thermal Burn. Alopecia and ulceration due to barn fire.

FROSTBITE

Features

Frostbite is an injury to the skin caused by excessive exposure to cold. Frostbite is rare in healthy animals that have been acclimatized to cold. It is more likely to occur in neonates; animals that are sick, debilitated, or dehydrated; animals having preexisting vascular insufficiency; animals recently removed from a warm climate to a cold one. Lack of shelter, blowing wind, and wetting decrease the amount of exposure time necessary for frostbite to develop.

Frostbite typically affects the pinnae, tail tip, teats, scrotum, and feet in variable combinations (Fig. 1.7-12). While frozen, the skin appears pale, is hypoesthetic, and is cool to the touch. After thawing, mild cases present with erythema, edema, scaling, and alopecia; severe cases present with necrosis, dry gangrene, and sloughing.

Differential Diagnosis

Ergotism, fescue toxicosis, vasculitis, other causes of gangrene (Box 1.7-1).

Box 1.7-1 Gangrene

Gangrene (Greek: consuming, gnawing) is a clinical term used to describe severe tissue necrosis and slough. *Moist* gangrene is produced by impairment of lymphatic and venous drainage plus infection (putrefaction) and is a complication of pressure sores. Moist gangrene presents as swollen, discolored areas with foul odor and progressive tissue decomposition. *Dry* gangrene occurs when arterial blood supply is occluded, but venous and lymphatic drainage remain intact and infection is absent (mummification). Dry gangrene assumes a dry, discolored, leathery appearance. Causes of gangrene include: (1) external pressure (e.g., pressure sores, ropes, constricting bands); (2) internal pressure (e.g., severe edema); (3) burns (thermal, chemical, frictional, electrical, radiational); (4) frostbite; (5) envenomation (snake, spider); (6) vasculitis; (7) ergotism; (8) fescue toxicosis; (9) photodermatitis; (10) various infections (*Clostridium, Staphylococcus, Streptococcus, Fusobacterium,* bovine herpes mammillitis, bovine lumpy skin disease).

Distal limb phlebitis, thrombosis, and sloughing in cattle has been associated with therapeutic procedures that incorporate various combinations of tourniquets, intravenous regional anesthesia, and intravenous regional antimicrobials. *Tail-tip necrosis* occurs in beef cattle housed on slatted floors, and is due to tramping injuries. Initially the tail tip is swollen, then becomes suppurative, necrotic, and sloughs.

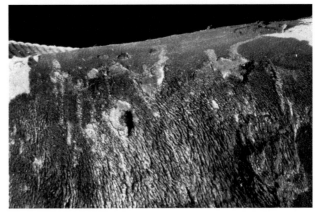

Figure 1.7-11 Close-up of Figure 1.7-10. Alopecia, necrosis, and ulceration over dorsolateral trunk.

Diagnosis

1. History and physical examination.

PRIMARY IRRITANT CONTACT DERMATITIS

Features

Primary irritant contact dermatitis is a common inflammatory skin reaction caused by direct contact with an offending substance. Moisture is an important predisposing factor, since it decreases the effectiveness of normal skin barriers and increases the

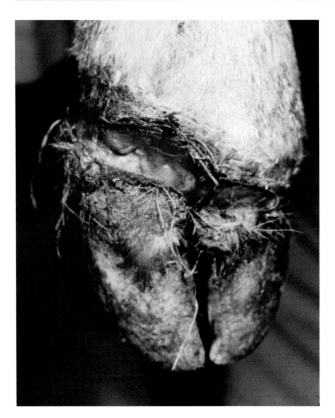

Figure 1.7-12 Frostbite. Necrosis, ulceration, and separation of the hoof.

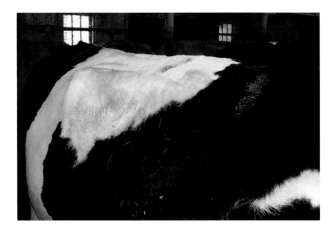

Figure 1.7-13 Contact Dermatitis. Erythema, alopecia, and crusts on rump due to pour-on parasiticide (courtesy M. Smith).

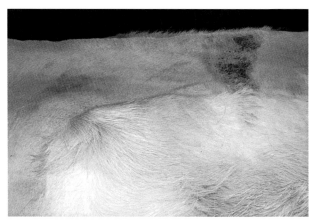

Figure 1.7-14 Close-up of Figure 1.7-13. Erythema, alopecia, and crusts.

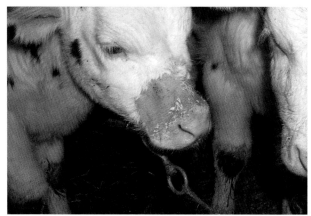

Figure 1.7-15 Contact Dermatitis. Alopecia and erythema on muzzle due to milk replacer fed from a bucket (courtesy M. Smith).

intimacy of contact between the contactant and the skin. Substances known to cause contact dermatitis in cattle include: body excretions and secretions (feces, urine, wound); caustics (acids, alkalis); crude oil, diesel fuel, turpentine; improper use of sprays, rinses, wipes; plants; wood preservatives; bedding; filth.

The dermatitis varies in severity from erythema, edema, papules and scale to vesicles, erosions, ulcers, necrosis, and crusts. Severe irritants, self-trauma, or secondary bacterial infections can result in alopecia, lichenification, and scarring. Leukotrichia and leukoderma can be transient or permanent sequelae. In most instances, the nature of the contactant can be inferred from the distribution of the dermatitis: muzzle and distal legs (plants, envi-

ronmental substances); face and dorsum (sprays, pour-ons, wipes) (Figs. 1.7-13 and 1.7-14); ventrum (bedding, filth); perineum and rear legs (urine, feces). Contact dermatitis is seen on the muzzle, lips, and ear tips of calves fed milk or milk replacers from pans and buckets (Fig. 1.7-15).

Immersion foot is a vasoneuropathy associated with prolonged exposure to moisture, cold temperatures, and impaired blood flow to the extremities (e.g., standing in cool water for >2 to 3 days). Early pain, stiffness, reluctance to move, edema, and erythema of submerged areas may progress to necrosis, sloughing, and ulceration (Figs. 1.7-16 and 1.7-17).

Diagnosis

1. History and physical examination.

ERGOTISM

Features

Ergotism is an uncommon disorder caused by alkaloids produced by the fungus *Claviceps purpurea* and characterized by dry gangrene and sloughing of distal extremities. *Claviceps purpurea* in-

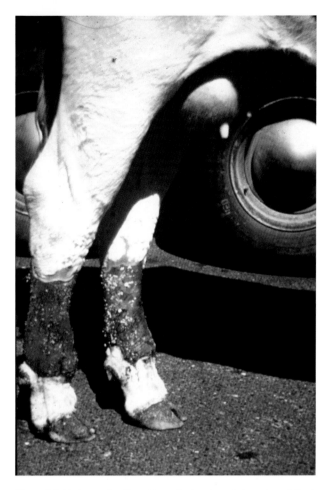

Figure 1.7-16 Immersion Foot. Necrosis, slough, and ulceration of distal hind legs (courtesy E. Guaguère).

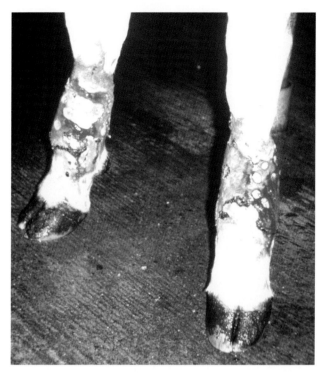

Figure 1.7-17 Immersion Foot. Necrosis, slough, and ulceration of distal front legs (courtesy E. Guaguère).

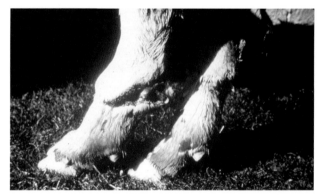

Figure 1.7-18 Ergotism. Necrosis and sloughing of distal limbs.

fects over 200 grasses and cultured cereals, especially wheat, barley, rye, and oats. The fungus is most abundant during wet seasons. Ergotism occurs in many parts of the world, and has no apparent age, breed, or sex predilections.

Initial clinical signs usually begin after 7 days of exposure to contaminated feed and include hind limb lameness, fever, poor appetite, weight loss, and decreased milk production. Swelling begins at the coronary bands and progresses to the fetlocks. The feet become cold, insensitive, necrotic, and a distinct line separates viable from dead tissue. Front feet, ears, tail, and teats may be similarly affected and, in severe cases, may slough (Figs. 1.7-18 to 1.7-20). Occasionally, large areas of skin (shoulder, lateral thorax, neck, muzzle) may be affected. Morbidity and mortality are usually low.

Differential Diagnosis

Fescue toxicosis, frostbite, vasculitis, septicemia, and other causes of gangrene (see Box 1.7-1).

Diagnosis

1. History and physical examination.
2. Feed analysis.

FESCUE TOXICOSIS

Features

Fescue toxicosis is an uncommon disorder caused by ingestion of tall fescue (*Festuca elatior [aruninacea]*) infected with the fungus *Neotyphodium (Acremonium) coenophialium*, and characterized by dry gangrene and sloughing of distal extremities. Tall fescue is a widely used grass in many parts of the world. There are no apparent age, breed, or sex predilections.

Initial clinical signs occur 1 week to 6 months after exposure and include: hind limb lameness, arched back, diarrhea, poor appetite, and emaciation. Erythema and edema begin at the coronary bands and may spread to the fetlocks. The feet become cold, insensitive, and necrotic (Fig. 1.7-21). The tail switch may be lost. Front feet, ears, tail, and teats are occasionally affected, and may

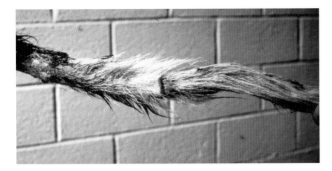

Figure 1.7-19 Ergotism. Necrosis of distal tail.

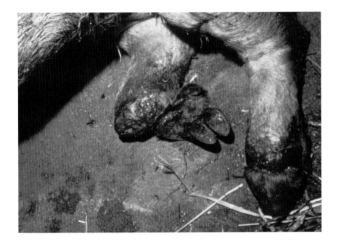

Figure 1.7-20 Ergotism. Necrosis, ulceration, and sloughing of hooves.

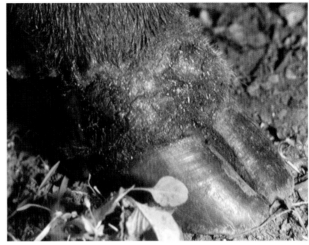

Figure 1.7-21 Fescue Toxicosis. Necrosis and ulceration of distal limb (courtesy L. George).

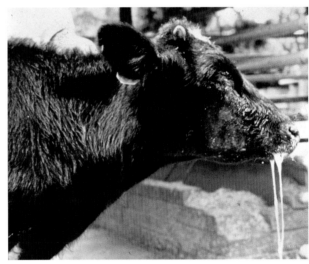

Figure 1.7-22 *Hyalomma* Toxicosis. Oozing, crusting, and alopecia of the head, in addition to naso- and sialorrhea (courtesy P. Bland).

slough. Morbidity varies from a single animal to most of the herd (usually about 10%).

Differential Diagnosis

Ergotism, frostbite, vasculitis, septicemia, and other causes of gangrene (see Box 1.7-1).

Diagnosis

1. History and physical examination.
2. Feed analysis.

HYALOMMA TOXICOSIS

Features

Hyalomma toxicosis ("sweating sickness") is an uncommon tick-borne disease in Africa, Sri Lanka, and southern India. It is caused by a toxin in certain strains of the tick, *Hyalomma truncatum (transiens)*. Disease prevalence is highest in rainy, warmer months when tick populations are high. There are no apparent breed or sex predilections, and cattle less than 1 year old are most commonly affected.

Clinical signs include the sudden onset of fever, depression, hyperemic mucous membranes and skin, hypersalivation, lacri-

mation, and nasal discharge (Fig. 1.7-22). A moist dermatitis is seen 48 to 72 hours later. The dermatitis may be confined to the pinnae, face, neck, axillae, flank, or groin, but is often generalized. Affected skin is erythematous, edematous, oozing, painful, and foul-smelling. Affected animals seek shade. Their hair coat becomes matted and easily epilated. When tufts of hair are epilated, erosions and ulcers are created (Figs. 1.7-23 and 1.7-24). The tips of the pinnae and tail may slough. Necrosis and ulceration may develop on oral, nasal, and vaginal mucosae. Myiasis is a frequent complication. If affected animals do not die, healing skin is dry, scaling, thickened, and alopecic. Mortality varies from 30% to 100%, with a course of 4 to 20 days.

Diagnosis

1. History and physical examination.

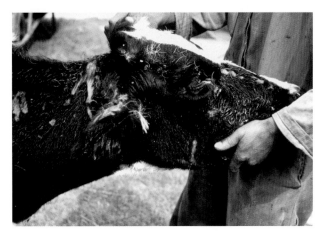

Figure 1.7-23 *Hyalomma* Toxicosis. Oozing, necrosis, sloughing, and ulceration of face and neck (courtesy P. Bland).

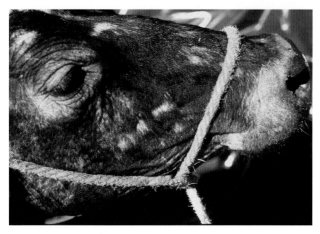

Figure 1.7-25 Dermatitis, Pyrexia, and Hemorrhage Syndrome. Papules, crusts, and alopecia on face (courtesy J. Ducroz, coll. J. Gourreau, AFSSA).

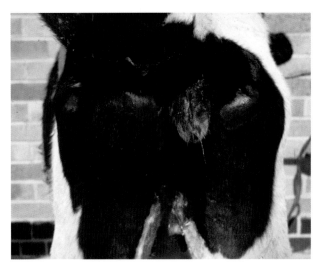

Figure 1.7-24 *Hyalomma* Toxicosis. Necrosis, sloughing, and ulceration of vulva and perineum (courtesy P. Bland).

DERMATITIS, PYREXIA, AND HEMORRHAGE SYNDROME

Features

The dermatitis, pyrexia, and hemorrhage syndrome (DPHS) is a toxicosis with unclear pathogenesis and multifactorial etiology. It typically occurs in silage-fed dairy cattle in winter. It has been reported in Europe. Outbreaks of DPHS have been attributed to feed additives such as diureidoisobutane or citrinin in some instances, and have been idiopathic in others.

Clinical signs typically occur 3 to 7 days after beginning the feed and initially include pyrexia and a pruritic papulocrustous dermatitis on the head (Fig. 1.7-25), neck (Fig. 1.7-26), tailhead, perineum, and udder (Fig. 1.7-27). Severe cases may also progress to involvement of the back legs. Animals rub, kick, and lick, producing alopecia, excoriation, and secondary bacterial infections. Affected animals are depressed, have variable appetites, lose weight, and have decreased milk production. Some animals have petechiation of mucous membranes and/or epistaxis, bloody diar-

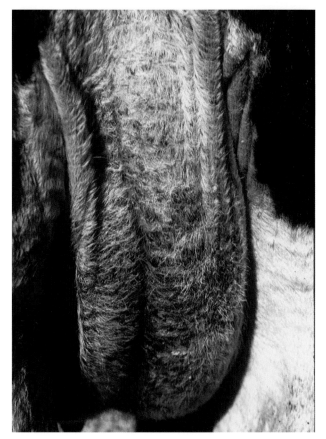

Figure 1.7-26 Dermatitis, Pyrexia, and Hemorrhage Syndrome. Erythema, papules, and crusts on scrotum (courtesy J. Ducroz, coll. J. Gourreau, AFSSA).

rhea, fecal blood clots, and subcutaneous hematomas. Morbidity varies from 1% to 90%, and mortality from 25% to 95%.

Diagnosis

1. History and physical examination.
2. Necropsy—Widespread hemorrhages and mild vasculitis.

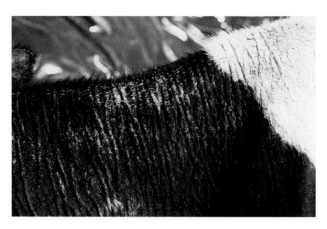

Figure 1.7-27 Dermatitis, Pyrexia, and Hemorrhage Syndrome. Crusts and alopecia over dorsum (courtesy J. Ducroz, coll. J. Gourreau, AFSSA).

PHOTODERMATITIS

Features

Photodermatitis (solar dermatitis, actinic dermatitis) is an inflammatory skin disease caused by exposure to ultraviolet light. *Phototoxicity* (sunburn) occurs on white skin, light skin, or damaged skin (e.g., depigmented or scarred) not sufficiently covered by hair. *Photosensitization* is classified according to the source of the photodynamic agents (Tables 1.7-1 and 1.7-2).

1. Primary photosensitization (a preformed or metabolically-derived photodynamic agent reaches the skin by ingestion, injection or contact.
2. Hepatogenous photosensitization (blood phylloerythrin levels are elevated in association with liver abnormalities).

3. Photosensitization due to aberrant pigment synthesis (porphyria).
4. Idiopathic photosensitization.

Skin lesions are usually restricted to light-skin, sparsely-haired areas (Figs. 1.7-28 and 1.7-29) but, in severe cases, can extend into the surrounding dark-skin areas too. Restlessness and discomfort often precede visible skin lesions. Erythema and edema may be followed by vesicles and bullae, ulceration, oozing, crusts, scales, and alopecia. Secondary bacterial infections are common.

Table 1.7-1 Causes of Primary Photosensitization

Source	Photodynamic Agent
Plants	
St. John's Wort (*Hypericum perforatum*)	Hypericin
Buckwheat (*Fagopyrum esculentum, Polygonum fagopyrum*)	Fagopyrin, photofagopyrin
Bishop's weed (*Ammi majus*)	Furocoumarins
Dutchman's breeches (*Thamnosma texana*)	Furocoumarins
Wild carrot (*Daucus carota*), spring parsley (*Cymopterus watsonii*)	Furocoumarins
Cooperia pedunculata	Furocoumarins
Smartweeds (*Polygonum* spp.)	Furocoumarins
Perennial ryegrass (*Lolium perenne*)	Perloline
Burr trefoil (*Medicago denticulata*)	Aphids
Alfalfa silage	
Chemicals	
Phenothiazines	
Thiazides	
Acriflavines	
Rose Bengal	
Methylene blue	
Sulfonamides	
Tetracyclines	

Table 1.7-2 Causes of Hepatogenous Photosensitization

Source	Hepatotoxin
Plants	
Burning bush, fireweed (*Kochia scoparia*)	?
Ngaio tree (*Myoporum* spp.)	Ngaione
Lechuguilla (*Agave lechuguilla*)	Saponins
Rape, kale (*Brassica* spp.)	?
Coal oil brush, spineless horsebrush (*Tetradynia* spp.)	?
Moldy alfalfa hay	?
Sacahuiste (*Nolina texana*)	?
Salvation Jane (*Echium lycopsis*)	Pyrrolizidine alkaloids
Lantana (*Lantana camara*)	Triterpene
Heliotrope (*Heliotropium europaeum*)	Pyrrolizidine alkaloids
Ragworts, groundsels (*Senecio* spp.)	Pyrrolizidine alkaloids
Tarweed, fiddle-neck (*Amsinckia* spp.)	Pyrrolizidine alkaloids
Crotalaria, rattleweed (*Crotalaria* spp.)	Pyrrolizidine alkaloids
Millet, panic grass (*Panicum* spp.)	?
Ganskweed (*Lasiopermum bipinnatum*)	?
Verrain (*Lippia rehmanni*)	Triterpenes
Bog asphodel (*Narthecium ossifragum*)	Saponins
Alecrim (*Holocalyx glaziovii*)	?
Vuusiektebossie (*Nidorella foetida*)	?
Anthanasia trifurcata	?
Asaemia axillaris	?
Fungi	
Pithomyces chartarum ("facial eczema")— on pasture, especially rye	Sporidesmin
Anacystis spp.—blue-green algae in water	Alkaloid
Periconia spp.—on Bermuda grass	?
Phomopsis leptostromiformis—on lupins	Phomopsin A
Fusarium spp.—on moldy corn	T-2 toxin
Aspergillus spp.—on stored feeds	Aflatoxin
Infections	
Leptospirosis	Leptospires
Liver abscess	Bacteria/toxins
Parasitic liver cysts (flukes, hydatids)	Parasite
Rift Valley fever	Virus
Neoplasia	
Lymphoma	Malignant lymphocytes
Hepatic carcinoma	Malignant hepatocytes
Chemicals	
Copper	
Phosphorus	
Carbon tetrachloride	
Phenanthridium	

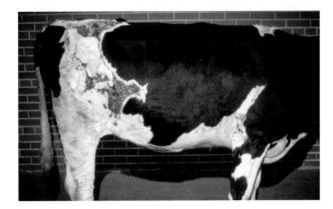

Figure 1.7-28 Photosensitization. Erythema, necrosis, and ulceration of white-haired skin associated with liver disease.

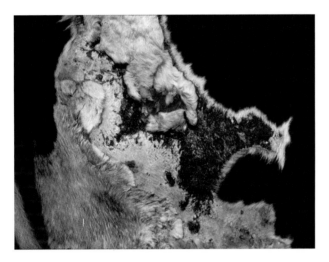

Figure 1.7-29 Close-up of Figure 1.7-28. Erythema, necrosis, ulceration, and alopecia.

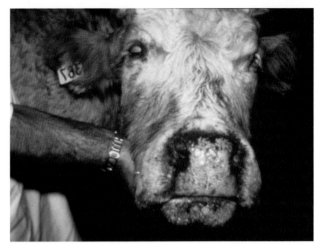

Figure 1.7-30 Photosensitization. Necrosis and ulceration of nasal planum associated with leptospirosis (courtesy S. Bouisset, coll. J. Gourreau, AFSSA).

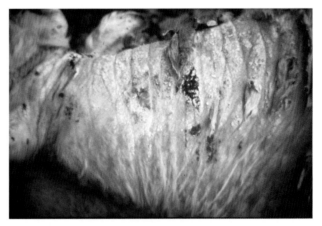

Figure 1.7-31 Photosensitization. Erythema, necrosis, ulceration, and alopecia over neck and trunk associated with leptospirosis (courtesy S. Bouisset, coll. J. Gourreau, AFSSA).

In severe cases, necrosis and sloughing may occur (Figs. 1.7-30 and 1.7-31). Variable degrees of pruritus and pain are present. The muzzle, eyelids, lips, face, pinnae, back, perineum, distal legs, teats (Figs. 1.7-32 and 1.7-33), and coronary bands are most commonly affected. In severe cases, pinnae, eyelids, tail, teats, and feet may slough. Affected animals often attempt to protect themselves from sunlight.

Although photosensitized animals rarely die, resultant weight loss, damaged udder and teats, refusal to allow young to nurse, and secondary infections/flystrike all may lead to appreciable economic loss.

Diagnosis

1. History and physical examination.
2. Liver function testing should always be performed whether or not clinical signs of liver damage are present.
3. Primary photodynamic agents can often be identified with various biological assay systems.
4. Measuring blood and tissue porphyrins.

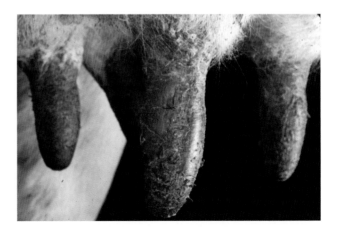

Figure 1.7-32 Photosensitization. Necrosis and ulceration of teats associated with liver disease.

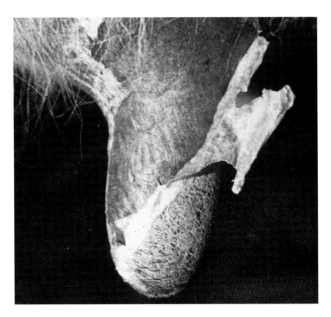

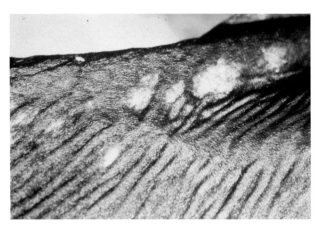

Figure 1.7-34 Chlorinated Naphthalene Toxicosis. Alopecia, scaling, and thickening of skin over back (courtesy D. Luquet, coll. J. Gourreau, AFSSA).

Figure 1.7-33 Photosensitization. Necrosis and sloughing on teat associated with liver disease.

MISCELLANEOUS DISEASES

Table 1.7-3 Miscellaneous Environmental Skin Diseases

Amanita toxicosis	Rare and cosmopolitan; eating mushroom *Amanita verna*; painful defecation and matting of feces around tail base and perineum; papules, vesicles, and necrotic foci in affected areas apparently due to irritating substance in feces
Arsenic toxicosis	Very rare and cosmopolitan; arsenic-containing dips, sprays, baits, wood preservatives, and medications; gastroenteritis, emaciation, variable appetite; dry, dull, easily epilated hair coat progresses to alopecia and exfoliative dermatitis; arsenic levels in liver or kidney
Chlorinated naphthalene toxicosis ("X-disease," "hyperkeratosis X") (Figs. 1.7-34 and 1.7-35)	Very rare and cosmopolitan; chlorinated naphthalene-containing industrial lubricants and wood preservatives; hypersalivation, lacrimation, proliferative stomatitis, variable appetite, weight loss, decreased milk production; progressive scaling, hyperkeratosis, thickening, fissuring, and alopecia of skin; initially withers and neck, with cranial/caudal/ventral extension; nonpruritic; tissue vitamin A levels and necropsy
Foreign bodies	See Box 1.7-2
Hairy vetch toxicosis	Rare and cosmopolitan; eating vetch plants (*Vicia villosa* and *V. benghalensis*); after two to several weeks of exposure; >3 years of age; papules, plaques, oozing, crusts, pruritus, alopecia; begins on tailhead, udder, and neck with spread to face, trunk, and limbs; conjunctivitis, anorexia, fever, weight loss, diarrhea; necropsy (systemic granulomatous disease); morbidity 6% to 8%; mortality as high as 50%
Iodism (Fig. 1.7-36)	Rare and cosmopolitan; excessive iodine-containing feeds or medicaments; nasal discharge, lacrimation, cough, variable appetite; severe skin scaling with or without partial alopecia, especially over dorsum, neck, head, and shoulders
Mercurialism	Very rare and cosmopolitan; eating mercury-containing feeds, fertilizers, sprays; gastroenteritis, nephrosis, lameness, oral ulceration, depression, anorexia, weight loss, and progressive generalized alopecia; mercury levels in kidney
Mimosine toxicosis	Rare; humid and subhumid tropical lowlands; eating mimosine-containing plants (*Mimosa* and *Leucaena*); gradual loss of long hairs (e.g., tail) and variable hoof dysplasias and laminitis
Oat straw toxicosis	Rare and cosmopolitan; eating oat straw contaminated with the fungus *Fusarium sporotrichoides* (type A trichothecene); fever, anorexia, respiratory distress; papules, plaques, and fissures on udder, hind quarters, lips, muzzle, and vulva; necropsy (extensive inflammation—especially eosinophils—of multiple organs)
Polybrominated biphenyl (PBB) toxicosis	Very rare; industrialized areas; eating PBBs, which have numerous industrial uses and serious environmental contamination potential; anorexia, weight loss, hematomas and abscesses over back, abdomen, and hind legs; hoof dysplasia; matted coat, alopecia, lichenification over lateral thorax, neck, and shoulders; PBB levels in tissues (especially fat)
Selenium toxicosis (Fig. 1.7-37)	Rare; associated with high levels of selenium in soil and/or presence of selenium-concentrating plants, low rainfall, alkaline soil (e.g., Great Plains and Rocky Mountain areas of United States); lameness in hind feet, coronary band painful, hoof dysplasias, progressive loss of long hairs (e.g., tail switch), and generalized alopecia; selenium levels in blood, liver, kidney, hair, and grasses

(continued)

Table 1.7-3 Miscellaneous Environmental Skin Diseases (*continued*)

Snake bite	Uncommon and cosmopolitan; especially rattlesnakes (*Crotalus* and *Sistrusus*) in the United States; especially spring and summer; especially nose, head, and legs; progressive edema, pain, discoloration, and necrosis and slough; variable systemic signs (fever, tachycardia, tachypnea, dyspnea, epistaxis)
Stachybotryotoxicosis	Rare; Europe; eating hay and straw contaminated by the fungus *Stachybotrys atra* (macrocyclic trichothecenes); initial necrotic ulcers in mouth and on lips and nostrils, conjunctivitis, and rhinitis; later fever, depression, anorexia, colic, diarrhea, weakness, lameness, bleeding diathesis; isolate fungus and toxins from feed
Subcutaneous emphysema	Rare and cosmopolitan; sequel to tracheal perforation, esophageal rupture, pulmonary emphysema, penetrating wounds (external or internal; rib fracture, traumatic reticuloperitonitis), clostridial infections, bovine ephemeral fever; soft, fluctuant, crepitant, subcutaneous swellings; usually nonpainful and not acutely ill (unless clostridial)
Vampire bat bite	Uncommon; where vampire bats found (e.g., South America); especially dorsum and legs; multiple bleeding, crusted ulcers

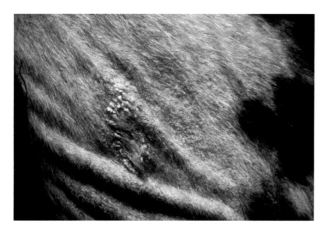

Figure 1.7-35 Chlorinated Naphthalene Toxicosis. Alopecia, thickening, and hyperkeratosis over withers (courtesy D. Luquet, coll. J. Gourreau, AFSSA).

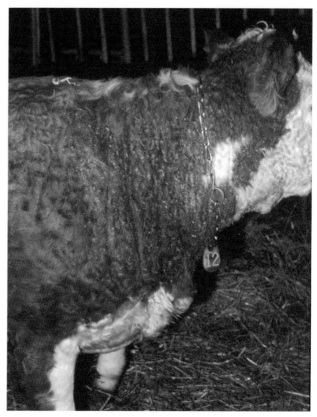

Figure 1.7-36 Iodism. Marked scaling and hypotrichosis associated with the administration of sodium iodide.

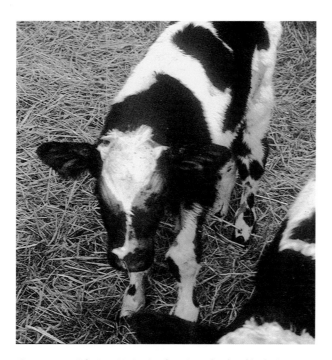

Figure 1.7-37 Selenium Toxicosis. Alopecia on head and limbs (courtesy J. Claessens, coll. J. Gourreau, AFSSA).

Box 1.7-2 Draining tracts

- A *fistula* is an abnormal passage or communication, usually between two internal organs or leading from an internal organ to the surface of the body.
- A *sinus* is an abnormal cavity or channel or fistula that permits the escape of pus to the surface of the body.
- Draining tracts are commonly associated with penetrating wounds that have left infectious agents and/or foreign material. Draining tracts may also result from infections of underlying tissues (e.g., bone, joint, lymph node) or previous injections.
- Foreign bodies include wood slivers, plant seeds and awns, cactus tines, fragments of wire, and suture material. Lesions include varying combinations of papules, nodules, abscesses, and draining tracts. Lesions occur most commonly on the legs, hips, muzzle, and ventrum.

REFERENCES

André-Fontaine G, et al. 1988. Photosensibilisation Leptospirosique: Mythe ou Réalité? *Point Vét* 20: 247.

Baines JR, et al. 2004. Ischaemic Necrosis of the Base of the Teat in Dairy Cows. *Vet Rec* 154: 443.

Botha CJ, et al. 2004. Gangrenous Ergotism in Cattle Grazing Fescue (*Festuca elatior* L.) in South Africa. *J S Afr Vet Assoc* 75: 45.

Coppock RW, et al. 1989. Cutaneous Ergotism in a Herd of Dairy Calves. *J Am Vet Med Assoc* 194: 549.

Griffiths IB, et al. 1991. Citrinin as a Possible Cause of the Pruritus, Pyrexia, Haemorrhagic Syndrome in Cattle. *Vet Rec* 129: 114.

Harper P, et al. 1993. Vetch Toxicosis in Cattle Grazing *Vicia villosa ssp dasycarpa* and *V. benghalensis. Aust Vet J* 70: 140.

House JK, et al. 1996. Primary Photosensitization Related to Ingestion of Alfalfa Silage by Cattle. *J Am Vet Med Assoc* 209: 1604.

Howard JL, Smith RA. 1999. Current Veterinary Therapy. Food Animal Practice. Ed 4. WB Saunders, Philadelphia, PA.

Johnson B, et al. 1992. Systemic Granulomatous Disease in Cattle in California Grazing Hairy Vetch (*Vicia villosa*). *J Vet Diagn Invest* 4: 360.

Kofler J, et al. 2004. Generalized Distal Limb Vessel Thrombosis in Two Cows with Digital and Inner Organ Infections. *Vet J* 167: 107.

Panciera RJ, et al. 1992. Hairy Vetch (*Vicia villosa* Roth) Poisoning in Cattle: Update and Experimental Induction of the Disease. *J Vet Diagn Invest* 4: 318.

Panciera RJ, et al. 1993. Bovine Hyperkeratosis: Historical Review and Report of an Outbreak. *Comp Cont Educ* 15: 1287.

Piccinii RS, et al. 1995. Comportamento do Morcego Hematofago *Desmodus Rotundus (Chiroptera)* Relacionado coma taxa de Ataque a Bovinos em Cativeiro. *Pesq Vet Bras* 5: 111.

Scruggs DW, et al. 1994. Toxic Hepatopathy and Photosensitization in Cattle Fed Moldy Alfalfa Hay. *J Am Vet Med Assoc* 204: 264.

Spickett AM, et al. 1991. Sweating Sickness: Relative Curative Effect of Hyperimmune Serum and a Precipitated Immunoglobulin Suspension and Immunoblot Identification of Proposed Immunodominant Tick Salivary Gland Proteins. *Onderstepoort J Vet Res* 58: 223.

Wu W, et al. 1997. Case Study of Bovine Dermatitis Caused by Oat Straw Infected with *Fusarium sporotrichoides. Vet Rec* 140: 399.

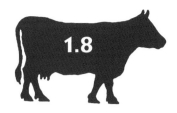

NUTRITIONAL SKIN DISEASES

Zinc-Responsive Dermatitis
Vitamin C–Responsive Dermatosis
Miscellaneous Nutritional Disorders
    Vitamin A Deficiency
    Riboflavin Deficiency
    Cobalt Deficiency
    Copper Deficiency
    Iodine Deficiency
    Selenium Deficiency
    High-Fat Milk Replacer Dermatosis

ZINC-RESPONSIVE DERMATITIS

Features

The characteristic dermatitis may be seen with true zinc deficiency or as an idiopathic zinc-responsive condition. Causes of deficiency include diets deficient in zinc; diets with excessive calcium, iron, phytates, and other chelating agents; drinking water with excessive iron and other chelating agents; genetic abnormality in zinc absorption (see Chapter 1.6). Zinc-responsive dermatoses are uncommon to rare. These are no apparent breed, sex, or age predilections.

More-or-less symmetrical erythema and scaling progress to crusting and alopecia. The face, pinnae, mucocutaneous junctions, pressure points, distal legs, flanks, and tail head are typically affected (Figs. 1.8-1 and 1.8-2). Some animals have a dull, rough, brittle hair coat. Pruritus may be intense or absent. Secondary bacterial skin infections are common. Truly zinc-deficient animals have accompanying systemic signs (decreased appetite and growth rate, weight loss, decreased milk production, depression, stiff joints, diarrhea), whereas animals with the idiopathic condition do not. With true zinc deficiency, multiple animals are often affected. With the idiopathic condition, a single animal is typically affected.

Differential Diagnosis

Dermatophytosis, dermatophilosis, staphylococcal folliculitis, demodicosis, stephanofilariasis, sterile eosinophilic folliculitis and furunculosis, and sarcoptic mange (when pruritic).

Diagnosis

1. Dermatohistopathology—Hyperplastic to spongiotic superficial perivascular-to-interstitial dermatitis with marked diffuse parakeratotic hyperkeratosis and a lymphoeosinophilic inflammatory infiltrate.
2. Analysis of diet.
3. Response to therapy.

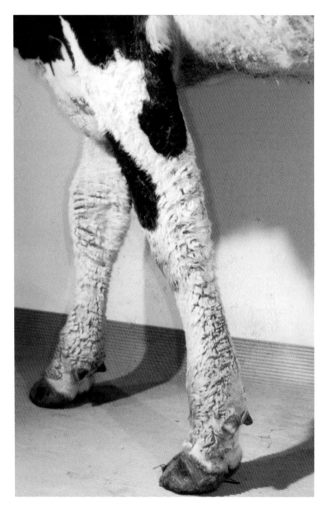

Figure 1.8-1 Zinc-Responsive Dermatitis. Fissured crusts on legs and ventrum.

VITAMIN C–RESPONSIVE DERMATOSIS

Features

Vitamin C–responsive dermatosis is an uncommon cosmopolitan disorder. It has been theorized that the condition may represent a temporary vitamin C deficiency in growing calves. The condition is most often seen in the fall and winter in temperate climates. The disorder is seen in dairy calves, 2 to 10 weeks of age, with no apparent sex predilection.

Moderate to severe scaling, alopecia, occasional crusts, and easy epilation of hairs begins on the head and/or limbs (Figs. 1.8-3 to 1.8-7). Extremities are erythematous, and petechiae and ecchy-

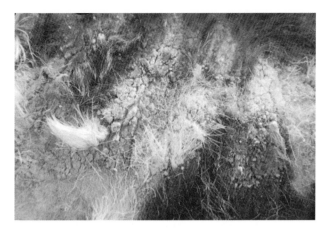

Figure 1.8-2 Zinc-Responsive Dermatitis. Thick crusts and alopecia over trunk.

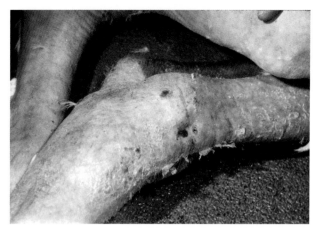

Figure 1.8-5 Vitamin C–Responsive Dermatosis. Alopecia, erythema, purpura, and scaling (peeling) of legs.

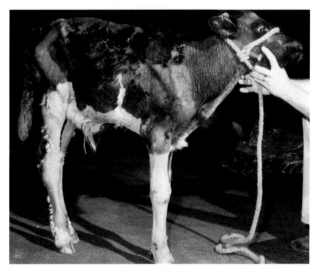

Figure 1.8-3 Vitamin C–Responsive Dermatosis. Widespread alopecia, scaling, and erythema of legs.

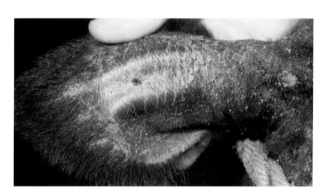

Figure 1.8-6 Vitamin C–Responsive Dermatosis. Alopecia and scaling of pinna.

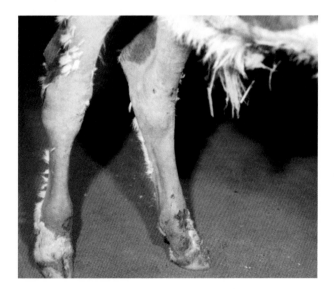

Figure 1.8-4 Vitamin C–Responsive Dermatosis. Alopecia, erythema, and purpura of legs.

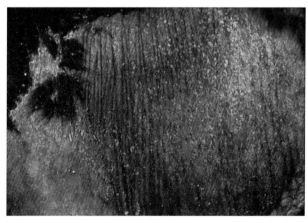

Figure 1.8-7 Vitamin C–Responsive Dermatosis. Alopecia and scaling over thorax.

moses are seen. Severely affected calves have widespread disease and may be depressed and grow slowly. Pruritus is absent.

Differential Diagnosis

Anagen defluxion.

Diagnosis

1. Dermatohistopathology—Diffuse orthokeratotic hyperkeratosis, curlicue hairs, vascular dilatation and congestion, and periadnexal hemorrhage.
2. Response to therapy.

MISCELLANEOUS NUTRITIONAL DISORDERS

Table 1.8-1 Miscellaneous Nutritional Disorders

Vitamin A deficiency	Very rare; deficient diet; rough, dry, faded hair coat and generalized seborrhea; systemic signs (night blindness, excessive lacrimation, corneal changes, neurologic disorders, skeletal abnormalities); serum and liver concentration of vitamin A
Riboflavin deficiency	Very rare; deficient diet; generalized alopecia; systemic signs (anorexia, poor growth, excessive lacrimation, hypersalivation, diarrhea); riboflavin levels in diet
Cobalt deficiency	Very rare; deficient diet; rough, brittle, faded hair coat; systemic signs (decreased growth and lactation); serum or liver concentration of cobalt and vitamin B_{12}
Copper deficiency (Figs. 1.8-8 and 1.8-9)	Rare; primary (deficient diet) or secondary (excess cadmium, molybdenum, or zinc diet); rough, brittle, faded hair coat with variable excessive licking; periocular hair coat fade and hair loss ("spectacles"); systemic signs (poor growth, diarrhea, anemia, bone disorders, infertility); serum and liver concentrations of copper
Iodine deficiency	Very rare; maternal dietary deficiency; newborn calves; generalized alopecia and thick, puffy skin (myxedema); systemic signs (weakness, neurologic disorders); serum concentration of thyroid hormone and thyroid gland pathology
Selenium deficiency	Rare and poorly documented; deficient diet; dermatitis over rump and tail base; systemic signs (infertility, retained placenta, respiratory disease, foot and leg problems); serum and liver concentrations of selenium
High-fat milk replacer dermatosis (Fig. 1.8-10)	Rare; calves; alopecia and scaling, especially muzzle, periocular area, base of pinnae and limbs

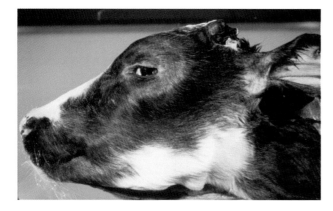

Figure 1.8-8 Copper Deficiency. Faded hairs on face and around eyes ("spectacles").

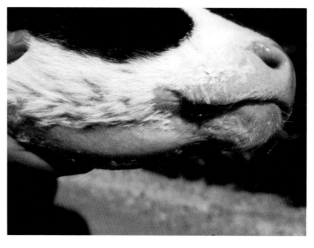

Figure 1.8-10 High-Fat Milk Replacer Dermatosis. Alopecia and scaling of muzzle and ventral neck.

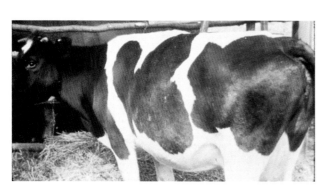

Figure 1.8-9 Copper Deficiency. Faded hairs in normally black hair coat (courtesy E. Meissonnier, coll. J. Gourreau, AFSSA).

REFERENCES

Abu Damir H, et al. 1988. Clinical Zinc and Copper Deficiencies in Cattle of Western Sudan. *Trop Anim Hlth Prod* 20: 52.

Anand KJ, et al. 2005. Zinc Deficiency in Two Calves. *Indian Vet J* 82: 768.

Howard JL, and Smith RA. 1999. Current Veterinary Therapy. Food Animal Practice. Ed 4. WB Saunders, Philadelphia, PA.

Radostits OM, et al. 2000. Veterinary Medicine. A Textbook of the Diseases of Cattle, Sheep, Pigs, Goats and Horses. Ed 9. WB Saunders, Philadelphia, PA.

Scott DW. 1988. Large Animal Dermatology. WB Saunders, Philadelphia, PA.

Singh AP, et al. 1994. Zinc Deficiency in Cattle. *Indian J Anim Sci* 64: 35.

Wikse SE, et al. 1992. Diagnosis of Copper Deficiency in Cattle. *J Am Vet Med Assoc* 200: 1625.

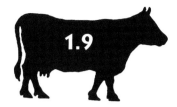

MISCELLANEOUS SKIN DISEASES

Sterile Eosinophilic Folliculitis and Furunculosis
Anagen Defluxion
Other Disorders
   Acral Lick Dermatitis
   Eosinophilic Granuloma
   Self-Destructive Behavior
   Sterile Panniculitis
   Telogen Defluxion
   Vitiligo

STERILE EOSINOPHILIC FOLLICULITIS AND FURUNCULOSIS

Features

Sterile eosinophilic folliculitis and furunculosis is a rare, idiopathic, cosmopolitan disorder. It occurs at any time of the year. There are no apparent breed or sex predilections, and adults are usually affected.

Lesions occur more-or-less symmetrically, and the head, neck, and trunk are commonly affected (Figs. 1.9-1 to 1.9-4). Early papules enlarge to plaques, and become alopecic and crusted. Some lesions exhibit central healing, others ooze. Lesions are neither pruritic nor painful, and affected animals are otherwise healthy. Only one animal in a herd is affected.

Differential Diagnosis

Dermatophytosis, dermatophilosis, staphylococcal folliculitis, demodicosis, and stephanofilariasis.

Diagnosis

1. Microscopy (direct smears)—Predominantly eosinophils, no phagocytosed bacteria (Fig. 1.9-5).
2. Culture—Sterile.
3. Dermatohistopathology—Eosinophilic luminal folliculitis with or without eosinophilic furunculosis.

ANAGEN DEFLUXION

Features

Anagen defluxion ("anagen effluvium") is uncommon and cosmopolitan. Various severe stressors (e.g., infectious diseases, metabolic diseases, high fevers) result in temporary growth defects in hair shafts. Calves are most commonly affected, and there are no apparent breed or sex predilections.

Hair loss occurs suddenly, within 7 to 10 days of the stressor.

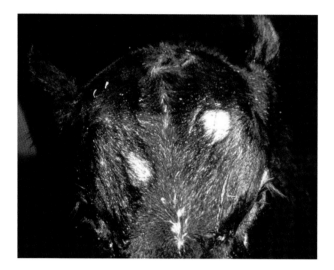

Figure 1.9-1 Sterile Eosinophilic Folliculitis and Furunculosis. Annular areas of alopecia and gray crusting on the head.

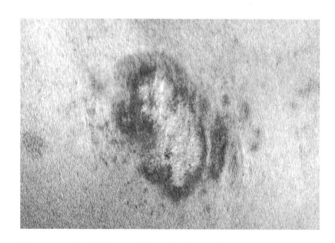

Figure 1.9-2 Sterile Eosinophilic Folliculitis and Furunculosis. Central thick crust with numerous peripheral tufted and crusted papules over lateral thorax.

The hair loss may be regional, multifocal, or fairly generalized, and is more-or-less bilaterally symmetric (Figs. 1.9-6 to 1.9-8). Skin in affected areas appears normal unless secondarily inflamed by trauma, contact dermatitis, or photodermatitis. Pruritus and pain are absent.

Differential Diagnosis

Hereditary hypotrichoses, follicular dysplasia, vitamin C-responsive dermatosis, and alopecia areata.

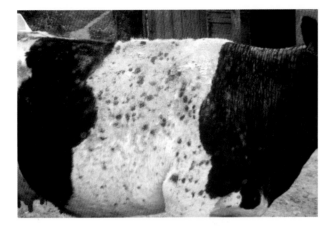

Figure 1.9-3 Sterile Eosinophilic Folliculitis and Furunculosis. Widespread erythematous papules and plaques (courtesy J. Gourreau).

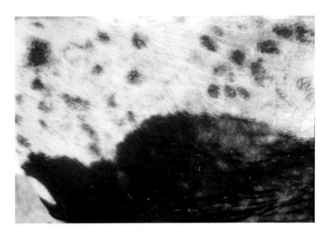

Figure 1.9-4 Sterile Eosinophilic Folliculitis and Furunculosis. Numerous erythematous oozing, crusted papules, and plaques over shoulder area (courtesy J. Gourreau).

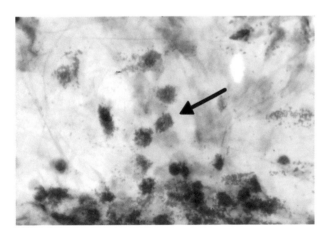

Figure 1.9-5 Sterile Eosinophilic Folliculitis and Furunculosis. Direct smear. Numerous eosinophils (arrow).

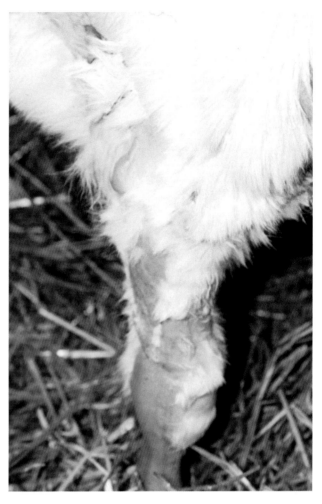

Figure 1.9-6 Anagen Defluxion. Alopecia on leg beginning several days after the onset of fever and pneumonia.

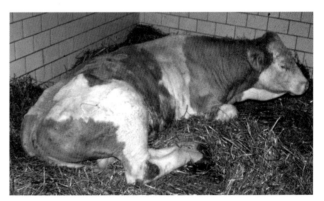

Figure 1.9-7 Anagen Defluxion. Widespread alopecia associated with pneumonia.

Diagnosis

1. Microscopy (plucked hairs in mineral oil)—Hair shaft diameters irregularly narrowed and deformed.
2. Dermatohistopathology—Apoptosis of hair matrix keratinocytes with or without dysplastic hair shafts.

OTHER DISORDERS

Table 1.9-1 Miscellaneous Skin Disorders

Acral lick dermatitis	Very rare; self-induced; ulcerated plaque over shoulder; preceded successive calvings by 2 to 3 weeks; dermatohistopathology
Eosinophilic granuloma	Very rare; adult dairy cattle; summer onset; multiple; widespread nodules; dermatohistopathology
Self-destructive behavior	Rare; Holsteins; especially first-calf heifers; severe udder edema precedes intense licking of skin between teats or base of teats; results in ulceration and necrosis
Sterile panniculitis	Very rare; one or multiple subcutaneous nodules and/or abscesses; especially neck, trunk, proximal limbs; culture (sterile) and dermatohistopathology
Telogen defluxion (Fig. 1.9-9)	Rare; 1 to 3 months after various stressors; regional or widespread, more-or-less bilaterally symmetric hair loss; skin normal; hair pluck
Vitiligo (Fig. 1.9-10)	Rare; cosmopolitan; probably hereditary (especially Holstein-Friesian, Hereford, Japanese Black, Bali, Madura); young animals; more-or-less symmetrical depigmentation of skin (leukoderma) and/or hairs (leukotrichia); especially face and neck, dermatohistopathology

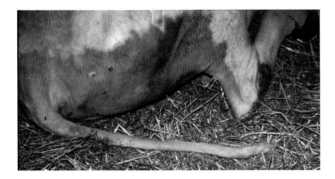

Figure 1.9-8 Close-up of Fig. 1.9-7. Note alopecic tail.

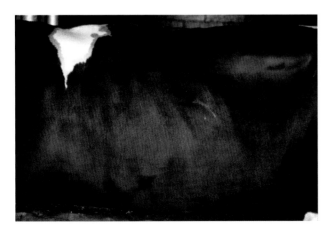

Figure 1.9-9 Telogen Defluxion. Widespread hypotrichosis three months after an undiagnosed illness and multiple drug administration.

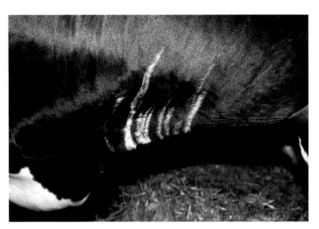

Figure 1.9-10 Vitiligo. Linear streak of leukotrichia on neck.

REFERENCES

Gourreau JM, et al. 1989. Cas de Dermo-folliculite à Éosinophiles chez un Bovin. *Point Vét* 21: 239.

Howard JO, and Smith RA. 1999. Current Veterinary Therapy. Food Animal Practice. Ed 4. WB Saunders, Philadelphia, PA.

Scott DW. 1988. Large Animal Dermatology. WB Saunders, Philadelphia, PA.

Scott PR, et al. 1996. Panniculitis in a Yearling Steer. *Vet Rec* 139: 252.

Wada T, and Okumura T. 1993. Three Cases of Eosinophilic Dermatitis in Holstein-Friesian Cattle. *J Jpn Vet Med Assoc* 46: 1018.

Yeruham I, et al. 1992. Acral Lick Dermatitis in a Dairy Cow. *Vet Rec* 130: 479.

Yeruham I, et al. 1996. Self-destructive Behaviour in Dairy Cattle. *Vet Rec* 138: 308.

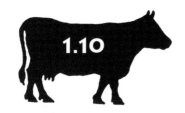

NEOPLASTIC AND NON-NEOPLASTIC GROWTHS

1.10

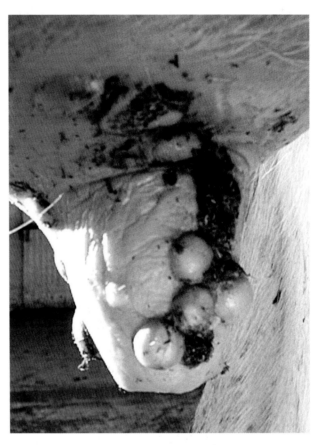

Figure 1.10-1 Papillomas. Typical papillomas on teat due to BPV 1 (courtesy L. Nicol, coll. J. Gourreau, AFSSA).

PAPILLOMA (PAPILLOMATOSIS, "WARTS")

Features

Papillomas are common cosmopolitan, benign neoplasms of keratinocytes. They are caused by papillomavirus. There are at least five types of bovine papillomavirus (BPV) that cause skin lesions in cattle. Infections follow direct or indirect contamination of various wounds (trauma, ectoparasites, ear marking, venepuncture, freeze- or heat-branding). In general, the five types of BPV produce different clinical syndromes with different biological behaviors.

BPV 1 causes typical fibropapillomas on the teats (Fig. 1.10-1) and penis (Fig. 1.10-2) of animals less than 2 years of age. These lesions often spontaneously regress within 1 to 12 months.

BPV 2 causes typical fibropapillomas on the head, neck, dewlap, shoulder, and occasionally the legs and teats of animals less than 2 years of age (Figs. 1.10-3 to 1.10-6). These lesions often spontaneously regress within 1 to 12 months.

BPV 1 and BPV 2 papillomas begin as multiple, small (2 to 5 mm diameter) firm papules with haired to smooth alopecic surfaces. Lesions become gray, firm, hyperkeratotic, often frond-like or cauliflower-like in appearance. Lesions may be pedunculated, digitate, or broad-based, and 1 mm to several cm in diameter.

BPV 3 causes so-called "atypical warts" in cattle of all ages. These lesions are low, flat, circular, and nonpedunculated, have delicate to thick frond-like projections on their surfaces, and may occur anywhere on the body, including the teats (Fig. 1.10-7). These papillomas rarely regress spontaneously.

BPV 5 causes so-called "rice grain warts" on the teats in cattle of all ages (Fig. 1.10-8). These lesions are small, white, elongated, hyperkeratotic, and do *not* regress spontaneously.

BPV 6 causes nonpedunculated, conical to branch-like papil-

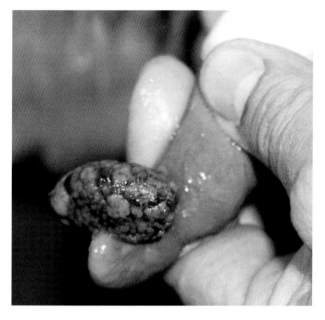

Figure 1.10-2 Papilloma. Typical cauliflower-like, hyperpigmented nodule on penis due to BPV 1.

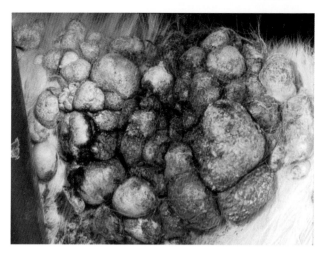

Figure 1.10-4 Close-up of Figure 1.10-3. Cluster of hyperkeratotic, broad-based to pedunculated nodules.

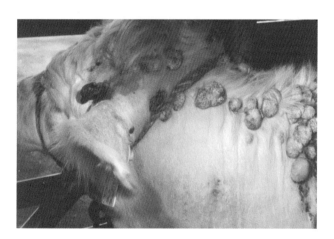

Figure 1.10-3 Papillomas. Typical hyperkeratotic, cauliflower-like nodules on head, neck, and shoulder due to BPV 2.

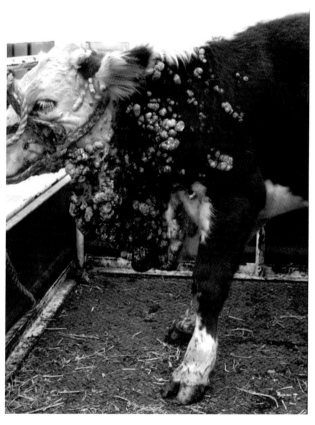

Figure 1.10-5 Papillomas. Severe papillomatosis due to BPV 2 in an immunosuppressed bovine.

lomas on the teats in cattle of all ages. These lesions are elongated and hyperkeratotic, with frond-like surface projections. They are frequently broken off, leaving ulcers that become secondarily infected by bacteria.

Congenital papillomas have been reported. However, viral causation has not been documented. All such lesions could actually be epidermal nevi (Fig. 1.10-9).

Differential Diagnosis

Squamous cell carcinoma (if solitary).

Diagnosis

1. Dermatohistopathology.

SQUAMOUS CELL CARCINOMA

Features

Squamous cell carcinoma is a common, cosmopolitan, malignant neoplasm of keratinocytes. It is especially common in subtropical and tropical climates, and at high altitudes. Ultraviolet light damage is important in the etiopathogenesis of this neoplasm, thus

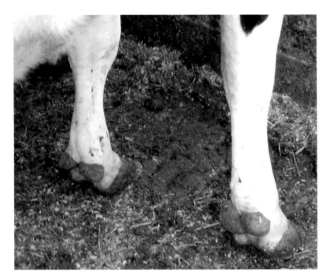

Figure 1.10-6 Papillomas. Typical papillomas on distal legs due to BPV 2 (courtesy E. Heinrich, coll. J. Gourreau, AFSSA).

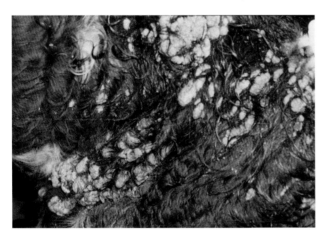

Figure 1.10-7 Papillomas. Flat, broad-based lesions with hyperkeratotic to frond-like surface due to BPV 3.

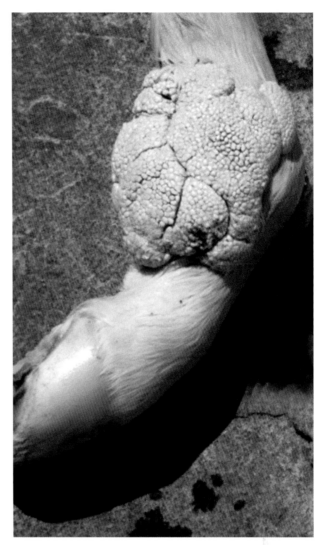

Figure 1.10-9 Congenital Papilloma (Probable Epidermal Nevus). Solitary cauliflower-like nodule on leg.

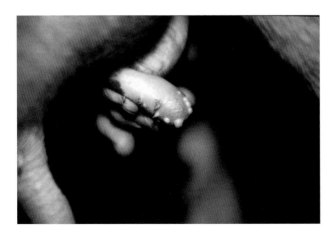

Figure 1.10-8 Papillomas. Thin, finger-like or "rice grain" lesions on teat due to BPV 5.

white skin that is lightly haired is at risk. Herefords and Ayrshires are at increased risk. Brand keratomas occasionally transform into squamous cell carcinomas. Adult to aged animals are most commonly affected, and there is no apparent sex predilection.

Lesions are usually solitary, and occur most commonly on the face (especially eyelids) (Figs. 1.10-10 to 1.10-12), pinnae, back, distal legs (Fig. 1.10-13), and vulva. Early lesions are erythematous, scaly, crusty, and hyperkeratotic (actinic keratosis). Invasive squamous cell carcinomas may be proliferative (verrucous or cauliflower-like) or ulcerative (granulating and nonhealing). Tumors may achieve a size of 50 cm diameter. Squamous cell carcinomas arising from brand keratomas (see Table 1.10-1) are heralded by ulceration and proliferation of previous hyperkeratotic lesions.

Differential Diagnosis

Papilloma, basal cell tumor (when ulcerated), various granulomas (infectious, foreign body).

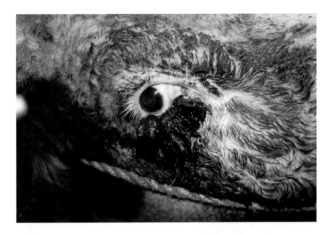

Figure 1.10-10 Squamous Cell Carcinoma. Ulcerated plaque covered by black crust on lower eyelid.

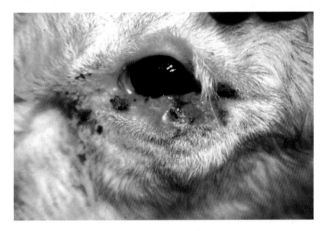

Figure 1.10-11 Squamous Cell Carcinoma. Multiple ulcers and crusts on lower eyelid (courtesy J. Nicol, coll. J. Gourreau, AFSSA).

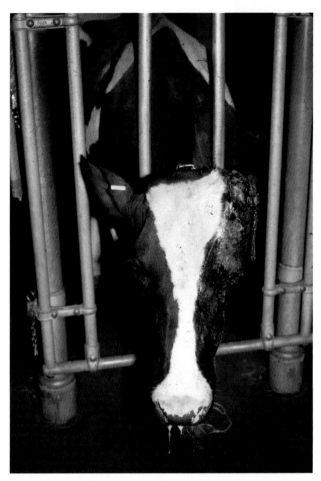

Figure 1.10-12 Squamous Cell Carcinoma. Ulcerated mass on head.

Diagnosis

1. Microscopy (direct smears). Keratinocytes showing various degrees of atypia.
2. Dermatohistopathology.

FIBROMA

Features

Fibroma is a common, cosmopolitan, benign neoplasm of fibroblasts. Adult or aged animals are affected. There are no apparent breed or sex predilections.

   Lesions are typically solitary, well-circumscribed, dome-shaped or pedunculated, and dermal or subcutaneous in location. They may be firm or soft, and may achieve a size of 50 cm diameter. Larger lesions may be alopecic, hyperpigmented, and ulcerated. Tumors can occur anywhere, especially on the head, neck, and shoulder (Figs. 1.10-14 to 1.10-16).

Differential Diagnosis

Fibrosarcoma, lymphoma, myxoma, myxosarcoma, neurofibroma, hemangiopericytoma.

Diagnosis

1. Microscopy (direct smears). Multiple fibroblasts.
2. Dermatohistopathology.

FIBROSARCOMA

Features

Fibrosarcoma is an uncommon, cosmopolitan, malignant neoplasm of fibroblasts. Adult or aged animals are affected. Congenital fibrosarcomas (solitary or multiple cutaneous lesions) have been reported. There are no apparent breed or sex predilections.

   Lesions are typically solitary, poorly circumscribed, round to irregular in shape, and dermal or subcutaneous in location. They may be firm or soft, and may achieve a size of 30 cm diameter. Larger lesions are often alopecic, edematous, necrotic, and ulcerated. Tumors can occur anywhere, especially on the head and neck (Figs. 1.10-17 to 1.10-19).

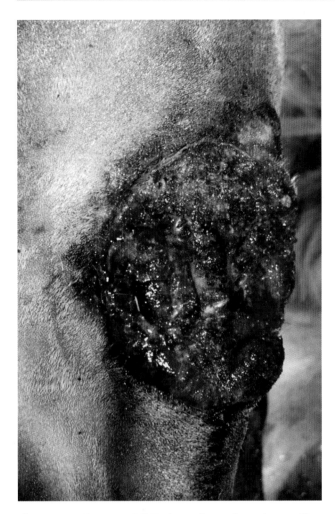

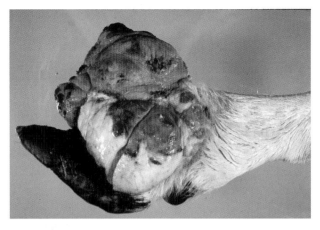

Figure 1.10-14 Fibroma. Large, ulcerated tumor on distal leg.

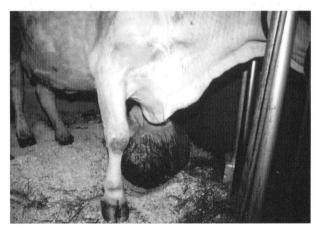

Figure 1.10-13 Squamous Cell Carcinoma. Large, ulcerated mass with a granular surface on the leg.

Figure 1.10-15 Fibroma. Huge, pedunculated, hyperpigmented, ulcerated tumor on brisket.

Differential Diagnosis.

Fibroma, lymphoma, myxoma, myxosarcoma, neurofibroma, hemangiopericytoma.

Diagnosis

1. Microscopy (direct smears). Fibroblasts showing various degrees of atypia.
2. Dermatohistopathology.

HEMANGIOMA

Features

Hemangioma is an uncommon, cosmopolitan, benign neoplasm of endothelial cells. Adult to aged animals develop solitary lesions. Solitary or multiple lesions may be seen congenitally or in young animals (Fig. 1.10-20). There are no apparent breed or sex predilections.

    Solitary hemangiomas are well-circumscribed, rounded, firm to soft, red-to-blue-to-black, 0.5 to 10 cm diameter lesions. Lesions can occur anywhere, especially on the head and legs.

    Cutaneous angiomatosis occurs predominantly in adult dairy

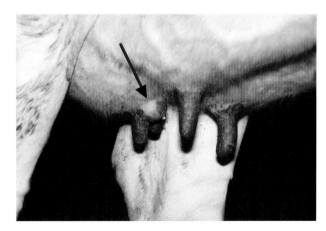

Figure 1.10-16 Fibroma. Nodule on udder.

cattle with no apparent sex predilection. Lesions are typically solitary and initially recognized due to profuse hemorrhage. They are circular, slightly raised, granular to wart-like in appearance, 0.5 to 2.5 cm diameter, and occur on the dorsal midline of the back. Intervals between hemorrhage vary from a few hours to several days. Animals occasionally become anemic, but rarely die.

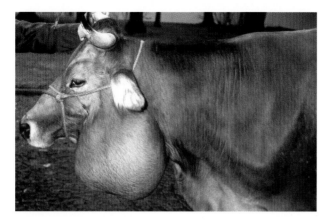

Figure 1.10-17 Fibrosarcoma. Huge tumor involving cheek and neck.

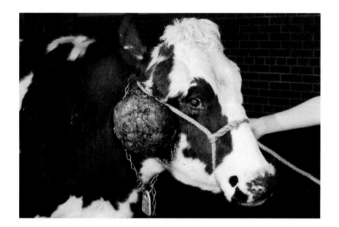

Figure 1.10-18 Fibrosarcoma. Ulcerated tumor on cheek.

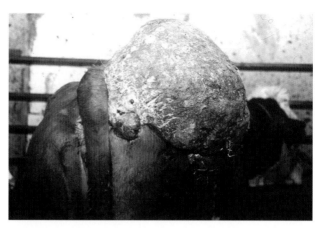

Figure 1.10-19 Fibrosarcoma. Huge tumor on hip (courtesy J. Trimaille, coll. J. Gourreau, AFSSA).

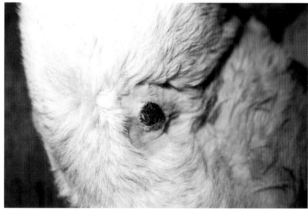

Figure 1.10-20 Congenital Hemangioma. Black, bleeding nodule in flank (area has been clipped).

Multiple hemangiomas occurring congenitally or in young animals (less than 1 year old) are often accompanied by widespread internal lesions ("angiomatosis," "angiomatous vascular malformation," "vascular hamartoma," "disseminated hemangioma").

Differential Diagnosis

Hemangiosarcoma, melanocytoma, melanoma.

Diagnosis

1. Dermatohistopathology.

MAST CELL TUMOR

Features

Mast cell tumors are uncommon to rare, cosmopolitan, benign or malignant neoplasms of mast cells. Adult to aged animals develop solitary (22% of cases) or multiple (78%) lesions. Multiple tumors are occasionally seen congenitally or in calves (Fig. 1.10-21).

Lesions begin as firm papules (0.2 to 1 cm diameter), and rapidly enlarge to firm to fluctuant nodules (up to 50 cm diameter),

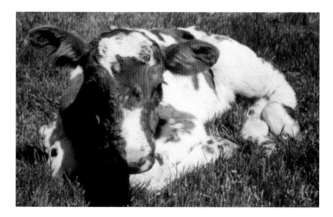

Figure 1.10-21 Congenital Mast Cell Tumors. Widespread erythematous, ulcerated nodules on a calf.

which are usually alopecic, erythematous, and ulcerated (Figs. 1.10-22 and 1.10-23). Lesions can occur anywhere. Multiple tumors are usually widespread, and about 60% of such animals have metastatic disease.

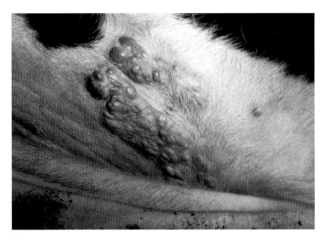

Figure 1.10-22 Mast Cell Tumors. Multiple erythematous papules and plaques on caudal thigh.

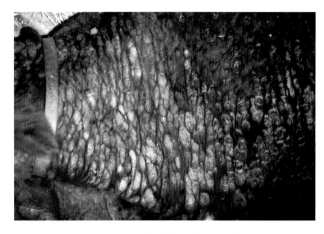

Figure 1.10-24 Lymphoma. Multiple hyperkeratotic plaques over neck and shoulder.

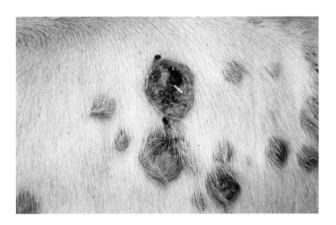

Figure 1.10-23 Mast Cell Tumors. Multiple erythematous, ulcerated papules and nodules on lateral thorax.

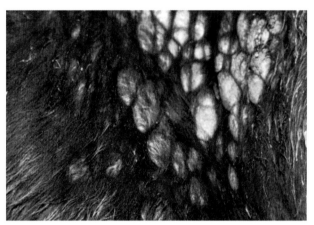

Figure 1.10-25 Lymphoma. Multiple hyperkeratotic plaques over thorax.

Differential Diagnosis

Lymphoma.

Diagnosis

1. Microscopy (direct smears). Mast cells showing various degrees of atypia.
2. Dermatohistopathology.

LYMPHOMA

Features

Cutaneous lymphoma is an uncommon to rare, cosmopolitan, malignant neoplasm of T lymphocytes. Enzootic lymphoma ("bovine leukemia," "lymphomatosis," "enzootic bovine leukosis") is caused by a retrovirus (bovine leukemia virus [BLV]), but most cases of cutaneous lymphoma are sporadic and not BLV-associated. Widespread lesions are seen in 6 month to 4 year old cattle, while solitary lesions are seen in 4 to 6 year olds. There are no apparent breed or sex predilections.

Multiple lesions typically involve a large area of the body, es-

pecially the neck and trunk (Fig. 1.10-24). Early lesions are dermal or subcutaneous papules and plaques. The overlying skin and hair coat are initially normal in appearance, but lesions enlarge (0.2 to 10 cm diameter) and become alopecic, crusted, hyperkeratotic, and ulcerated (Figs. 1.10-25 and 1.10-26). There may be one or more periods of spontaneous regression of lesions—lasting for several days or weeks—prior to persistent skin lesions and internal lymphoma.

Solitary lesions are typically firm, rounded, subcutaneous nodules (2 to 6 cm diameter). These cattle have internal lesions and are BLV-positive.

Differential Diagnosis

Multiple lesions: mast cell tumor, papilloma, urticaria (early lesions). Solitary lesions: lipoma, granuloma (infectious or sterile).

Diagnosis

1. Microscopy (direct smears). Lymphocytes showing various degrees of atypia.
2. Dermatohistopathology.

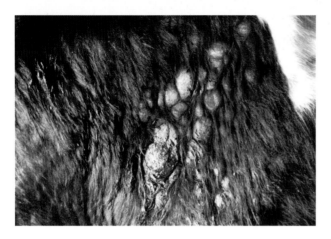

Figure 1.10-26 Lymphoma. Multiple hyperkeratotic papules and plaques, the largest of which is ulcerated.

MELANOCYTIC NEOPLASMS

Features

Melanocytic neoplasms are common, cosmopolitan, benign (melanocytoma) or malignant (melanoma) proliferations of melanocytes. About 80% to 90% of these neoplasms are benign. Melanocytic neoplasms occur in all ages of cattle, with over 50% of the cattle being less than 18 months old. Lesions also occur congenitally. Darkly colored cattle, especially Angus, may be at risk. There is no apparent sex predilection.

Lesions are usually solitary and can occur anywhere (especially the legs) (Figs. 1.10-27 and 1.10-28). Tumors are dermal or subcutaneous, round-to-pedunculated-to-multilobulated, gray-to-black in color, firm to fluctuant, and 5 to 50 cm in diameter. Larger tumors are often alopecic, necrotic, and ulcerated.

Differential Diagnosis

Hemangioma, hemangiosarcoma.

Diagnosis

1. Microscopy (direct smears). Melanocytes showing various degrees of atypia.
2. Dermatohistopathology.

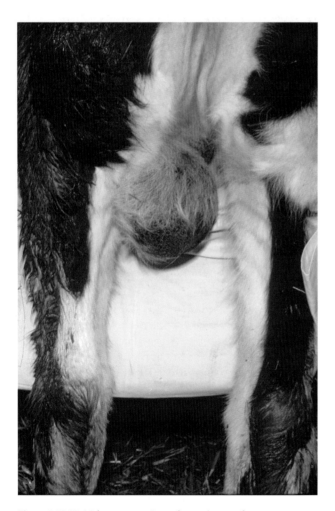

Figure 1.10-27 Melanocytoma. Large, hyperpigmented tumor on caudomedial thigh.

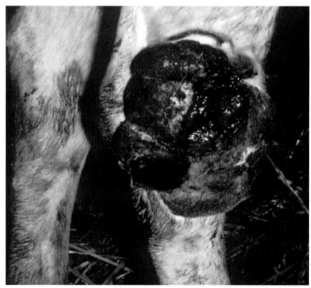

Figure 1.10-28 Melanocytoma. Large, multilobulated, hyperpigmented tumor with focal ulceration on lateral hock.

MISCELLANEOUS NEOPLASTIC AND NON-NEOPLASTIC GROWTHS

Table 1.10-1 Miscellaneous Neoplastic and Non-Neoplastic Growths

Basal cell tumor	Very rare, adult to aged; solitary firm to fluctuant nodule, often alopecic and ulcerated; anywhere; benign; direct smears and dermatohistopathology
Trichoepithelioma	Very rare; adult to aged; solitary firm to fluctuant nodule, often alopecic and ulcerated; anywhere; benign; dermatohistopathology
Sebaceous adenoma	Rare; adult to aged; solitary nodule; anywhere (especially eyelid); benign; direct smears and dermato-histopathology
Sebaceous adenocarcinoma	Very rare; adult to aged; solitary nodule; anywhere (especially jaw); malignant; direct smears and dermato-histopathology
Epitrichial (apocrine) adenoma	Very rare; adult to aged; solitary nodule; tail; benign; direct smears and dermatohistopathology
Myxoma	Very rare; congenital to aged; solitary soft nodule; anywhere (especially pinna, leg); benign; dermatohisto-pathology
Myxosarcoma	Very rare; adult to aged; solitary, poorly circumscribed nodule; anywhere; malignant; dermatohistopathology
Hemangiopericytoma	Very rare; adult to aged; solitary nodule, 5 to 10 cm diameter; anywhere (especially jaw); benign; dermato-histopathology
Hemangiosarcoma	Very rare; adult to aged; solitary nodule; often necrotic/ulcerated/bleeding; red/blue/black in color; 1 to 10 cm diameter; anywhere (especially leg); malignant; dermatohistopathology
Lymphangioma	Very rare; congenital or young; solitary, soft nodule; anywhere (especially leg, brisket); benign; dermato-histopathology
Neurofibroma (Schwannoma; neurofibromatosis)	Rare; congenital to adult; probably hereditary; usually multiple firm papules and nodules (0.5 to 8 cm diameter), unilateral or bilateral; anywhere (especially muzzle, face, eyelids, neck, brisket); multiple nodules may coalesce in clusters and chains; usually benign, though most animals have extracutaneous lesions too (especially heart, brachial plexus, intercostal nerves); dermatohistopathology
Leiomyosarcoma	Very rare; adult to aged; solitary nodule; anywhere; malignant; dermatohistopathology
Rhabdomyosarcoma	Very rare; adult to aged; solitary nodule; anywhere; malignant; dermatohistopathology
Lipoma (Fig. 1.10-29)	Rare; adult (rarely congenital) to aged; solitary subcutaneous nodules, up to 50 cm diameter; occasionally infiltrative ("lipomatosis"); anywhere (especially trunk); benign; direct smears and dermatohistopathology
Dermoid cyst	Very rare; probably congenital; solitary nodule; midline of neck, eyelid, and periocular; benign; dermato-histopathology
Branchial cyst	Very rare; congenital; solitary, firm to fluctuant swelling in ventral neck area; benign; dermatohistopathology
Actinic keratosis (Fig. 1.10-30)	Common; adult to aged; ultraviolet light damaged white skin; solitary or multiple erythematous, scaly crusted, hyperkeratotic plaques; premalignant; dermatohistopathology
Linear keratosis (epidermal nevus) (Fig. 1.10-31)	Very rare; probably congenital; numerous vertically-oriented, linear, hyperkeratotic bands on thorax/abdomen; unilateral; benign; dermatohistopathology
Cutaneous horn	Rare; horn-like hyperkeratosis; usually overlying epithelial neoplasms (papilloma, squamous cell carcinoma, actinic keratosis, basal cell tumor); benign or malignant; dermatohistopathology
Brand keratoma	1% to 8% of heat-branded cattle; adult to aged; follows contour of original brand; hard, dry, raised, hyperkera-totic, depigmented lesion; premalignant (can transform to squamous cell carcinoma); dermatohistopathology

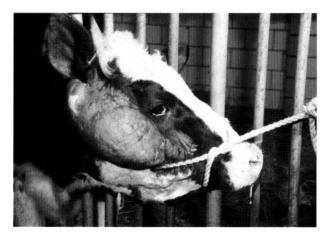

Figure 1.10-29 Infiltrative Lipoma. Large subcutaneous tumor on cheek.

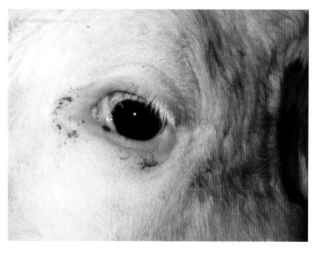

Figure 1.10-30 Actinic Keratosis. Multiple crusts on lower eyelid (courtesy J. Franc, coll. J. Gourreau, AFSSA).

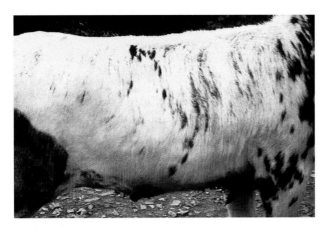

Figure 1.10-31 Linear Epidermal Nevus. Multiple, vertically-oriented hyperpigmented, hyperkeratotic plaques (courtesy P. Deprez, coll. J. Gourreau, AFSSA).

REFERENCES

Antony P. 1988. Horn Growth From the Upper Eyelid of a Crossbred Heifer. *Indian Vet J* 65: 83.

Baird AN, et al. 1993. Dermoid Cyst in a Bull. *J Am Vet Med Assoc* 202: 298.

Dakshinkar NP, et al. 1991. Trichoepithelioma in Cattle. *Indian Vet J* 68: 688.

Deprez P, et al. 1995. A Case of Bovine Linear Keratosis. *Vet Dermatol* 6: 45.

Gourreau JM, et al. 1995. Les Tumeurs Mélaniques Cutanées des Bovins. *Point Vét* 26: 785.

Hill JE, et al. 1991. Prevalence and Location of Mast Cell Tumors in Slaughter Cattle. *Vet Pathol* 28: 449.

Howard JO, Smith RA. 1999. Current Veterinary Therapy. Food Animal Practice. Ed 4. WB Saunders, Philadelphia, PA.

Loupal G, Schlerka G. 1988. Maligne Hämangioendotheliome beim Rind-2 Fallberichte. *Wien Tierärztl Mschr* 74: 102.

Matovelo JA, et al. 2005. Gross and Microscopic Pathological Findings in a Sebaceous Gland Carcinoma of the Perineum and Vulva in a Friesian Cow. *Vet Rec* 156: 612.

Meyers SA, Read WK. 1990. Squamous Cell Carcinoma of the Vulva in a Cow. *J Am Vet Med Assoc* 196: 1644.

Miller MA, et al. 1995. Cutaneous Melanocytomas in 10 Young Cattle. *Vet Pathol* 32: 479.

Misdorp W. 2002. Congenital Tumours and Tumour-Like Lesions in Domestic Animals. 1. Cattle. A Review. *Vet Quart* 24: 1.

Mitarai Y, et al. 1998. Haemangiopericytoma in a Calf. *Res Vet Sci* 65: 265.

Munro R, et al. 1994. Bovine Disseminated Haemangioma. *Vet Rec* 135: 333.

O'Toole D, Fox JD. 2003. Chronic Hyperplastic and Neoplastic Lesions (Marjolin's Ulcer) in Hot-Brand Sites in Adult Beef Cattle. *J Vet Diagn Invest* 15: 64.

Piercy DWT, et al. 1994. Mixed Apocrine (Sweat Gland) Adenocarcinoma in the Tail of a Cow. *Vet Rec* 134: 473.

Raoofi A, et al. 2004. Auricular Mast Cell Tumour in a Cow. *Vet Rec* 155: 124.

Sartin EA, et al. 1994. Characterization of Naturally Occurring Cutaneous Neurofibromatosis in Holstein Cattle. A Disorder Resembling Neurofibromatosis Type 1 in Humans. *Am J Pathol* 145: 1168.

Sartin EA, et al. 1996. Invasive Malignant Fibrous Histiocytoma in a Cow. *J Am Vet Med Assoc* 208: 1709.

Sasani F, Bazargani TT. 2005. Bovine Cutaneous Schwannoma. *Indian Vet J* 82: 716.

Scott DW. 1988. Large Animal Dermatology. WB Saunders, Philadelphia, PA.

Scott DW, Anderson WI. 1992. Bovine Cutaneous Neoplasms: Literature Review and Retrospective Analysis of 62 Cases (1978 to 1990). *Comp Cont Educ* 14: 1405.

Scott DW, Gourreau JM. 1992. Fibromes, Fibrosarcomes et Mastocytomes Cutanés Chez les Bovins. *Point Vét* 24: 539.

Scott DW, Gourreau JM. 1996. Les Tumeurs des Vaisseaux Sanguins Cutanés Chez les Bovins. *Point Vét* 27: 941.

Wapf P, Nuss K. 2005. Dentigerous Cyst in a Calf. *Vet Rec* 156: 580.

Watson TDG, Thompson H. 1990. Juvenile Bovine Angiomatosis: A Syndrome of Young Cattle. *Vet Rec* 127: 279.

Yeruham I, et al. 1996. Skin Tumours in Cattle and Sheep After Freeze- or Heat-Branding. *J Comp Pathol* 114: 101.

Yeruham I, et al. 1999. Congenital Skin Neoplasia in Cattle. *Vet Dermatol* 10: 149.

Yeruham I, et al. 1999. Tumours of the Vulva in Cattle—A 10 Year Survey. *Vet J* 158: 237.

Yeruham I, Perl S. 2002. Melanocytoma and Myxoma—Tumours of the Limbs in Cattle. *Berl Munch Tierärztl Wschr* 115: 425.

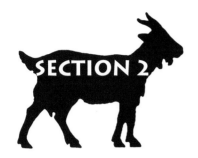

CAPRINE

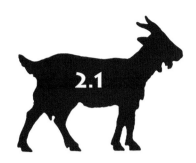

BACTERIAL SKIN DISEASES

IMPETIGO

Features

Impetigo ("goat pox") (Latin: an attack; scabby eruption) is a common, cosmopolitan superficial pustular dermatitis that does not involve hair follicles. It is caused by *Staphylococcus aureus*—less commonly *S. hyicus* or *S. chromogenes*—and predisposing factors include trauma, moisture, and the stress of parturition. Kids and lactating does are predisposed.

    Lesions are most commonly seen on the udder (especially the base of the teats and the intramammary sulcus), teats, ventral abdomen, medial thighs, vulva, perineum, and ventral tail (Figs. 2.1-1 and 2.1-2). Superficial vesicles rapidly become pustular, rupture, and leave annular erosions and yellow-brown crusts. Lesions are neither pruritic nor painful, and affected animals are otherwise healthy. Single or multiple animals may be affected. Staphylococcal mastitis is a possible, but uncommon complication.

Differential Diagnosis

Other bacterial infections, dermatophilosis, dermatophytosis, and viral infections.

Diagnosis

1. Microscopy (direct smears)—Degenerate neutrophils, nuclear streaming, and phagocytosed cocci (Gram-positive, about 1 μm diameter)(see Figs. 2.1-6 and 2.1-7).
2. Culture (aerobic).
3. Dermatohistopathology—Subcorneal pustular dermatitis with degenerate neutrophils and intracellular cocci.

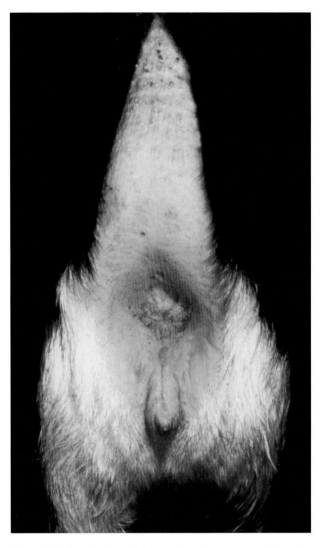

Figure 2.1-1 Impetigo. Superficial pustules and crusts on ventral surface of tail and perineum.

FOLLICULITIS AND FURUNCULOSIS

Features

Folliculitis and furunculosis (hair follicle rupture) ("acne") are common, cosmopolitan, caused by *Staphylococcus aureus*—less commonly *S. hyicus* or *S. intermedius*—and predisposing factors include trauma and moisture. There are no apparent breed, sex, or age predilections.

    Lesions can be seen anywhere, most commonly on the face, pinnae, back, and distal legs (Figs. 2.1-3 to 2.1-5). Tufted papules

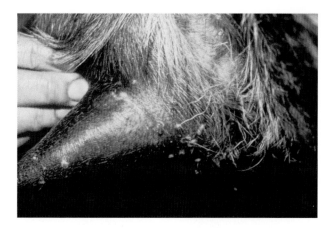

Figure 2.1-2 Impetigo. Superficial pustules on teat and udder.

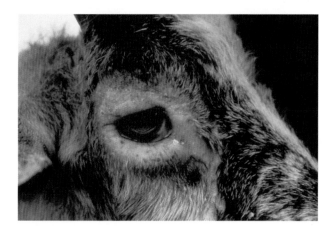

Figure 2.1-3 Staphylococcal Folliculitis. Periocular edema, erythema, crusts and erosions.

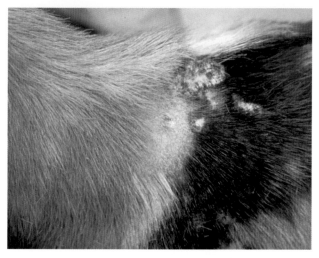

Figure 2.1-4 Staphylococcal Furunculosis. Crusts and draining tracts over back.

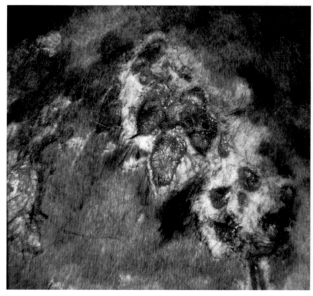

Figure 2.1-5 Staphylococcal Furunculosis. Multiple ulcers and draining tracts over trunk (area has been clipped).

and pustules become crusted, then alopecic. Furuncles are characterized by nodules, draining tracts, and ulcers. Lesions are rarely pruritic but furuncles may be painful. Affected animals are usually otherwise healthy. Pending the inciting cause(s), single or multiple animals may be affected.

Differential Diagnosis

Dermatophilosis, dermatophytosis, demodicosis, and contagious viral pustular dermatitis ("orf").

Diagnosis

1. Microscopy (direct smears)—Degenerate neutrophils, nuclear streaming, and phagocytosed cocci (Gram-positive, about 1 µm diameter) with folliculitis (Figs. 2.1-6 and 2.1-7). Furunculosis is characterized by numerous macrophages, lymphocytes, eosinophils, and plasma cells in addition to the findings described for folliculitis (Fig. 2.1-8).
2. Culture (aerobic).
3. Dermatohistopathology—Suppurative luminal folliculitis with intracellular cocci; pyogranulomatous furunculosis.

DERMATOPHILOSIS

Features

Dermatophilosis ("streptothricosis") is a common, cosmopolitan skin disease. *Dermatophilus congolensis* proliferates under the influence of moisture (especially rain) and skin damage (especially ticks, insects, prickly vegetation, ultraviolet light and white skin). The disease is more common and more severe in tropical and subtropical climates and in outdoor animals. There are no apparent breed, sex, or age predilections.

Lesions may occur anywhere, especially the face, pinnae, dorsum, tail, distal legs, udder, and scrotum (Figs. 2.1-9 to 2.1-14). Tufted papules and pustules coalesce and become exudative, which results in large ovoid to linear ("run-off" or "scald-line") groups of hairs being matted together in thick crusts ("paint

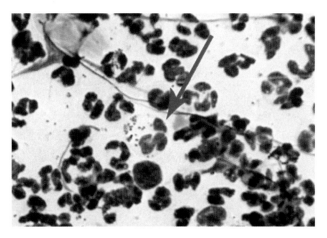

Figure 2.1-6 Staphylococcal Folliculitis. Direct smear (Diff-Quik stain). Suppurative inflammation with degenerate neutrophils, nuclear streaming, and phagocytosed cocci (arrow).

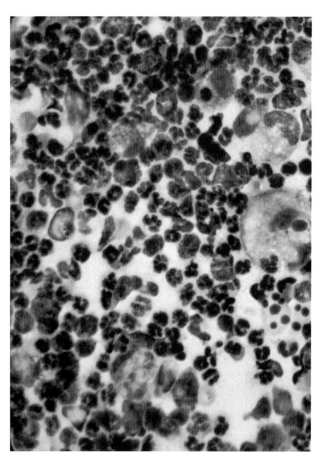

Figure 2.1-8 Staphylococcal Furunculosis. Direct smear (Diff-Quik stain). Pyogranulomatous inflammation with degenerate and nondegenerate neutrophils, macrophages, lymphocytes, and plasma cells.

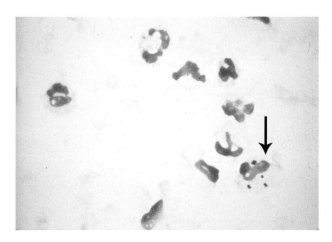

Figure 2.1-7 Staphylococcal Folliculitis. Direct smear (Gram stain). Degenerate neutrophils and phagocytosed Gram-positive cocci (arrow).

brush"). Erosions, ulcers, and thick, creamy yellowish to greenish pus underlie the crusts. Acute lesions are painful, but not pruritic. Chronic lesions consist of dry crust, scale, and alopecia. Typically multiple animals are affected.

Dermatophilosis is a zoonosis. Human skin infections are uncommon and characterized by pruritic or painful pustular lesions in contact areas (Fig. 2.1-15).

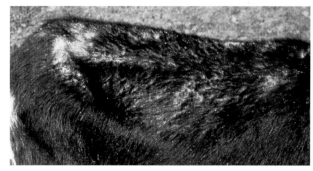

Figure 2.1-9 Dermatophilosis. Crusts, scales, and alopecia over back and rump.

Differential Diagnosis

Staphylococcal folliculitis, dermatophytosis, contagious viral pustular dermatitis ("orf"), and zinc-responsive dermatitis.

Diagnosis

1. Microscopy (direct smears)—Degenerate neutrophils, nuclear streaming, and Gram-positive cocci in two to eight parallel rows forming branching filaments ("railroad tracks")(Fig. 2.1-16).

2. Culture (aerobic).
3. Dermatohistopathology—Suppurative luminal folliculitis and epidermitis with palisading crusts containing Gram-positive cocci in branching filaments.

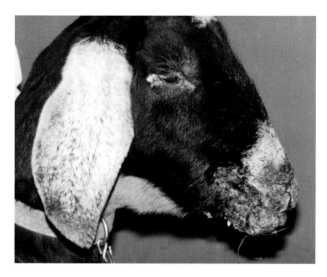

Figure 2.1-10 Dermatophilosis. Thick crusts on muzzle.

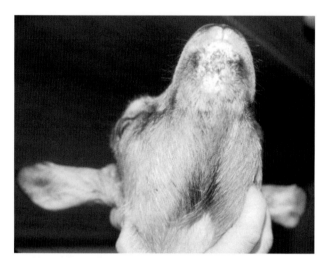

Figure 2.1-11 Dermatophilosis. Thick crusts on chin.

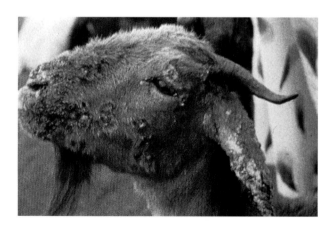

Figure 2.1-12 Dermatophilosis. Thick crusts on face and pinna (courtesy S. Torres).

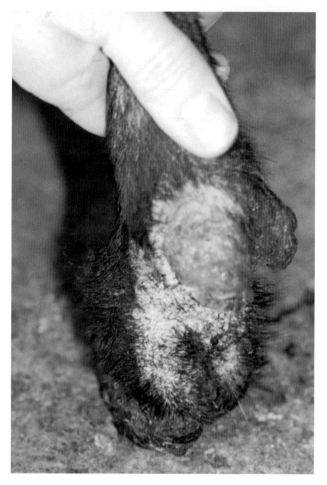

Figure 2.1-13 Dermatophilosis. Thick crust on caudal pastern.

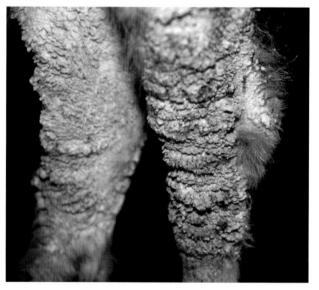

Figure 2.1-14 Dermatophilosis. Thick crusts on pelvic limbs.

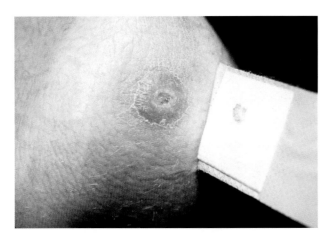

Figure 2.1-15 Dermatophilosis in a Human. Ruptured pustule and surrounding erythema on the elbow.

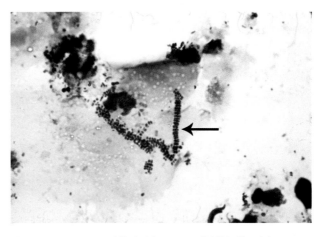

Figure 2.1-16 Dermatophilosis. Direct smear (Diff-Quik stain). Branching filaments composed of cocci ("railroad tracks," arrow).

MISCELLANEOUS BACTERIAL DISEASES

Table 2.1-1 Miscellaneous Bacterial Diseases	
Abscess (Figs. 2.1-17 and 2.1-18)	Common and cosmopolitan; anywhere (especially face [associated with tooth root abscess or cheek biting], neck [post-injection], and sternum [lameness and prolonged recumbency]); subcutaneous ± underlying bone involvement; especially *Arcanobacterium pyogenes, Corynebacterium pseudotuberculosis, Staphylococcus aureus*; culture
Clostridial cellulitis ("big head")	Uncommon and cosmopolitan; especially in summer/early fall when fighting is common in bucks; head and neck; edema, exudation, rare crepitus; *Clostridium novyi* and *C. oedematiens*; systemic signs; culture and necropsy
Ulcerative lymphangitis (Fig. 2.1-19)	Rare and cosmopolitan; firm to fluctuant nodules, draining tracts, corded lymphatics, and regional lymphadenopathy; especially *A. pyogenes, C. pseudotuberculosis,* and *S. aureus*; culture
Actinomycosis ("lumpy jaw")	Very rare and cosmopolitan; face and udder; firm nodules, abscesses, draining tracts with yellowish-white granules; *Actinomyces* sp.; culture and dermatohistopathology
Actinomycetic mycetoma	Very rare (Asia); leg and shoulder; solitary nodules, draining tracts with variably-colored granules; *Actinomadura madurae* and *A. pelletierii;* culture and dermatohistopathology
Actinobacillosis	Very rare and cosmopolitan; face and neck; nodules, abscesses, draining tracts with grayish-white to brownish-white granules; *Actinobacillus* sp.; culture and dermatohistopathology
Nocardiosis (Fig. 2.1-20)	Very rare and cosmopolitan; face; subcutaneous nodules and abscesses; *Nocardia* sp.; culture and dermatohistopathology

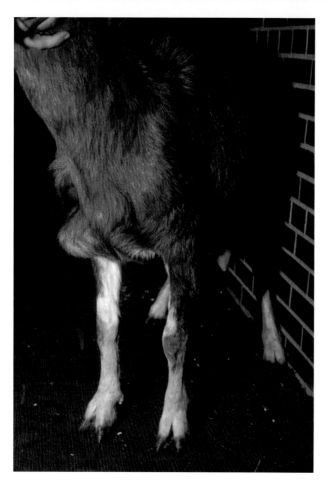

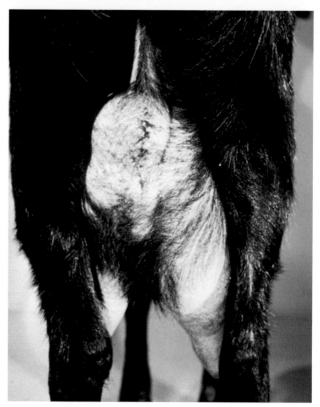

Figure 2.1-18 Subcutaneous Abscess on caudal aspect of udder due to *Corynebacterium pseudotuberculosis.*

Figure 2.1-17 Subcutaneous Abscess on chest due to *Corynebacterium pseudotuberculosis.*

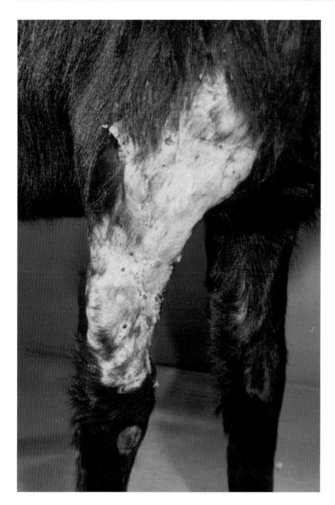

Figure 2.1-19 Lymphangitis. Multiple papules, nodules, and draining tracts due to *Corynebacterium pseudotuberculosis*.

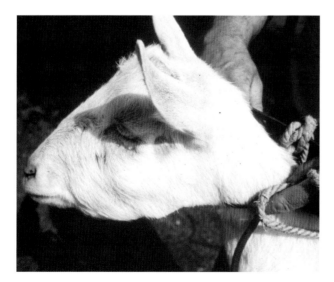

Figure 2.1-20 Nocardial Abscess. Large abscess on side of face (courtesy P. Jackson).

REFERENCES

Andrews AH, Lamport A. 1997. Isolation of *Staphylococcus chromogenes* from an Unusual Case of Impetigo in a Goat. *Vet Rec* 140: 584.

Baby PG, et al. 2000. Actinomycosis in Goat—A Case Report. *Indian J Vet Med* 20: 52.

Gezon HM, et al. 1991. Epizootic of External and Internal Abscesses in a Large Goat Herd over a 16-Year Period. *J Am Vet Med Assoc* 198: 257.

Hotter A, Buchner A. 1995. Euteraktinomykose bei einer Ziege. *Wiener Tierärz Monat* 82: 225.

Howard JL, Smith RA. 1999. Current Veterinary Therapy. Food Animal Practice. Ed 4. WB Saunders, Philadelphia, PA.

Loria GR, et al. 2005. Dermatophilosis in Goats in Sicily. *Vet Rec* 156: 120.

Mahanta PN, et al. 1997. Identification and Characterization of Staphylococci Isolated from Cutaneous Lesions in Goats. *J Vet Med B* 44: 309.

Matthews JG. 1999. Diseases of the Goat. Ed 2. Blackwell Science, Oxford, United Kingdom.

Radostits OM, et al. 2000. Veterinary Medicine. A Textbook of the Diseases of Cattle, Sheep, Pigs, Goats and Horses. Ed 9. WB Saunders, Philadelphia, PA.

Smith MC, Sherman DM. 1994. Goat Medicine. Lea & Febiger, Philadelphia, PA.

Yeruham I, et al. 2003. Dermatophilosis in Goats in the Judean Foothills. *Rev Méd Vét* 154: 785.

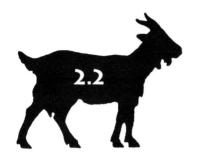

FUNGAL SKIN DISEASES

Dermatophytosis
Malassezia Dermatitis
Miscellaneous Fungal Diseases
   Aspergillosis
   Cryptococcosis
   Phaeohyphomycosis

DERMATOPHYTOSIS

Features

Dermatophytosis (ringworm) is a common cosmopolitan disease. It is most commonly caused by *Trichophyton verrucosum*, and less frequently by *T. mentagrophytes* and *Microsporum canis*. In temperate climates the disease is most common in fall and winter, especially in confined animals. There are no apparent breed or sex predilections, and young animals are most commonly affected.

Lesions can occur anywhere, but are most common on the face, head, pinnae, neck, and legs (Figs. 2.2-1 to 2.2-4). Annular to uneven to diffuse areas of alopecia, scaling, erythema, and yellowish crusts are seen. Pain and pruritus are rare, and affected animals are otherwise healthy. Typically multiple animals are affected.

Caprine dermatophytosis is a zoonosis. *T. verrucosum* infection in humans causes typical ringworm lesions or kerions in contact areas, especially hands, arms, neck, face, and scalp (Fig. 2.2-5).

Differential Diagnosis

Dermatophilosis, staphylococcal folliculitis, contagious viral pustular dermatitis ("orf"), zinc-responsive dermatitis, and pemphigus foliaceus.

Diagnosis

1. Microscopy (trichography)—Plucked hairs placed in mineral oil or potassium hydroxide contain hyphae and arthroconidia (spores) (Figs. 2.2-6 and 2.2-7).
2. Culture.
3. Dermatohistopathology—Suppurative luminal folliculitis with fungal hyphae and arthroconidia in hairs.

MALASSEZIA DERMATITIS

Features

Malassezia dermatitis is probably an uncommon, cosmopolitan disease. Inadequate nutrition and disease-related debilitation (e.g.,

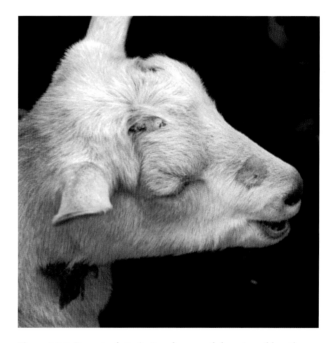

Figure 2.2-1 Dermatophytosis. Annular area of alopecia, mild erythema, and mild scaling on face.

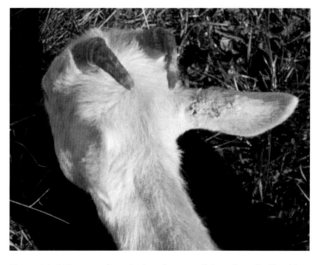

Figure 2.2-2 Dermatophytosis. Annular area of alopecia and yellowish-grey crust on right pinna.

severe enteritis with weight loss) appear to be predisposing factors. There are no apparent breed, sex, or age predilections.

Lesions begin multifocally over the back and trunk, become fairly generalized and tend to spare the head and legs (Figs. 2.2-8

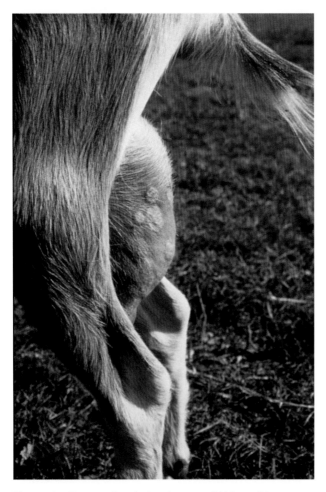

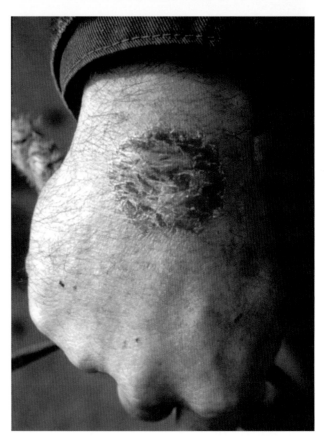

Figure 2.2-5 Dermatophytosis. Severely inflamed lesions on the hand caused by *Trichophyton verrucosum*.

Figure 2.2-3 Dermatophytosis. Annular areas of thick, greyish crusts on udder.

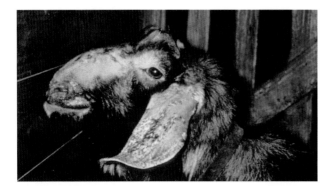

Figure 2.2-4 Dermatophytosis. Well-circumscribed areas of alopecia, erythema, and scaling on face and pinna.

to 2.2-10). Variable combinations of erythema, hyperpigmentation, greasiness, scaling, yellowish waxy crusts, alopecia, and lichenification are seen. The condition is neither pruritic nor painful.

Differential Diagnosis

Staphylococcal dermatitis, dermatophilosis, dermatophytosis, and vitamin E-selenium-responsive dermatitis.

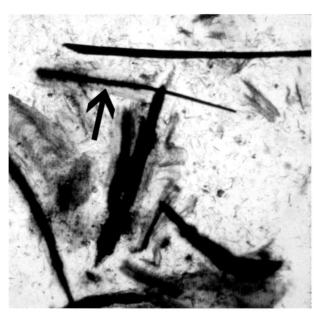

Figure 2.2-6 Dermatophytosis. Plucked hairs in mineral oil. Note thickened, irregular appearance of infected hair (arrow).

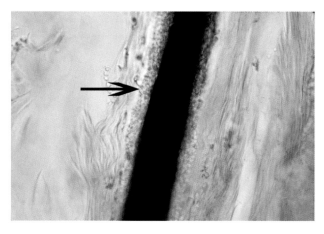

Figure 2.2-7 Dermatophytosis. Numerous arthroconidia (arrow) on surface of infected hair.

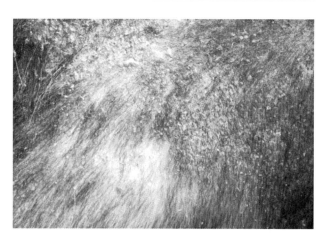

Figure 2.2-9 *Malassezia* Dermatitis. Severe scaling, patchy alopecia, and occasional yellowish waxy crusts on thorax of protein-deficient goat.

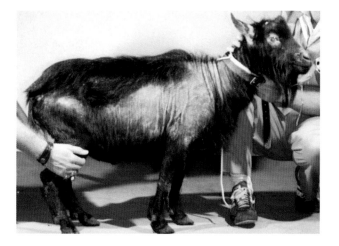

Figure 2.2-8 *Malassezia* Dermatitis. Marked alopecia and lichenification over trunk of protein-deficient goat.

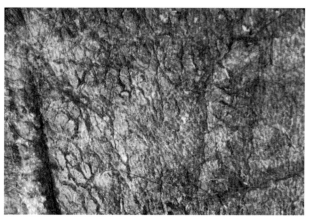

Figure 2.2-10 *Malassezia* Dermatitis. Alopecia, lichenification, and yellowish-brown waxy crusts over thorax of protein-deficient goat.

Diagnosis

1. Microscopy (direct smears)—Numerous unipolar budding yeasts (3 to 8 μm diameter) ("peanut" or "footprint" shaped) (Fig. 2.2-11).
2. Culture.
3. Dermatohistopathology—Marked surface and follicular hyperkeratosis (orthokeratotic and parakeratotic) with numerous budding yeasts.

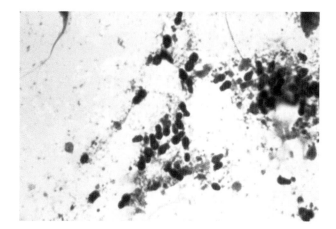

Figure 2.2-11 *Malassezia* Dermatitis (direct smear). Numerous budding yeasts.

MISCELLANEOUS FUNGAL DISEASES

Table 2.2-1 Miscellaneous Fungal Diseases	
Aspergillosis	Very rare; ulcerated nodules on scrotum and medial thighs; *Aspergillus fumigatus*; culture and dermatopathology
Cryptococcosis	Very rare; solitary erythematous nodule on nostril; solitary ulcerated plaque on top of head; *Cryptococcus neoformans*; culture and dermatohistopathology
Phaeohyphomycosis	Very rare; hyperkeratotic papules and plaques on pinnae; *Peyronellaea glomerata*; culture and dermatohistopathology

REFERENCES

Chapman HM, et al. 1990. *Cryptococcus neoformans* Infection in Goats. *Aust Vet J* 67: 263.

Howard JL, Smith RA. 1999. Current Veterinary Therapy. Food Animal Practice. Ed 4. WB Saunders, Philadelphia, PA.

Matthews JG. 1999. Diseases of the Goat. Ed 2. Blackwell Science, Oxford, United Kingdom.

Pin D. 2004. Seborrhoeic Dermatitis in a Goat due to *Malassezia pachydermatis*. *Vet Dermatol* 15: 53.

Radostits OM, et al. 2000. Veterinary Medicine. A Textbook of the Diseases of Cattle, Sheep, Pigs, Goats and Horses. Ed 9. WB Saunders, Philadelphia, PA.

Scott DW. 1988. Large Animal Dermatology. WB Saunders, Philadelphia, PA.

Smith MC, Sherman DM. 1994. Goat Medicine. Lea & Febiger, Philadelphia, PA.

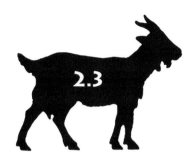

PARASITIC SKIN DISEASES

CHORIOPTIC MANGE

Features

Chorioptic mange is a common, cosmopolitan infestation caused by the mite *Chorioptes caprae*. There are no apparent breed, age, or sex predilections. Mite populations are usually much larger during cold weather. Thus clinical signs are usually seen, or are more severe, in winter. Transmission occurs by direct and indirect contact.

Lesions are most commonly seen on the feet and hind legs (Figs 2.3-1 and 2.3-2), but may also be present on the front legs, perineum, tail, udder and teats (Fig. 2.3-3), scrotum, and ventrum. Erythema and papules progress to scaling, oozing, crusts, and alopecia. Pruritus varies from marked to absent. Typically multiple animals are affected. Humans are not affected.

Differential Diagnosis

Sarcoptic mange, zinc-responsive dermatitis.

Diagnosis

1. Microscopy (Skin Scrapings in Mineral Oil)—Psoroptid mites, 0.3 to 0.5 mm in length (Figs 2.3-4 and 2.3-5).
2. Dermatohistopathology—Hyperplastic eosinophilic perivascular-to-interstitial dermatitis with eosinophilic epidermal microabscesses and parakeratotic hyperkeratosis (mites rarely seen).

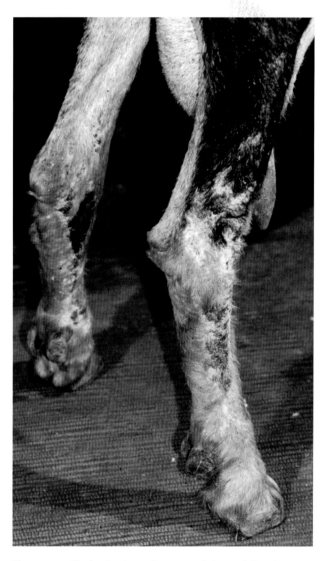

Figure 2.3-1 Chorioptic Mange. Crusts, excoriation, and alopecia over hind legs.

PSOROPTIC MANGE

Features

Psoroptic mange is an uncommon, cosmopolitan infestation caused by, perhaps, two different mites: *Psoroptes cuniculi* and *P. caprae*. There are no apparent breed, age, or sex predilections. Transmission occurs by direct and indirect contact.

P. cuniculi is found in the ear canal. Many affected animals appear to be clinically normal, whereas others manifest head shak-

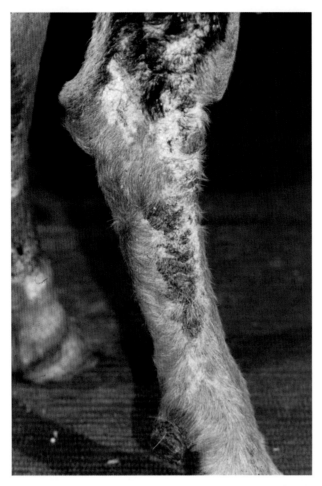

Figure 2.3-2 Close-up of Figure 2.3-1. Alopecia, scale, crust, and excoriation on hind leg.

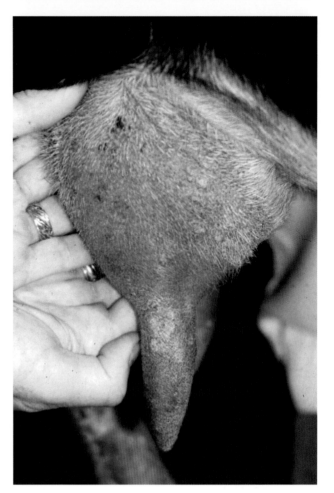

Figure 2.3-3 Chorioptic Mange. Papules, crusts, and scales on udder and teat.

ing, ear scratching, and variable degrees of excessive cerumen accumulation and/or crusts and alopecia on the pinnae. If the tympanic membrane ruptures, otitis media and interna are potential complications. *P. caprae* can also cause otitis externa, along with crusts, scales, and alopecia on the pinnae, head, face, pasterns, and interdigital areas (Figs. 2.3-6 and 2.3-7). Pruritus is variable. Typically multiple animals are affected. Humans are not affected.

Differential Diagnosis

Sarcoptic mange, zinc-responsive dermatitis, pemphigus foliaceus.

Diagnosis

1. Microscopy (Ear Swabs and or Skin Scrapings in Mineral Oil)—Psoroptid mites, 0.4 to 0.8 mm in length (Fig. 2.3-8).

SARCOPTIC MANGE

Features

Sarcoptic mange (scabies) is a common, cosmopolitan infestation caused by the mite *Sarcoptes scabiei var caprae*. There are no apparent breed, age, or sex predilections. Transmission occurs by direct and indirect contact.

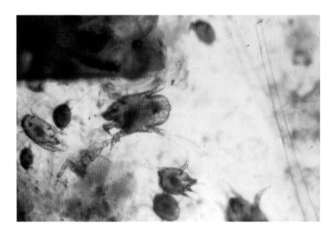

Figure 2.3-4 Chorioptic Mange. Multiple mites in a skin scraping.

Lesions are most commonly seen on the face, pinnae, neck, and legs, but may become generalized (Figs. 2.3-9 through 2.3-13). Erythema and papules progress to scaling, oozing, crusts, and alopecia. Pruritus is intense. Excoriation, lichenification, and hyperkeratosis are prominent in chronic cases. Peripheral lymphadenopathy is usually moderate to marked. Typically, multiple

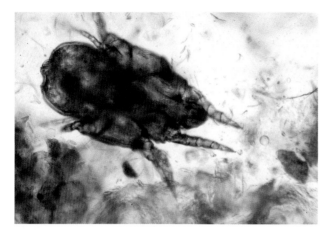

Figure 2.3-5 Chorioptic Mange. Adult mite in a skin scraping.

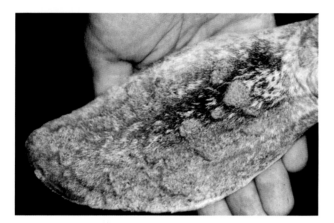

Figure 2.3-6 Psoroptic Mange. Crusts and scales on pinna.

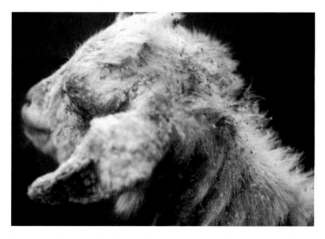

Figure 2.3-7 Psoroptic Mange. Crusts, alopecia, and erythema on pinnae, head, face, and neck (courtesy J. King).

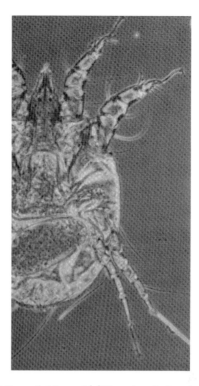

Figure 2.3-8 Psoroptic Mange. Adult *Psoroptes* mite (courtesy J. Georgi).

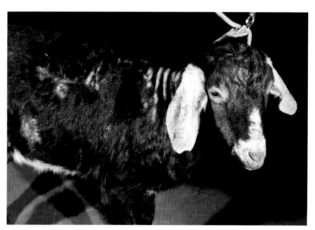

Figure 2.3-9 Sarcoptic Mange. Crusts, scales, and alopecia on face, pinnae, neck, and thorax.

velop pruritic erythematous papules with crusts and excoriations on the arms, chest, abdomen, and legs (Fig. 2.3-14). In addition, although *Sarcoptes* mites tend to be species-specific, cross-infestation is possible, especially between goats and sheep.

Differential Diagnosis

Psoroptic mange, zinc-responsive dermatitis, pemphigus foliaceus, insect hypersensitivity, and atopic dermatitis.

Diagnosis

1. Microscopy (Skin Scrapings in Mineral Oil)—Sarcoptic mites, 0.25 to 0.6 mm in length (Figs. 2.3-15 and 2.3-16). Ova

animals are affected. Weight loss, decreased milk production, hide damage, and secondary bacterial (usually staphylococcal) pyoderma can occur due to the intense pruritus and irritation. Typically multiple animals are affected.

Sarcoptic mange is a potential zoonosis. Affected humans de-

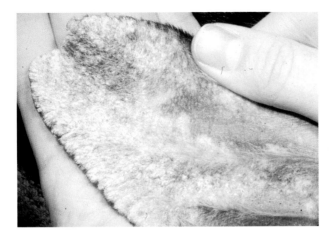

Figure 2.3-10 Sarcoptic Mange. Crusts and scale on pinnae.

(eggs) and scyballa (fecal pellets) may also be found (Fig. 2.3-17). Mites are often difficult to find, especially in chronic cases.

2. Dermatohistopathology—Hyperplastic eosinophilic perivascular-to-interstitial dermis with eosinophilic epidermal microabscesses and parakeratotic hyperkeratosis (mites rarely seen).

DEMODECTIC MANGE

Features

Demodectic mange (demodicosis) is a common, cosmopolitan dermatosis caused by the mite *Demodex caprae*. This mite is a normal resident of hair follicles, transmitted from the dam to nursing neonates during the first few days of life. It is assumed that all animals experiencing disease due to the excessive replication of this normal resident mite are in some way immunocompromised (e.g., concurrent disease, poor nutrition, debilitation, stress, genetic predilection). There are no apparent breed, age, or sex predilections. Demodectic mange is not a contagious disease.

Lesions are most commonly seen on the face, neck, and shoulders, but may occasionally be widespread. Deep-seated, firm papules and nodules (up to 2 cm in diameter) are more easily felt than seen, as the overlying hair coat is usually normal (Fig. 2.3-18). The overlying skin initially is normal in appearance, and the lesions are neither painful nor pruritic. Occasionally, draining tracts, crusts, and abscesses may be present, wherein follicular rupture (furunculosis), secondary bacterial infection (usually staphylococcal), or both of these have occurred (Fig. 2.3-19). At this point, lesions may be painful, pruritic, or both of these. Typically, only an individual animal is affected.

Differential Diagnosis

Bacterial and fungal infections (see Chapters 1 and 2).

Diagnosis

1. History and physical examination.
2. Microscopy (Incision and Manual Evacuation of a Thick, Caseous, Whitish to Yellowish Material From a Lesion)—

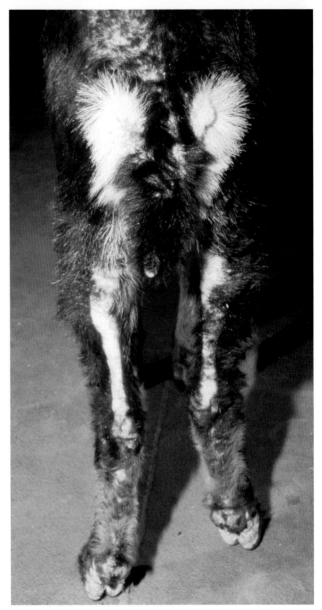

Figure 2.3-11 Sarcoptic Mange. Alopecia, crusts, and excoriation on hind legs and rump.

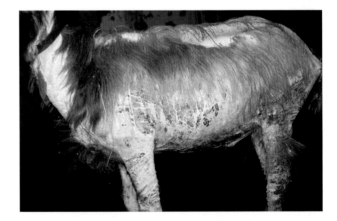

Figure 2.3-12 Sarcoptic Mange. Alopecia, erythema, scales, and crusts on legs, trunk, and neck.

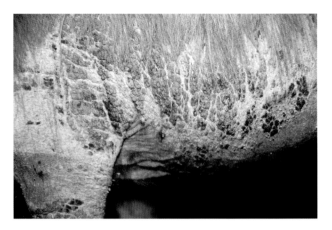

Figure 2.3-13 Close-up of Figure 2.3-12. Erythema, scales, crusts, alopecia, and excoriation on trunk and front leg.

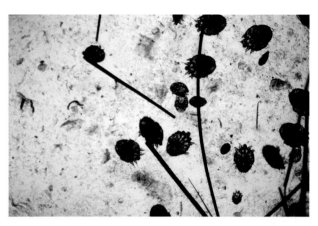

Figure 2.3-15 Sarcoptic Mange. Multiple mites in a skin scraping.

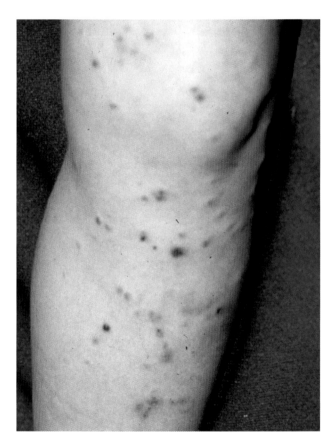

Figure 2.3-14 Sarcoptic Mange. Erythematous and crusted papules on the leg of a human with animal-origin scabies.

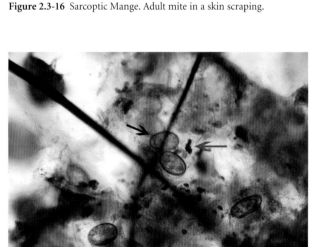

Figure 2.3-16 Sarcoptic Mange. Adult mite in a skin scraping.

Figure 2.3-17 Sarcoptic Mange. Multiple eggs (black arrow) and fecal pellets (red arrow) in a skin scraping.

Multiple demodicid mites (0.2 to 0.3 mm in length) (Fig. 2.3-20).

PEDICULOSIS

Features

Pediculosis (lice) is a common, cosmopolitan infestation caused by various lice. In the United States, recognized goat lice include *Damalinia (Bovicola) caprae, D. crassipes,* and *D. limbata* (biting lice, order Mallophaga) and *Linognathus stenopsis* and *L. africanus* (sucking lice, order Anoplura). There are no apparent breed, age, or sex predilections. Louse populations are usually much larger during cold weather. Thus clinical signs are usually

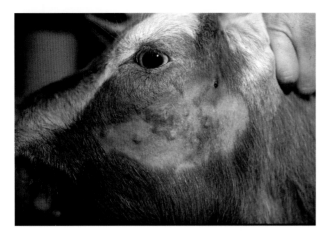

Figure 2.3-18 Demodectic Mange. Papules and nodules on face (area has been clipped).

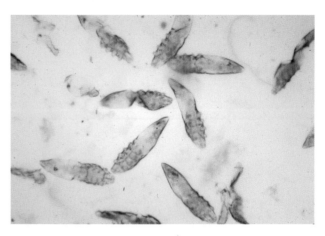

Figure 2.3-20 Demodectic Mange. Numerous mites from an incised and squeezed lesion.

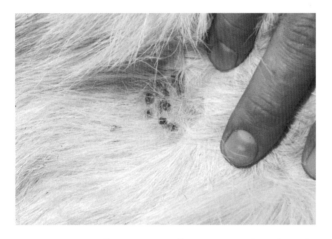

Figure 2.3-19 Demodectic Mange. Erythematous, crusted papules, and nodules (due to secondary bacterial infection) on neck.

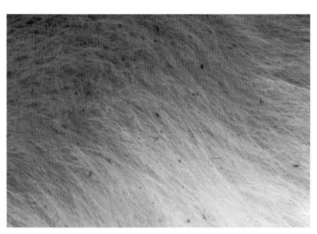

Figure 2.3-21 Pediculosis. Numerous biting lice in the hair coat of a goat with no clinical signs of skin disease.

seen, or are more severe in winter. Transmission occurs by direct and indirect contact.

Lice are most commonly seen on the head, neck, dorsum, and groin. Some animals will show no clinical signs (Fig. 2.3-21). Others will have variable combinations of scaling, crusting, erythema, excoriation, and hair loss (Figs. 2.3-22 and 2.3-23). Pruritus may be marked or absent. Louse infestations can be heavy in debilitated animals. Large populations of lice can cause anemia, especially in kids. Damage to skin and wool can cause considerable economic losses in Angoras. Typically, multiple animals are affected. Humans are not affected. *D. ovis* can be transmitted between goats and sheep.

Diagnosis

1. History and Physical Examination—Sucking lice are bluish gray in color. Biting lice are pale to brownish in color.
2. Microscopy (Lice and Hairs Placed in Mineral Oil)—Adult lice are large (3 to 6 mm in length) (Figs. 2.3-24 and 2.3-25). Ova (nits) are 1 to 2 mm in length and may be found attached to hair shafts (Fig. 2.3-26).

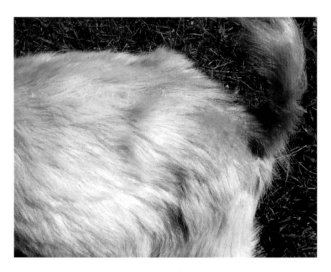

Figure 2.3-22 Pediculosis. Alopecia and erythema over the rump (courtesy M. Smith).

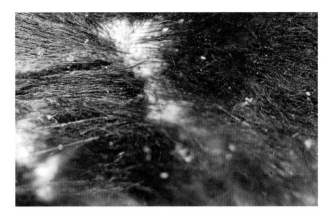

Figure 2.3-23 Pediculosis. Alopecia, crusts, scales, nits, and lice.

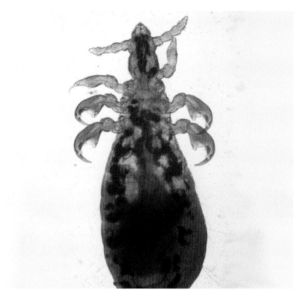

Figure 2.3-25 Pediculosis. Sucking louse.

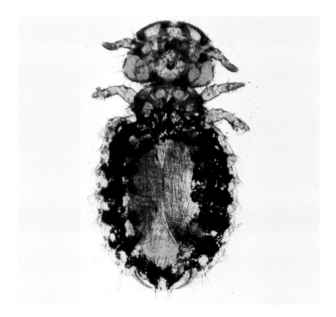

Figure 2.3-24 Pediculosis. Biting louse.

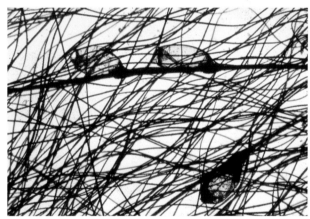

Figure 2.3-26 Pediculosis. Nits on hair shaft.

PRZHEVALSKIANA SILENUS INFESTATION

Features

Przhevalskiana silenus (P. crossi, P. aegagi, Hypoderma silenus, H. crossi) infestation ("warbles") is common in certain parts of Asia and Europe. Adult *P. silenus* flies lay eggs on the hairs of the legs and chest, and larvae migrate by a subcutaneous route to the back. There are no apparent breed, age, or sex predilections.

Lesions appear in the spring and early summer as numerous subcutaneous nodules and cysts over the back (Fig. 2.3-27). The lesions develop a central pore in which the third-stage larvae may be seen. Typically multiple animals are affected. Serious hide damage can occur.

Diagnosis

1. History and Physical Examination—Third-stage larvae extracted from skin lesions are typically 10 to 12 mm in length.

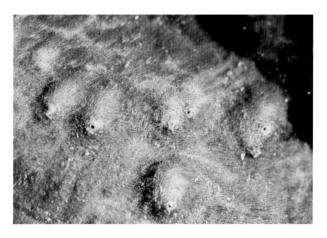

Figure 2.3-27 *Przhevalskiana silenus* Infestation. Numerous nodules with central pores on back (area has been clipped) (courtesy J. King).

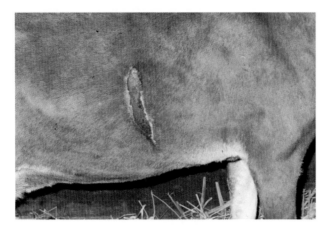

Figure 2.3-28 *Parelaphostrongylus tenuis* Infestation. Linear, vertically-oriented, well-circumscribed area of alopecia, ulceration, and crusting over lateral thorax.

PARELAPHOSTRONGYLUS TENUIS INFESTATION

Features

Parelaphostrongylus tenuis is a common parasite of white-tailed deer in North America, and a common cause of neurologic diseases in goats. Infestation of goats occurs through ingestion of intermediate hosts (terrestrial snails and slugs) containing larvae passed in deer feces. There are no apparent breed, age, or sex predilections.

Some goats—with or without concurrent neurologic disease—develop linear, vertically-oriented skin lesions over the neck, shoulder, thorax, or flank. Lesions are usually unilateral and alopecic, ulcerated, crusted, or scarred (Figs. 2.3-28 and 2.3-29). Goats produce the lesions by biting or rubbing, possibly because migrating larvae irritate dorsal nerve roots supplying individual dermatomes.

Diagnosis

1. History and physical examination.
2. Analysis of Cerebrospinal Fluid—Eosinophilia, increased protein, or both of these.
3. Necropsy examination.

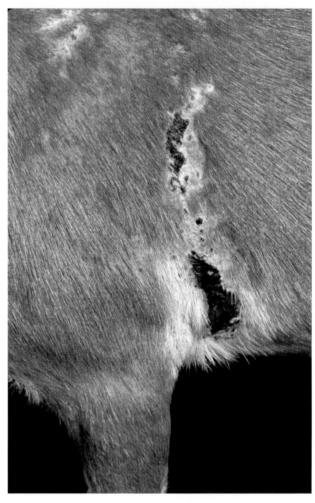

Figure 2.3-29 *Parelaphostrongylus tenuis* Infestation. Linear, vertically-oriented, well-circumscribed area of alopecia, scarring, and crusts caudal to shoulder.

MISCELLANEOUS PARASITIC DISEASES

Table 2.3-1 Miscellaneous Parasitic Diseases

Trombiculosis ("chiggers," "harvest mite")	Rare and cosmopolitan; late summer and fall; infested woods and fields; legs, face, and ventrum; papulocrustous dermatitis with variable pruritus; trombiculid larvae (0.2 to 0.4 mm in length, red to orange in color); e.g., *Trombicula (Eutrombicula) alfreddugesi, T. (Neotrombicula) autumnalis, T. sarcina*
Dermanyssus gallinae dermatitis ("poultry mite")	Rare and cosmopolitan; proximity to poultry roosts; especially late summer; especially legs and ventrum; pruritic, papulocrustous dermatitis; *D. gallinae* (0.6 to 1 mm in length)
Raillietia caprae infestation ("ear mites")	Uncommon; *R. caprae (R. manfredi)* 0.5 to 0.8 mm in length; North and South America and Australia, usually no clinical signs, but occasionally otitis externa
Ticks	Common and cosmopolitan; most in spring and summer; especially ears, face, neck, axillae, groin, distal legs, and tail; minimal lesions or papules and nodules centered around attached ticks; variable pain and pruritus; e.g., *Otobius megnini, Ixodes scapularis, I. cookei, I. pacificus, Rhipicephalus sanguineous, Dermacentor andersonii,* and *D. variabilis* in the United States
Keds ("sheep ticks")	Uncommon and cosmopolitan; *Melophagus ovinus* (4 to 7 mm in length); usually fall and winter; especially neck, sides, rump, and abdomen; intense pruritus results in broken hairs, alopecia, and excoriations; heavy infestations can cause anemia
Fleas	Uncommon and cosmopolitan; *Ctenocephalides felis* ("cat flea"), *C. canis* ("dog flea"), and *Pulex irritans* ("human flea"), 2 to 4 mm in length; especially summer and fall; variable degrees of pruritus and papulocrustous dermatitis; especially legs and ventrum; some animals may develop hypersensitivity (allergy) to flea salivary antigens (see Chapter 5); heavy infestations in kids and debilitated animals may cause anemia and even death
Dermatobia hominis infestation	Uncommon; Central and South America; painful subcutaneous nodules with a central pore containing third-stage larvae (about 20 mm in length)
Calliphorine myiasis ("maggots," flystrike)	Common and cosmopolitan; especially *Lucilia* spp., *Calliphora* spp., and *Phormia* spp.; especially late spring, summer, and early fall; any wounded/damaged skin; foul-smelling ulcers with scalloped margins and a "honeycombed" appearance, teeming with larvae ("maggots"); usually painful and pruritic
Screw-worm myiasis	Uncommon; Central and South America (*Callitroga hominivorax* and *C. macellaria*); Africa and Asia (*Chrysomyia bezziana* and *C. megacephala*); especially late spring, summer, and early fall; any wounded/damaged skin; foul-smelling ulcers with scalloped margins and "honeycombed" appearance, teeming with larvae; painful and pruritic; humans are also susceptible (e.g., skin, genitalia, ears, sinuses)
Stephanofilariasis	Rare; Malaysia (*Stephanofilaria kaeli*); India and Indonesia (*S. assamensis* and *S. dedoesi*); pruritic crusting dermatitis of face, neck, shoulders, and feet; dermatohistopathology
Elaphostrongylus rangiferi infestation	Rare; Norway; *Elaphostrongylus rangiferi*; pruritus and neurologic disease; necropsy
Strongyloidosis	Rare and cosmopolitan; *Strongyloides papillosus*; pruritic, pustular, crusted dermatitis of feet, legs, and ventrum; fecal flotation

REFERENCES

Abo-Shehada MN. 2005. Incidence of *Chrysomyia bezziana* screw-worm myiasis in Saudi Arabia, 1999/2000. *Vet Rec* 156: 354.

Alexander JL. 2006. Screwworms. *J Am Vet Med Assoc* 228: 357.

Baker AS. 1999. Mites and Ticks of Domestic Animals. An Identification Guide and Information Source. The Stationary Office, London, UK.

Bates P, et al. 2001. Observations on the Biology and Control of the Chewing Louse (*Bovicola limbata*) of Angora Goats in Great Britain. *Vet Rec* 149: 675.

Bowman DD. 1999. Georgis' Parasitology for Veterinarians. Ed 7. WB Saunders, Philadelphia, PA.

Christodoulopoulos G, Theodoropoulos G. 2003. Infestation of Dairy Goats with the Human Flea, *Pulex irritans*, in Central Greece. *Vet Rec* 152: 371.

Handeland K, and Sparboe O. 1991. Cerebrospinal Elaphostrongylosis in Dairy Goats in Northern Norway. *J Vet Med B* 38: 755.

Ibrahim KEE, et al. 1987. Experimental Transmission of a Goat Strain of *Sarcoptes scabiei* to Desert Sheep and Its Treatment with Ivermectin. *Vet Parasitol* 26: 157.

Matthews JG. 1999. Diseases of the Goat. Ed 2. Blackwell Science, Malden, MA.

Radostits OM, et al. 2000. Veterinary Medicine. A Textbook of the Diseases of Cattle, Sheep, Pigs, Goats, and Horses. Ed 9. WB Saunders, Philadelphia, PA.

Scott DW. 1988. Large Animal Dermatology. WB Saunders, Philadelphia, PA.

Smith MC, and Sherman DM. 1994. Goat Medicine. Lea & Febiger, Philadelphia, PA.

Soulsby EJL. 1982. Helminths, Arthropods, and Protozoa of Domesticated Animals. Ed 7. Lea & Febiger, Philadelphia, PA.

Wall R, et al. 2001. Veterinary Ectoparasites. Ed 2. Blackwell Scientific, Oxford, UK.

Zahler M, et al. 1998. Genetic Evidence Suggests that *Psoroptes* Isolates of Different Phenotypes, Hosts, and Geographic Origins are Conspecific. *Int J Parasitol* 28: 1713.

Zahler M, et al. 1999. Molecular Analyses Suggest Monospecificity of the Genus *Sarcoptes* (Acari: Sarcoptidae). *Int J Parasitol* 29: 759.

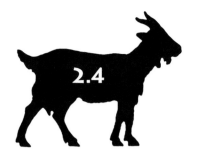

VIRAL AND PROTOZOAL SKIN DISEASES

2.4

CONTAGIOUS VIRAL PUSTULAR DERMATITIS

Features

Contagious viral pustular dermatitis ("contagious ecthyma," "orf," "soremouth," "scabby mouth," "contagious pustular dermatitis") is a common, cosmopolitan disease caused by *Parapoxvirus ovis*. Transmission occurs through contamination of skin abrasions. There are no apparent breed or sex predilections. Although all ages can be affected, the disease is primarily seen in 3 to 6 month old kids. The disease tends to be seasonal, occurring most commonly during kidding season.

Lesions progress from papules to vesicles, and to pustules, which become umbilicated and thickly crusted. In some instances, lesions become large and papillomatous due to masses of infected granulation tissue proliferating beneath the crusts. Lesions are often painful, but not pruritic. The lips, muzzle, nostrils, eyelids, and pinnae are most commonly affected (Figs. 2.4-1 through 2.4-3). The oral cavity, coronets, interdigital spaces, scrotum, teats, vulva, perineum, and distal legs are less commonly involved (Figs. 2.4-4 through 2.4-7). Oral lesions are raised, red-to-gray-to-yellowish papules and plaques with a surrounding zone of hyperemia (Figs. 2.4-8 through 2.4-10). Lesions may occur at the sites of various injuries and some outbreaks are characterized by unusual distribution of lesions (e.g., head, neck, and chest). Generalized lesions may occur in animals debilitated for other reasons.

Severe, generalized, persistent disease has been seen in Boer and Boer cross goats. Moderate to severe lymphadenopathy was present in all animals. Suppurative arthritis, chronic fibrinous pneumonia, and premature thymic involution were found in many goats. Breed genetic susceptibility and immune defects may be involved in these unusual outbreaks.

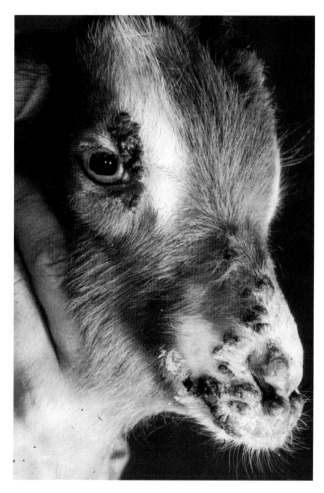

Figure 2.4-1 Contagious Viral Pustular Dermatitis. Multiple thick brown crusts on lips, nostrils, muzzle, and periocular region of a kid.

Signs of systemic illness may include fever, depression, and decreased food consumption. Significant economic losses occur through loss of condition (failure to suck or eat, mastitis), abandonment, and secondary bacterial infections and myiasis. Morbidity in kids often approaches 100%, while mortality is usually around 1%, although it can be as high as 20%. Sheep are susceptible.

Contagious viral pustular dermatitis is a zoonosis. In humans, the condition is often called "ecthyma contagiosum," "orf," or "farmyard pox". Transmission can be direct, indirect, and even human-to-human. Lesions are often solitary, and occur most commonly on the fingers, arm, face, and leg (Figs. 2.4-11 and 2.4-12). Erythematous papules evolve into nodules with a red

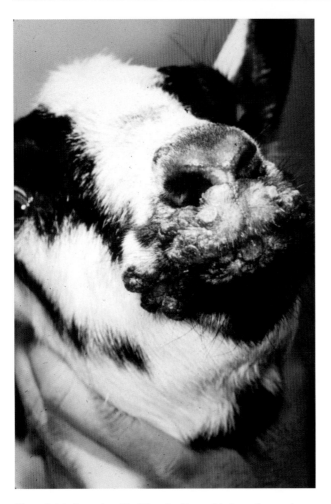

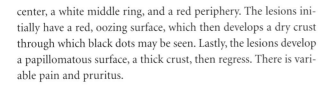

Figure 2.4-2 Contagious Viral Pustular Dermatitis. Extensive crusting on the muzzle and medial canthus region of a kid.

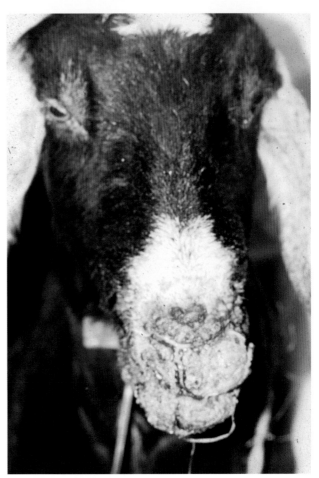

Figure 2.4-3 Contagious Viral Pustular Dermatitis. Extensive fissured crusts on the muzzle and periocular regions of an adult goat.

center, a white middle ring, and a red periphery. The lesions initially have a red, oozing surface, which then develops a dry crust through which black dots may be seen. Lastly, the lesions develop a papillomatous surface, a thick crust, then regress. There is variable pain and pruritus.

Differential Diagnosis

Dermatophilosis, staphylococcal folliculitis, *Capripoxvirus* infection, and zinc-responsive dermatitis.

Diagnosis

1. History and physical examination.
2. Dermatohistopathology—Eosinophilic intracytoplasmic inclusion bodies in epithelial keratinocytes.
3. Viral isolation.
4. Viral antigen detection.

CAPRIPOXVIRUS INFECTION

Features

Capripoxvirus infections (goat pox) vary in severity, presumably because of differences in viral strains, host susceptibility, or both of these. Severe ("malignant") infections occur in the Middle East, Asia, Africa, and parts of Europe. Mild ("benign") infections have been reported in the United States and parts of Europe. Transmission occurs through contamination of skin abrasions, aerosol, or insect vectors. There are no apparent breed or sex predilections. Although all ages are susceptible, the disease is more severe in the young.

In the severe form, initial pyrexia, anorexia, rhinitis, and conjunctivitis are followed by skin lesions. Erythematous papules, pustules, and crusts appear on the lip, nostrils, and in the mouth. Oral cavity lesions rapidly become ulcerated. Lesions often spread to involve the head, pinnae, neck, axillae, groin, perineum, and ventral tail. In some outbreaks, lesions only occur on the muzzle and lips. In other outbreaks, lesions only occur on the udder, teats, scrotum, prepuce, perineum, and ventral tail. Occasionally, only nodular lesions are seen ("stone pox"), resembling lumpy skin disease of cattle. Morbidity may be up to 90%, while mortality is usually about 5%, although it can be as high as 50%. Eco-

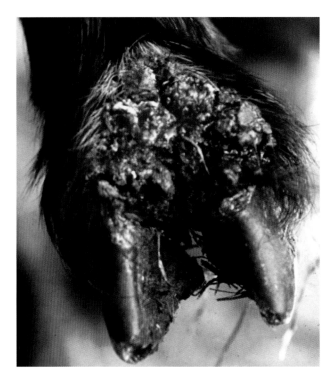

Figure 2.4-4 Contagious Viral Pustular Dermatitis. Thick crust overlying ulcerated, proliferative granulation tissue on the foot (Courtesy B. Fiocre, coll. J. Gourreau, AFSSA).

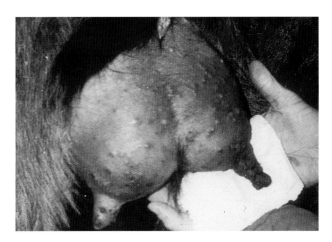
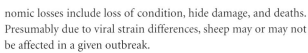

Figure 2.4-5 Contagious Viral Pustular Dermatitis. Pustules and crusts on the udder and teats (courtesy P. Bonnier, coll. J. Gourreau, AFSSA).

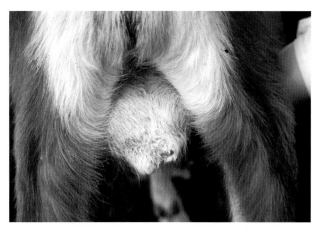

Figure 2.4-6 Contagious Viral Pustular Dermatitis. Crusts on the scrotum (courtesy M. Smith).

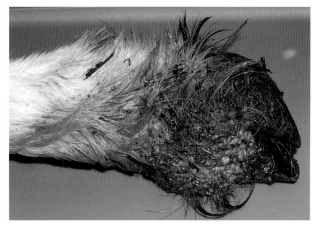

Figure 2.4-7 Contagious Viral Pustular Dermatitis. Papilloma-like crusting on foot (courtesy M. Smith).

nomic losses include loss of condition, hide damage, and deaths. Presumably due to viral strain differences, sheep may or may not be affected in a given outbreak.

In mild forms of the infection, papules, vesicles, pustules, and crusts are seen on the lips, udder, and teats, and occasionally the perineum and medial thighs (Fig. 2.4-13). Systemic signs are usually not present.

Although a few literature reports indicate that caprine *Capripoxvirus* infection can be transmitted to humans (see contagious viral pustular dermatitis), current literature discounts this possibility.

Differential Diagnosis

Dermatophilosis, staphylococcal folliculitis, contagious viral pustular dermatitis and zinc-responsive dermatitis.

Diagnosis

1. History and physical examination.
2. Dermatohistopathology—Eosinophilic intracytoplasmic inclusion bodies in epithelial keratinocytes.
3. Viral isolation.
4. Viral antigen detection.

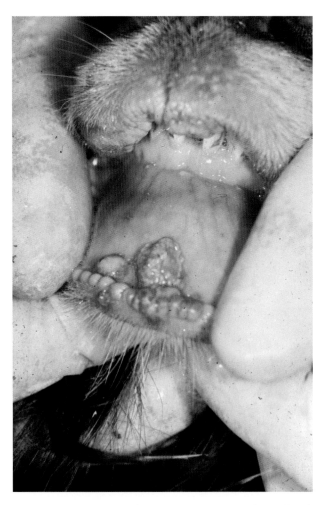

Figure 2.4-8 Contagious Viral Pustular Dermatitis. Whitish-to-yellowish papule and plaque with hyperemic haloes on lower lip mucosa.

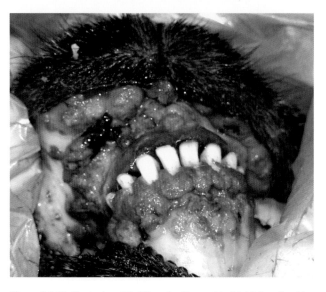

Figure 2.4-10 Contagious Viral Pustular Dermatitis. Multiple yellowish-brown papules and plaques on oral mucosa (courtesy J. Lessirand, coll. J. Gourreau, AFSSA).

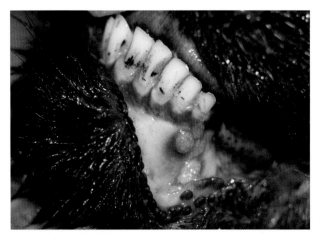

Figure 2.4-9 Contagious Viral Pustular Dermatitis. Whitish- yellow papules with hyperemic haloes on lower gingival mucosa (courtesy J. Lessirand, coll. J. Gourreau, AFSSA).

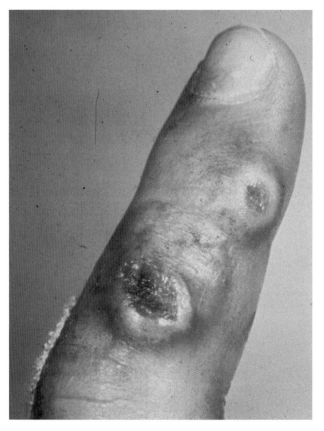

Figure 2.4-11 Contagious Viral Pustular Dermatitis. Two umbilicated pustules with erythematous haloes on the finger of a veterinary student ("orf").

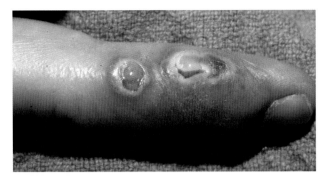

Figure 2.4-12 Contagious Viral Pustular Dermatitis. Two umbilicated, oozing pustules with erythematous haloes on the finger of a veterinary student.

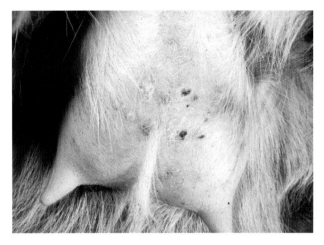

Figure 2.4-13 *Capripoxvirus* Infection. Pustules and crusts on the udder.

MISCELLANEOUS VIRAL AND PROTOZOAL DISEASES

Table 2.4-1 Miscellaneous Viral and Protozoal Diseases

Besnoitiosis (globidiosis, "dimple")	Uncommon; Africa, Asia, parts of Europe and South America; *Besnoitia caprae*; thickened lichenified, hypotrichotic, fissured, oozing skin over legs, ventrum, scrotum and hindquarters; occasionally subcutaneous papules (about 1 mm diameter); granular conjunctivitis; dermatohistopathology (parasitic cysts—up to 600 μm diameter—containing bradyzoites 2 to 7 μm in length)
Bluetongue (*Orbivirus*)	Rarely clinical; worldwide; *Culicoides* spp. are major vectors; occasionally erythema and edema of legs and muzzle; fever; viral isolation and viral antigen detection
Caprine *Herpesvirus* infection	Rare; worldwide; experimental inoculation produces vesicles, ulcers, and crusts on muzzle, feet; erythema, edema, and ulcers on vulva and prepuce of adults; one spontaneous case of necrotic foci in skin of a kid; neonates also show weakness, anorexia, dyspnea, and diarrhea; adult does show abortion and stillbirths; viral isolation
Caprine viral dermatitis	Uncommon; Asia; unclassified pox virus; pyrexia and nodules that become necrotic and develop crateriform ulcers; entire skin surface including lips, gums, and tongue; necropsy examination
Foot-and-mouth disease ("aphthous fever") (*Aphthovirus*) (Fig. 2.4-14)	Uncommon; Africa, Asia, South America, and parts of Europe; usually mild; lameness and vesicles, bullae, and ulcers in mouth, interdigital spaces, and on coronets; humans rarely get vesicles on hands and/or oral mucosa; viral isolation, viral antigen detection
Peste des petits ruminants ("goat plague," "kata") (*Morbillivirus*)	Uncommon; Africa, South-East Asia, and Middle East; edematous, ulcerated, crusted lips; fever, ocular discharge, necrotic stomatitis, enteritis, and pneumonia; viral isolation, viral antigen detection
Pseudorabies (Aujeszky's disease, "mad itch") (porcine *Herpesvirus* 1)	Very rare; cosmopolitan; intense, localized, unilateral pruritus with frenzied, violent licking, chewing, rubbing, and kicking at affected area; especially head, neck, thorax, flank, and perineum; fever, excitement, circling, convulsions, paralysis; sheep and cattle are susceptible; necropsy, viral antigen detection
Rabies (*Lyssavirus*)	Very rare; cosmopolitan; intense, localized, unilateral pruritus with licking, chewing, rubbing, and kicking at affected area; aggression, continuous bleating, incoordination and paralysis; viral antigen detection
Rinderpest (cattle plague) (*Morbillivirus*)	Rare; Africa and Asia; erythema, papules, oozing, crusts and alopecia over perineum, flanks, medial thighs, neck, scrotum, udder, and teats; fever, oculonasal discharge, hypersalivation, ulcerative stomatitis, and diarrhea; viral isolation, viral antigen detection
Sarcocystosis	Rare; cosmopolitan; *Sarcocystis capricanis*; anecdotal reports indicate poor hair coat and patchy alopecia; necropsy examination
Scrapie	Rare; North America, Europe and Asia; prion protein; intermittent, bilaterally symmetrical pruritus: especially tailhead, progressing cranially to flanks, thorax, and occasionally head and pinnae; chronic rubbing and biting results in alopecia, excoriation, and even occasional hematomas; behavioral change, tremor, ataxia, emaciation, and paresis; brain histopathology, various immunohistochemical and Western blot procedures
Vesicular Stomatitis (*Vesiculovirus*)	North, Central, and South America; especially summer and fall; goats considered resistant; anecdotal reports indicate vesicles and ulcers on the lips, especially at the commissures; viral isolation, viral antigen detection

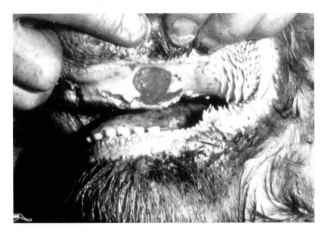

Figure 2.4-14 Foot-and-Mouth Disease. Ulcers on the upper lip (courtesy C. Rees).

REFERENCES

Abraham SS, et al. 2005. An Outbreak of Peste des Petits Ruminants Infection in Kerala. *Indian Vet J* 82: 815.

Cam Y, et al. 2005. Peste des Petits Ruminants in a Sheep and Goat Flock in Kayseri Province, Turkey. *Vet Rec* 157: 523.

Capucchio MT, et al. 1998. Natural Occurrence of Scrapie in Goats in Italy. *Vet Rec* 143: 452.

Coates JW, and Hoff S. 1990. Contagious Ecthyma: an Unusual Distribution of Lesions in Goats. *Can Vet J* 31: 209.

de la Concha-Bermejillo A, et al. 2003. Severe Persistent Orf in Young Goats. *J Vet Diag Invest* 15: 423.

Gavier-Widén D, et al. 2005. Diagnosis of Transmissible Spongiform Encephalopathies in Animals: A Review. *J Vet Diagn Invest* 17: 509.

Hajer I, et al. 1988. *Capripoxvirus* in Sheep and Goats in Sudan. *Rév Elev Méd Vét Pay Trop* 41: 125.

Njenga JM, et al. 1995. Comparative Ultrastructural Studies on *Besnoitia besnoiti* and *Besnoitia caprae*. *Vet Res Comm* 19: 295.

Radostits OM, et al. 2000. Veterinary Medicine. A Textbook of the Diseases of Cattle, Sheep, Pigs, Goats and Horses. Ed 9. WB Saunders, Philadelphia, PA.

Scott DW. 1988. Large Animal Dermatology. WB Saunders, Philadelphia, PA.

Shakya S, et al. 2004. Characterization of *Capripoxvirus* Isolated From Field Outbreak in Goats. *Indian Vet J* 81:241.

Smith MC, and Sherman DM. 1994. Goat Medicine. Lea & Febiger, Philadelphia, PA.

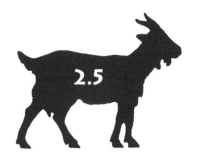

IMMUNOLOGICAL SKIN DISEASES

Pemphigus Foliaceus
Miscellaneous Immunological Diseases
    Flea Bite Hypersensitivity
    Insect Hypersensitivity
    Toxic Epidermal Necrolysis

PEMPHIGUS FOLIACEUS

Features

Pemphigus foliaceus is a rare, idiopathic, cosmopolitan autoimmune dermatosis. Autoantibodies target desmosomal proteins (desmoglein 1) in the epidermis. There are no apparent age, sex, or breed predilections.

Skin lesions are more-or-less bilaterally symmetric and usually begin on the ventrum and perineum. The condition becomes widespread, and is often very severe on the face and pinnae (Figs. 2.5-1 to 2.5-6). Initial lesions are pustules or vesicles. Erosions, oozing, crusts, scales, and alopecia are the dominant lesions found. Pruritus is mild to severe. Occasional animals are systemically ill (pyrexia, lethargy, depression, inappetence). Only one animal in a group is affected.

Differential Diagnosis

Staphylococcal folliculitis, dermatophilosis, dermatophytosis, zinc-responsive dermatitis.

Diagnosis

1. Microscopy (direct smears)—Nondegenerate neutrophils and/or eosinophils with numerous acantholytic keratinocytes (Fig. 2-5-7).
2. Dermatohistopathology—Intragranular to subcorneal pustular epidermitis with numerous acantholytic keratinocytes.

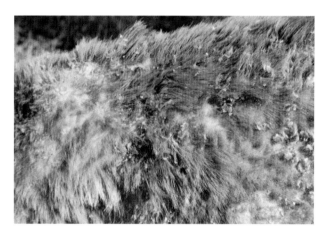

Figure 2.5-2 Pemphigus Foliaceus. Thick crusts over lateral thorax.

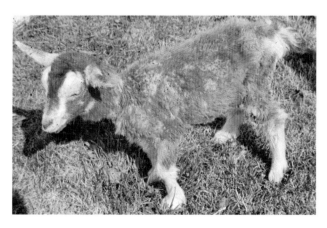

Figure 2.5-1 Pemphigus Foliaceus. Generalized crusts.

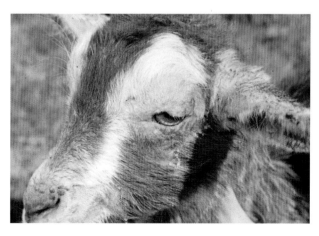

Figure 2.5-3 Pemphigus Foliaceus. Crusts on nose, eyelids, and pinna.

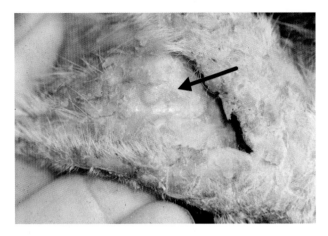

Figure 2.5-4 Pemphigus Foliaceus. Crusts, alopecia, and pustules (arrow) on pinna.

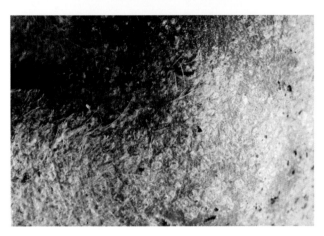

Figure 2.5-6 Pemphigus Foliaceus. Alopecia, erythema, and scale over lateral thorax.

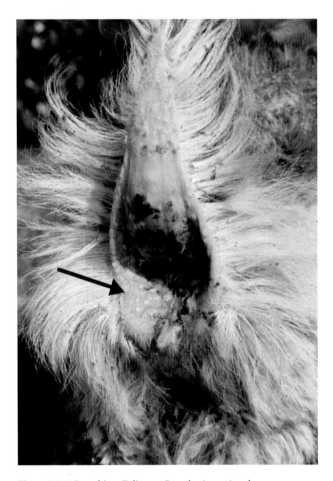

Figure 2.5-5 Pemphigus Foliaceus. Pustules (arrow) and crusts on perineum and ventral tail.

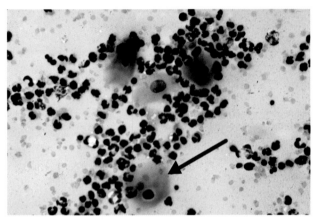

Figure 2.5-7 Pemphigus Foliaceus. Direct smear. Nondegenerate neutrophils and acantholytic keratinocytes (arrow).

MISCELLANEOUS IMMUNOLOGICAL DISEASES

Table 2.5-1 Miscellaneous Immunological Diseases

Flea bite hypersensitivity	Rare; presumed hypersensitivity to *Ctenocephalides felis felis* salivary antigens; seasonal (spring to fall); pruritic dermatitis on ventrum and legs; especially kids; can be anemic
Insect hypersensitivity (Figs. 2.5-8 to 2.5-11)	Rare; presumed hypersensitivity to *Culicoides* spp. salivary antigens; seasonal (spring to summer); pruritic dermatitis, especially dorsum
Toxic epidermal necrolysis	Very rare; host-specific cell-mediated response associated with various antigens (drugs, infections); reported case anecdotal with no supportive dermatohistopathology; generalized mucocutaneous ulcerative dermatitis with pyrexia and depression

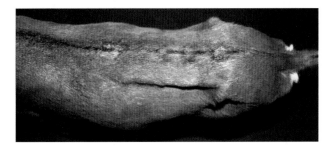

Figure 2.5-8 Insect Hypersensitivity. Alopecia and hyperpigmentation on dorsal midline.

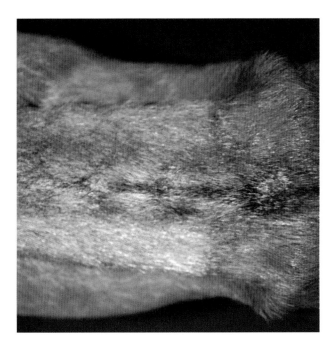

Figure 2.5-9 Insect Hypersensitivity. Alopecia, hyperpigmentation, and crust on dorsal midline.

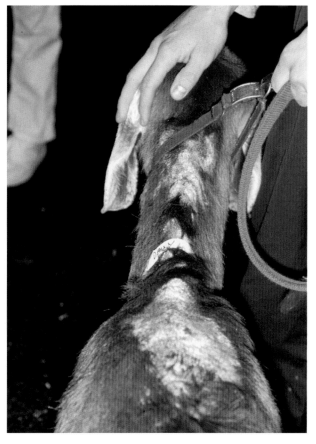

Figure 2.5-10 Insect Hypersensitivity. Alopecia, crust, and scale on dorsal midline.

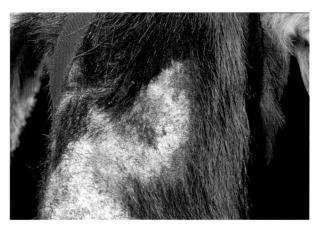

Figure 2.5-11 Insect Hypersensitivity. Alopecia, crust, and scale on dorsal neck.

REFERENCES

Jackson P. 1986. Skin Diseases in Goats. *In Pract* 8: 5.

Pappalardo E, et al. 2002. Pemphigus Foliaceus in a Goat. *Vet Dermatol* 13: 331.

Scott DW. 1988. Large Animal Dermatology. WB Saunders, Philadelphia, PA

Valdez RA, et al. 1995. Use of Corticosteroids and Aurothioglucose in a Pygmy Goat with Pemphigus Foliaceus. *J Am Vet Med Assoc* 208: 761.

Yeruham I, et al. 1997. An Apparent Flea-Allergy Dermatitis in Kids and Lambs. *J Vet Med A* 44: 391.

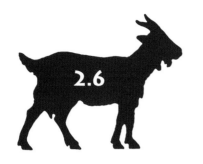

2.6

CONGENITAL AND HEREDITARY SKIN DISEASES

Hypotrichosis
Sticky Kid Syndrome
Congenital Goiter and Hypothyroidism

HYPOTRICHOSIS

Hypotrichosis implies *clinically* a less than normal amount of hair that is hereditary and often congenital; and *histopathologically* a hypoplasia of hair follicles. All reports of hypotrichosis in goats are anecdotal. Hair loss is symmetrical and exposed skin is initially normal in appearance. Exposed skin is susceptible to sunburn, infections, and contact dermatitis. Affected animals are often intolerant to cold.

The diagnosis is based on history, physical examination, and dermatohistopathology (hypoplastic hair follicles).

STICKY KID SYNDROME

This syndrome has been reported anecdotally in Golden Guernseys. It is believed to be an autosomal recessive trait. There is no sex predilection. Affected kids are born with sticky, matted hair coats that do not dry normally. The coat remains harsh and sticky in older goats.

Diagnosis is based on history and physical examination.

CONGENITAL GOITER AND HYPOTHYROIDISM

Congenital goiter and hypothyroidism is rare and associated with maternal dietary iodine deficiency. Kids are born weak and die within a few hours or weeks. The haircoat varies from short and fuzzy to completely absent. The skin is often thickened and puffy (myxedema).

Congenital goiter and hypothyroidism due to defective thyroglobulin synthesis has been reported in Saanen-Dwarf Crossbreds. The disorder is presumed to be an autosomal recessive trait. There is no sex predilection. Affected goats exhibit retarded growth, decreased ruminations with a tendency for recurrent bloat, thick and scaly skin, and a sparse hair coat.

Diagnosis is based on history, physical examination and thyroid function testing.

REFERENCES

Matthews JG. 1999. Diseases of the Goat. Ed 2. Blackwell Science, Malden, MA.
Scott DW. 1988. Large Animal Dermatology. WB Saunders, Philadelphia, PA.
Smith MC, and Sherman DM. 1994. Goat Medicine. Lea & Febiger, Philadelphia, PA.

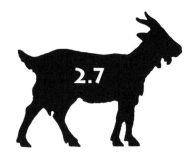

ENVIRONMENTAL SKIN DISEASES

Frostbite
Primary Irritant Contact Dermatitis
Photodermatitis
Miscellaneous Diseases
    Ergotism
    Foreign Bodies
    Intertrigo
    Kaalsiekte
    Pressure Sores
    Selenium Toxicosis
    Stachybotryotoxicosis
    Subcutaneous Emphysema

FROSTBITE

Features

Frostbite is an injury to the skin caused by excessive exposure to cold. Frostbite is rare in healthy animals that have been acclimatized to cold. It is more likely to occur in neonates; animals that are sick, debilitated, or dehydrated; animals having pre-existing vascular insufficiency; animals recently moved from a warm climate to a cold one. Lack of shelter, blowing wind, and wetting decrease the amount of exposure time necessary for frostbite to develop.

Frostbite typically affects the pinnae, tail tip, teats, scrotum, and feet in variable combinations (Figs. 2.7-1 and 2.7-2). While frozen, the skin appears pale, is hypoesthetic, and is cool to the touch. After thawing, mild cases present with erythema, edema, scaling, and alopecia: severe cases present with necrosis, dry gangrene, and sloughing.

Differential Diagnosis

Ergotism, vasculitis, other causes of gangrene (Box 2.7-1).

Diagnosis

1. History and physical examination.

PRIMARY IRRITANT CONTACT DERMATITIS

Features

Primary irritant contact dermatitis is a common inflammatory skin reaction caused by direct contact with an offending substance. Moisture is an important predisposing factor, since it decreases the effectiveness of normal skin barriers and increases the intimacy of contact between the contactant and the skin.

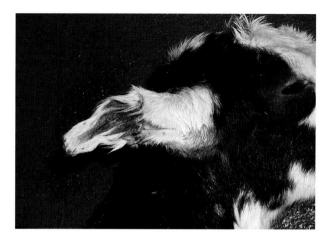

Figure 2.7-1 Frostbite. Necrosis of distal pinna (courtesy M. Smith).

Box 2.7-1 Gangrene

Gangrene (Greek: consuming, gnawing) is a clinical term used to describe severe tissue necrosis and slough. *Moist* gangrene is produced by impairment of lymphatic and venous drainage plus infection (putrefaction) and is a complication of pressure sores. Moist gangrene presents as swollen, discolored areas with foul odor and progressive tissue decomposition. *Dry* gangrene occurs when arterial blood supply is occluded, but venous and lymphatic drainage remain intact and infection is absent (mummification). Dry gangrene assumes a dry, discolored, leathery appearance. Causes of gangrene include: (1) external pressure (e.g., pressure sores, ropes, constricting bands); (2) internal pressure (e.g., severe edema); (3) burns (thermal, chemical, frictional, electrical, radiational); (4) frostbite; (5) envenomation (snake, spider); (6) vasculitis; (7) ergotism; (8) fescue toxicosis; (9) photodermatitis; (10) various infections (*Clostridium, Staphylococcus, Streptococcus, Fusobacterium*).

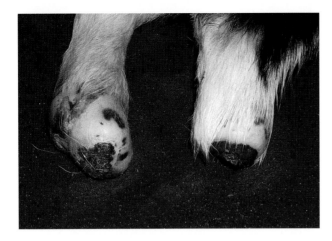

Figure 2.7-2 Frostbite. Slough of feet (courtesy M. Smith).

Substances known to cause contact dermatitis in goats include: body excretions and secretions (feces, urine, wounds); caustics (acids, alkalis); crude oil, diesel fuel, turpentine; improper use of sprays, rinses, wipes; plants; wood preservatives; bedding; filth.

The dermatitis varies in severity from erythema, edema, papules, and scale to vesicles, erosions, ulcers, necrosis, and crusts. Severe irritants, self-trauma, or secondary bacterial infections can result in alopecia, excoriation, lichenification, and scarring. Leukotrichia and leukoderma can be transient or permanent sequelae. In most instances, the nature of the contactant can be inferred from the distribution of the dermatitis: muzzle and distal legs (plants, environmental substances); face and dorsum (sprays, pour-ons, wipes); ventrum (bedding, filth); perineum and rear legs (urine, feces). Contact dermatitis is seen on the

muzzle, lips, and ear tips of kids fed milk or milk replacers from pans and buckets.

Buck goats urinate on their own face, beard, and forelimbs as a result of sexual excitation during breeding season, resulting in contact dermatitis due to urine scald (Figs. 2.7-3 and 2.7-4).

Diagnosis

1. History and physical examination.

PHOTODERMATITIS

Features

Photodermatitis (solar dermatitis, actinic dermatitis) is an inflammatory skin disease caused by exposure to ultraviolet light. *Phototoxicity* (sunburn) occurs on white skin, light skin, or damaged skin (e.g., depigmented or scarred) not sufficiently covered by hair. *Photosensitization* is classified according to the source of photodynamic agents (Tables 2.7-1 and 2.7-2): (1) primary photosensitization (a preformed or metabolically-derived photodynamic agent reaches the skin by ingestion, injection, or contact; (2) hepatogenous photosensitization (blood phylloerythrin levels are elevated in association with liver abnormalities); and (3) idiopathic photosensitization.

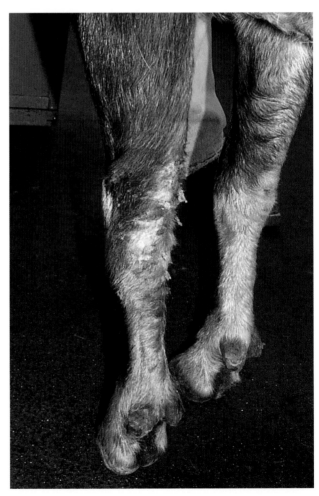

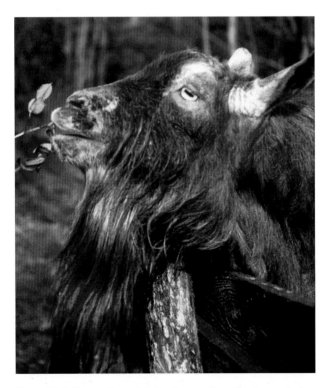

Figure 2.7-3 Contact Dermatitis. Erythema and crusting on muzzle due to urine scald (courtesy M. Smith).

Figure 2.7-4 Contact Dermatitis. Erythema and crusting on caudal aspect of front limbs due to urine scald (courtesy M. Smith).

Table 2.7-1 Causes of Primary Photosensitization

Source	Photodynamic Agent
Plants	
St. John's Wort (*Hypericum perforatum*)	Hypericin
Buckwheat (*Fagopyrum esculentum,* *Polygonum fagopyrum*)	Fagopyrin, photofagopyrin
Bishop's Weed (*Ammi majus*)	Furocoumarins
Dutchman's Breeches (*Thamnosma texana*)	Furocoumarins
Wild Carrot (*Daucus carota*), spring parsley (*Cymopterus watsonii*)	Furocoumarins
Cooperia pedunculata	Furocoumarins
Smartweeds (*Polygonum* spp.)	Furocoumarins
Perennial ryegrass (*Lolium perenne*)	Perloline
Burr trefoil (*Medicago denticulata*)	Aphids
Alfalfa silage	?
Chemicals	
Phenothiazines	
Thiazides	
Acriflavines	
Rose Bengal	
Methylene blue	
Sulfonamides	
Tetracyclines	

Table 2.7-2 Causes of Hepatogenous Photosensitization

Source	Hepatotoxin
Plants	
Burning bush, fireweed (*Kochia scoparia*)	?
Ngaio tree (*Myoporum* spp.)	Ngaione
Lechuguilla (*Agave lechuguilla*)	Saponins
Rape, kale (*Brassica* spp.)	?
Coal oil brush, spineless horsebrush (*Tetradynia* spp.)	?
Moldy alfalfa hay	?
Sacahuiste (*Nolina texana*)	?
Salvation Jane (*Echium lycopsis*)	Pyrrolizidine alkaloids
Lantana (*Lantana camara*)	Triterpene
Heliotrope (*Heliotropium europaeum*)	Pyrrolizidine alkaloids
Tarweed, fiddle-neck (*Amsinckia* spp.)	Pyrrolizidine alkaloids
Crotalaria, rattleweed (*Croatalaria* spp.)	Pyrrolizidine alkaloids
Millet, panic grass (*Panicum* spp.)	?
Ganskweed (*Lasiopermum bipinnatum*)	?
Verrain (*Lippia rehmanni*)	Triterpenes
Bog asphodel (*Narthecium ossifragum*)	Saponins
Alecrim (*Holocalyx glaziovii*)	?
Vuusiektebossie (*Nidorella foetida*)	?
Anthanasia trifurcata	?
Asaemia axillaris	?
Fungi	
Anacystis spp.—blue-green algae in water	Alkaloid
Periconia spp.—on Bermuda grass	?
Phomopsis leptostromiformis—on lupins	Phomopsin A
Infections	
Liver abscess	Bacteria/toxins
Neoplasia	
Lymphoma	Malignant lymphocytes
Hepatic carcinoma	Malignant hepatocytes
Chemicals	
Copper	
Phosphorus	
Carbon tetrachloride	
Phenanthridium	

Skin lesions are usually restricted to light-skin, sparsely-haired areas but, in severe cases, can extend into the surrounding dark-skin areas too. Restlessness and discomfort often precede visible skin lesions. Erythema and edema may be followed by vesicles and bullae, ulceration, oozing, crusts, scales, and alopecia. Secondary bacterial infections are common. In severe cases, necrosis and sloughing may occur. Variable degrees of pruritus and pain are present. The muzzle, eyelids, lips, face, pinnae, back, perineum, distal legs, teats, and coronary bands are most commonly affected. In severe cases, pinnae, eyelids, tail, teats, and feet may slough. Affected animals often attempt to protect themselves from sunlight.

Although photosensitized animals rarely die, resultant weight loss, damaged udders and teats, refusal to allow young to nurse, and secondary infections/flystrike all may lead to appreciable economic loss.

Diagnosis

1. History and physical examination.
2. Liver function testing should always be performed, whether or not clinical signs of liver disease are present.
3. Primary photodynamic agents can often be identified with various biological assay systems.

MISCELLANEOUS DISEASES

Table 2.7-3 Miscellaneous Environmental Diseases

Ergotism	Rare and cosmopolitan; eating grasses contaminated by the fungus *Claviceps pupurea* (alkaloids); gangrene and sloughing of distal limbs, ears, tail, teats; feed analysis
Foreign bodies	See Box 2.7-2
Intertrigo	Uncommon and cosmopolitan; dairy goats, especially in association with the udder edema of parturition; dermatitis at the junction of the lateral aspects of the udder and medial thighs
Kaalsiekte	Rare; South Africa; nursing kids ingest toxin in milk of does eating bitterkarro bush (*Chrysocoma tenuifola*); diarrhea, haircoat shedding, pruritus when exposed to sunlight
Pressure sores	Uncommon and cosmopolitan; especially emaciated or recumbent animals; especially over elbows, hocks, and sternum; deep ulcers undermined at the edges
Selenium toxicosis	Rare; associated with high levels of selenium in soil and/or presence of selenium-concentrating plants, low rainfall, alkaline soil (e.g. Great Plains areas of United States); suspected cause of loss of hair in flanks and beard; selenium levels in blood, liver, kidney, grasses
Stachybotryotoxicosis	Rare; Europe; eating hay and straw contaminated by the fungus *Stachybotrys atra* (macrocyclic trichothecenes); initial necrotic ulcers in mouth and on lips and nostrils; conjunctivitis and rhinitis; later fever, depression, anorexia, diarrhea, weakness, bleeding diathesis; isolate fungus and toxins from feed
Subcutaneous emphysema	Rare and cosmopolitan; sequel to tracheal perforation, esophageal rupture, pulmonary emphysema, penetrating wounds (external or internal; rib fracture), clostridial infections; soft, fluctuant, crepitant, subcutaneous swellings; usually nonpainful and not acutely ill (unless clostridial)

Box 2.7-2 Draining Tracts

- A *fistula* is an abnormal passage or communication, usually between two internal organs or leading from an internal organ to the surface of the body.
- A *sinus* is an abnormal cavity or channel or fistula that permits the escape of pus to the surface of the body.
- Draining tracts are commonly associated with penetrating wounds that have left infectious agents and/or foreign material. Draining tracts may also result from infections of underlying tissues (e.g., bone, joint, lymph node) or previous injections.
- Foreign bodies include wood slivers, plant seeds and awns, cactus tines, fragments of wire, and suture material. Lesions include varying combinations of papules, nodules, abscesses, and draining tracts. Lesions occur most commonly on the legs, hips, muzzle, and ventrum.

REFERENCES

Howard JL, Smith RA. 1999. Current Veterinary Therapy. Food Animal Practice. Ed 4. WB Saunders, Philadelphia, PA.

Radostits OM, et al. 2000. Veterinary Medicine. A Textbook of the Diseases of Cattle, Sheep, Pigs, Goats and Horses. Ed 9. WB Saunders, Philadelphia, PA.

Scott DW. 1988. Large Animal Dermatology. WB Saunders, Philadelphia, PA.

Smith MC, and Sherman DM. 1994. Goat Medicine. Lea & Febiger, Philadelphia, PA.

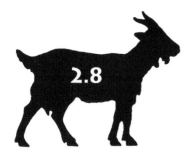

NUTRITIONAL SKIN DISEASES

2.8

Vitamin E- and Selenium-Responsive Dermatosis
Zinc-Responsive Dermatitis
Miscellaneous Nutritional Disorders
    Vitamin A Deficiency
    Iodine Deficiency
    Sulfur Deficiency

VITAMIN E- AND SELENIUM-RESPONSIVE DERMATOSIS

Features

Vitamin E- and selenium-responsive dermatosis is rare. There are no apparent breed, sex, or age predilections.

Affected animals develop periocular alopecia and generalized scaling (Fig. 2.8-1). Multifocal greasy crusts can be present. The haircoat is dry to waxy, dull, brittle, and easily epilated. Patchy hypotrichosis may be present. The condition is not pruritic, and affected animals are usually otherwise healthy.

Differential Diagnosis

Other nutritional imbalances, *Malassezia* dermatitis.

Diagnosis

1. Dermatohistopathology—Mild superficial lymphohistiocytic perivascular dermatitis with marked, diffuse orthokeratotic hyperkeratosis.
2. Analysis of diet.
3. Response to therapy.

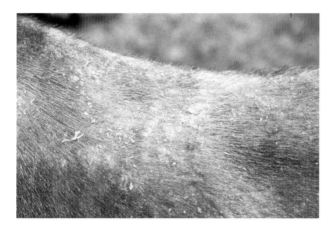

Figure 2.8-1 Vitamin E- and Selenium-Responsive Dermatosis. Scaling, waxy crusts, and patchy hypotrichosis over trunk.

ZINC-RESPONSIVE DERMATITIS

Features

The characteristic dermatitis may be seen with true zinc deficiency or as an idiopathic zinc-responsive condition. Causes of deficiency include diets deficient in zinc; diets with excessive calcium, iron, phytates, and other chelating agents; drinking water with excessive iron and other chelating agents. Zinc-responsive dermatoses are uncommon to rare. There are no apparent breed, sex, or age predilections.

More-or-less symmetrical erythema and scaling progress to crusting and alopecia. The face, pinnae, mucocutaneous junctions, pressure points, and distal legs are typically affected (Figs. 2.8-2 to 2.8-4). Some animals have a dull, rough, brittle haircoat. Pruritus may be intense or absent. Secondary bacterial (and

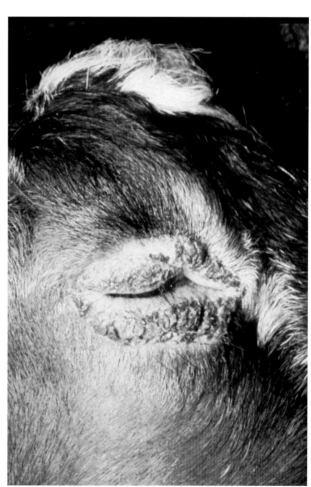

Figure 2.8-2 Zinc-Responsive Dermatitis. Thick brown crusts around eye.

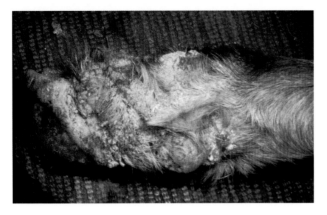

Figure 2.8-3 Zinc-Responsive Dermatitis. Thick crusts and ulceration of distal leg.

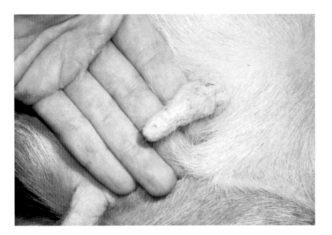

Figure 2.8-4 Zinc-Responsive Dermatitis. Crusts and erythema on teat.

possibly *Malassezia*) skin infections are common. Truly zinc-deficient animals have accompanying systemic signs, whereas animals with the idiopathic condition do not. With true zinc-deficiency, multiple animals are often affected. With the idiopathic condition, a single animal is typically affected.

Differential Diagnosis

Dermatophytosis, dermatophilosis, staphylococcal folliculitis, sarcoptic mange (when pruritic).

Diagnosis

1. Dermatohistopathology—Hyperplastic to spongiotic superficial perivascular-to-interstitial dermatitis with marked diffuse parakeratotic hyperkeratosis and a lymphoeosinophilic inflammatory infiltrate.
2. Analysis of diet and water.
3. Response to therapy.

MISCELLANEOUS NUTRITIONAL DISORDERS

Table 2.8-1 Miscellaneous Nutritional Disorders	
Vitamin A deficiency	Very rare; deficient diet; rough, dry, faded haircoat and generalized seborrhea; systemic signs; serum and liver concentrations of vitamin A, and vitamin A levels in diet
Iodine deficiency	Very rare; maternal dietary deficiency; newborn kids; generalized alopecia and thick puffy skin (myxedema); systemic signs; serum concentration of thyroid hormone and thyroid gland pathology
Sulfur deficiency	Rare; deficient diet; fleece-or-hair biting and alopecia, especially hips, abdomen, and shoulder; systemic signs; serum and liver concentrations of sulfur

REFERENCES

Howard JL, Smith RA. 1999. Current Veterinary Therapy. Food Animal Practice. Ed 4. WB Saunders, Philadelphia, PA.

Krametter-Froetscher R, et al. 2005. Zinc-Responsive Dermatitis in Goats Suggestive of Hereditary Malabsorption: Two Field Cases. *Vet Dermatol* 16: 269.

Radostits OM, et al. 2000. Veterinary Medicine. A Textbook of the Diseases of Cattle, Sheep, Pigs, Goats and Horses. Ed 9. WB Saunders, Philadelphia, PA.

Reuter R, et al. 1987. Zinc Responsive Alopecia and Hyperkeratosis in Angora Goats. *Aust Vet J* 64: 351.

Scott DW. 1988. Large Animal Dermatology. WB Saunders, Philadelphia, PA.

Singh JL, et al. 2003. Clinicobiochemical Profile and Therapeutic Management of Congenital Goitre in Kids. *Indian J Vet Med* 23: 83.

Smith ME, Sherman DM. 1994. Goat Medicine. Lea & Febiger, Philadelphia, PA.

Youde H. 2001. Preliminary Epidemiological and Clinical Observations on *Shimao zheng* (fleece-eating) in Goats and Sheep. *Vet Res Commun* 125: 585.

Youde H. 2002. An Experimental Study on the Treatment and Prevention of *Shimao zheng* (fleece-eating) in Sheep and Goats in the Haizi Area of Akesai County in China. *Vet Res Commun* 26: 39.

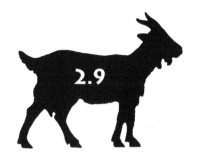

MISCELLANEOUS SKIN DISEASES

Psoriasiform Dermatitis
Other Miscellaneous Disorders
  Idiopathic Lichenoid Dermatitis

PSORIASIFORM DERMATITIS

Features

Psoriasiform dermatitis is rare and cosmopolitan. The cause is unknown, and genetics may play a role. Pygmy goats and Alpine goats have been most commonly described. The condition often begins in three to five month old animals, but may occur in young adults as well. There is no apparent sex predilection.

Lesions begin on the face and pinnae and commonly involve the neck, distal legs, and ventrum (Figs. 2.9-1 to 2.9-4). Early erythema and scaling progress to crusting, thickened skin, and variable degrees of hair loss. The condition is neither pruritic, nor painful, and affected animals are otherwise healthy. Spontaneous waxing and waning of the disorder is seen, but complete resolution does not occur.

Differential Diagnosis

Zinc-responsive dermatitis, vitamin E- and selenium-responsive dermatosis, dermatophytosis, and *Malassezia* dermatitis.

Diagnosis

1. Dermatohistopathology—Psoriasiform perivascular dermatitis with neutrophils; spongiform and Munro microabscesses in epidermis; prominent orthokeratotic and parakeratotic hyperkeratosis.

Figure 2.9-1 Psoriasiform Dermatitis. Alopecia, scaling, and crusting over face, legs, and withers.

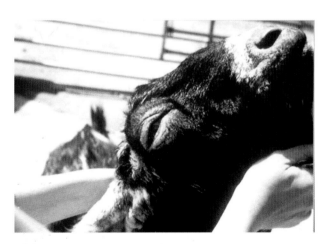

Figure 2.9-2 Psoriasiform Dermatitis. Alopecia and crusting on muzzle and around eye.

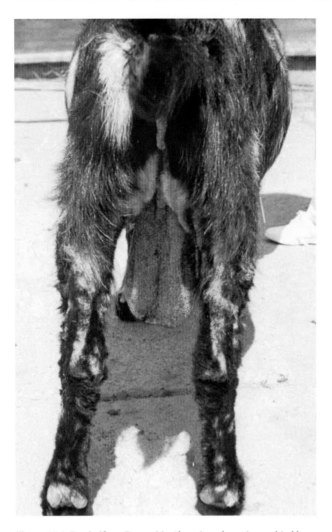

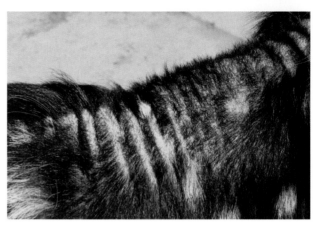

Figure 2.9-4 Psoriasiform Dermatitis. Alopecia, crusting, and thickening of skin over dorsal neck and withers.

Figure 2.9-3 Psoriasiform Dermatitis. Alopecia and crusting on hind legs.

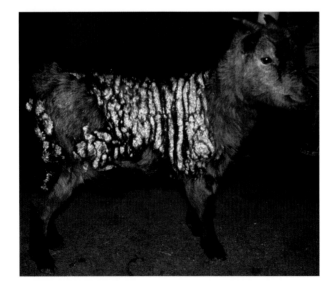

Figure 2.9-5 Idiopathic Lichenoid Dermatitis. Flat-topped papules and plaques, covered with adherent grey hyperkeratosis, over trunk and proximal limbs. The condition was not pruritic, and the goat was otherwise healthy.

OTHER MISCELLANEOUS DISORDERS

Table 2.9-1 Other Miscellaneous Disorders	
Idiopathic lichenoid dermatitis (Fig. 2.9-5)	One reported case; Boer billy goat with hyperkeratotic papules and plaques over back, groin, scrotum, perineum, tail, head, pinnae; dermatohisto-pathology

REFERENCES

Jeffries AR, et al. 1991. Seborrheic Dermatitis in Pigmy Goats. *Vet Dermatol* 2: 109.

Yeruham I, et al. 2002. Apparent Idiopathic Interface Disease in a Boer Billy Goat. *J S Afr Vet Assoc* 73: 77.

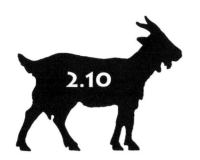

NEOPLASTIC AND NON-NEOPLASTIC GROWTHS

2.10

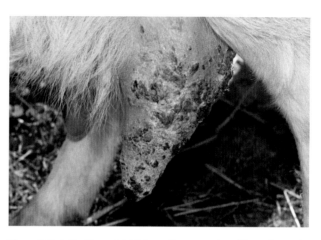

Figure 2.10-1 Papilloma. Multiple papillomas on the udder and teat of a Saanen doe.

PAPILLOMA

Features

Papillomas are uncommon, cosmopolitan, benign neoplasms of keratinocytes. They are caused by papillomavirus. Infections follow direct or indirect contamination of various wounds. Given the different reported localizations and biological behaviors for papillomas in goats, it is probable that multiple types of caprine papillomavirus are involved.

In one form, papillomas occur on the face, pinnae, neck, shoulder, and forelegs with no apparent age, breed, or sex predilections. Lesions are multiple, hyperkeratotic, and verrucous. Multiple animals in a herd are affected, and spontaneous regression usually occurs within 1 to 12 months.

In the second form, papillomas occur on the udder and teats (Fig 2.10-1), especially in white goats (Saanen, Angora) that have lactated at least once. Lesions are multiple, hyperkeratotic, and verrucous. Cutaneous horns may develop on some lesions. Spontaneous regression does not occur. Some lesions may undergo transformation into squamous cell carcinomas (Fig. 2.10-2).

Differential Diagnosis

Squamous cell carcinoma (if solitary).

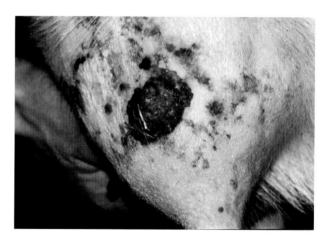

Figure 2.10-2 Squamous Cell Carcinoma. Ulcerated mass on udder along with multiple papillomas (courtesy J. Gourreau).

Diagnosis

1. Dermatohistopathology.

SQUAMOUS CELL CARCINOMA

Features

Squamous cell carcinoma is a common, cosmopolitan, malignant neoplasm of keratinocytes. They are especially common in subtropical and tropical climates, and at high altitudes. Ultraviolet

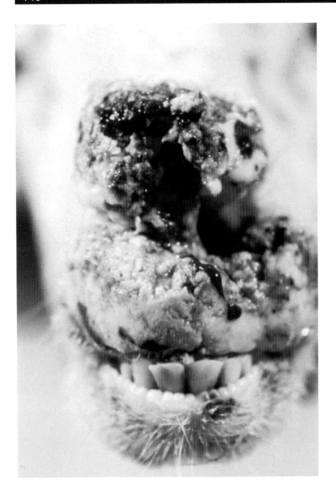

Figure 2.10-3 Squamous Cell Carcinoma. Large, infiltrative, ulcerative, destructive mass on muzzle.

light damage is important in the etiopathogenesis of this neoplasm, thus white skin that is lightly haired is at risk. Udder papillomas can undergo transformation into squamous cell carcinomas. Adult to aged animals are most commonly affected, and Angoras and Boers may be at risk. There is no apparent sex predilection.

Lesions are usually solitary and occur most commonly on the pinnae, horn stumps, muzzle, perineum, vulva, and udder (Figs. 2.10-2 and 2.10-3). Early lesions are erythematous, scaly, crusty, and hyperkeratotic (actinic keratosis). Invasive squamous cell carcinomas may be proliferative (verrucous or cauliflower like) or ulcerative (granulating and nonhealing).

Differential Diagnosis

Papilloma, basal cell tumor (when ulcerated), various granulomas (infectious, foreign body).

Diagnosis

1. Microscopy (direct smears)—Keratinocytes showing various degrees of atypia.
2. Dermatohistopathology.

MISCELLANEOUS NEOPLASTIC AND NON-NEOPLASTIC GROWTHS

Table 2.10-1 Miscellaneous Neoplastic and Non-Neoplastic Growths

Sebaceous adenoma	Very rare; adult; solitary nodule; anywhere; benign; direct smears and dermatohistopathology
Fibroma	Very rare; adult; solitary nodule; anywhere; benign; direct smears and dermatohistopathology
Fibrosarcoma	Very rare; adult; solitary nodule; anywhere; malignant; dermatohistopathology
Leiomyoma	Very rare; adult; solitary nodule on pinnae; benign; dermatohistopathology
Hemangioma	Rare; adult to aged; solitary and nodular; pedunculated or multilobular; often bleeding; anywhere; benign; dermatohistopathology
Hemangiosarcoma	Very rare; adult to aged; solitary nodule; often bleeding; anywhere; malignant; dermatohistopathology
Histiocytoma (Fig. 2.10-4)	Very rare; adult; solitary nodule on scrotum; benign; direct smears and dermatohistopathology
Melanoma	Uncommon; adult to aged; especially Angoras; solitary or multiple nodules; especially perineum, vulva, tail, udder, and pinnae; malignant; direct smears and dermatohistopathology
Wattle cyst (Figs. 2.10-5 to 2.10-7)	Rare; probably hereditary branchial cleft cyst; Nubians and Nubian crossbreeds; birth to 3 months old; unilateral or bilateral at base of wattles; round, soft, fluctuant, painless; benign; needle aspiration (thin or thick clear fluid) and dermatohistopathology
Salivary mucocele	Very rare; few weeks to few months old; especially Nubians; cystic parotid salivary gland ducts; unilateral, painless cyst on cheek or submandibular area; benign; needle aspiration (saliva) and histopathology
Thyroglossal duct cyst	Very rare; congenital; painless cyst on ventral neck midline (area of thyroid gland); benign; histopathology
Goiter	Very rare; bilateral, firm, painless mass slightly behind larynx (enlarged thyroid gland); histopathology
Thymus	Rare; 2 to 4 weeks old; bilaterally symmetric swelling in upper neck; benign (spontaneous regression at 4 months old); histopathology
Udder cyst	Rare; older ewes; frequently multiple, 1 to 5 cm diameter, soft, reducible cysts on udder; benign; needle aspiration (milk)
Ectopic mammary gland tissue	Rare; adult female; bilateral firm, lobular swellings in vulvar lips (distended for 3 months post-partum); benign; needle aspiration (milk); histopathology
Actinic keratosis	Common; adult to aged; ultraviolet light damaged white skin; solitary or multiple erythematous, scaly, crusty, hyperkeratotic plaques, pre-malignant; dermatohistopathology
Cutaneous horn (Fig. 2.10-8)	Rare; hornlike hyperkeratosis; usually overlying neoplasms (papilloma, squamous cell carcinoma, actinic keratosis, basal cell tumor); benign or malignant; dermatohistopathology

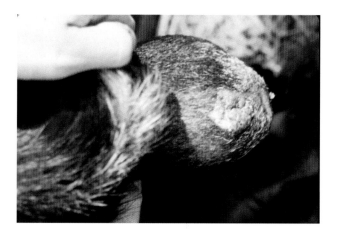

Figure 2.10-4 Histiocytoma. Hyperkeratotic nodule on scrotum.

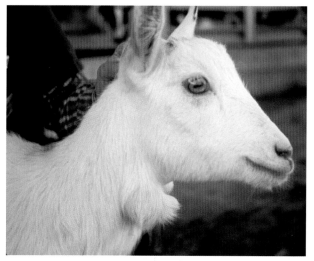

Figure 2.10-5 Wattle Cyst. Fluctuant cyst at base of wattle.

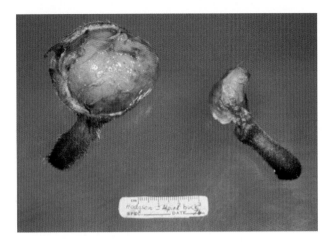

Figure 2.10-6 Wattle Cysts. Two cysts in amputated wattles.

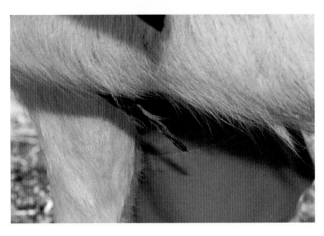

Figure 2.10-8 Cutaneous Horn. Hornlike growth on sternum.

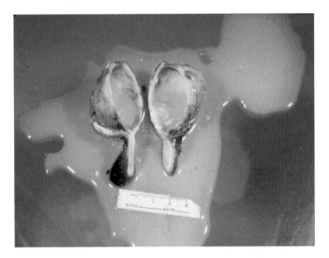

Figure 2.10-7 Wattle Cysts. Bisected cyst and liberated liquid content.

REFERENCES

Bildfell RJ, et al. 2002. Cutaneous Vasoproliferative Lesions in Goats. *Vet Pathol* 39: 273.

Brown PJ, et al. 1989. Developmental Cysts in the Upper Neck of Anglo-Nubian Goats. *Vet Rec* 125: 256.

Howard JO, Smith RL. 1999. Current Veterinary Therapy. Food Animal Practice. Ed 4. WB Saunders, Philadelphia, PA.

Manni V, et al. 1998. Presence of Papillomavirus-like DNA Sequences in Cutaneous Fibropapillomas of the Goat Udder. *Vet Microbiol* 61: 1.

Rajguru DN, et al. 1988. A Clinical Report on Cutaneous Caprine Papillomatosis. *Indian Vet J* 65: 827.

Ramadan RO, et al. 1988. Malignant Melanomas in Goats: A Clinicopathological Study. *J Comp Pathol* 98: 237.

Scott DW. 1988. Large Animal Dermatology. WB Saunders, Philadelphia, PA.

Smith MC, Sherman DM. 1994. Goat Medicine. Lea & Febiger, Philadelphia, PA.

Yeruham I, et al. 1993. Perianal Squamous Cell Carcinoma in Goats. *J Vet Med A* 40: 432.

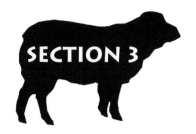

OVINE

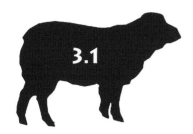

BACTERIAL SKIN DISEASES

3.1

Impetigo
Folliculitis and Furunculosis
Dermatophilosis
Miscellaneous Bacterial Diseases
    Abscess
    Actinobacillosis
    Clostridial Cellulitis
    Anthrax
    Pseudomonas aeruginosa Infection
    "Staphylococcal Scalded Skin Syndrome"

IMPETIGO

Features

Impetigo (Latin: an attack; scabby eruption) is a common, cosmopolitan superficial pustular dermatitis that does not involve hair follicles. It is caused by *Staphylococcus aureus*, and predisposing factors include trauma, moisture, and the stress of parturition. Lambs and lactating ewes are predisposed.

Lesions are most commonly seen on the udder (especially the base of the teats and the intramammary sulcus), teats, ventral abdomen, medial thighs, vulva, perineum, and ventral tail (Fig. 3.1-1). Superficial vesicles rapidly become pustular, rupture, and leave annular erosions and yellow-brown crusts. Lesions are neither pruritic nor painful, and affected animals are otherwise healthy. Single or multiple animals may be affected. Staphylococcal mastitis is a possible, but uncommon complication.

Differential Diagnosis

Other bacterial infections, dermatophilosis, dermatophytosis, and viral infections.

Diagnosis

1. Microscopy (direct smears)—Degenerate neutrophils, nuclear streaming, and phagocytosed cocci (Gram-positive; about 1 μm diameter)(see Fig. 3.1-5).
2. Culture (aerobic.)
3. Dermatohistopathology—Subcorneal pustular dermatitis with degenerate neutrophils and intracellular cocci.

FOLLICULITIS AND FURUNCULOSIS

Features

Folliculitis (hair follicle inflammation) and furunculosis (hair follicle rupture) are common and cosmopolitan, and caused by *Staphylococcus aureus*, and predisposing factors include trauma and moisture. There are no apparent breed, sex, or age predilections.

Lesions can be seen anywhere, most commonly on the muzzle, tail, and perineum of three-to-four week old lambs ("plooks"); bony prominence of face, pinnae, and horn base of adults ("eye scab," "periorbital/facial eczema"); legs; and occasionally the prepuce or vulva (Figs. 3.1-2 to 3.1-4). Tufted papules and pustules become crusted, then alopecic. Furuncles are characterized by nodules, draining tracts, and ulcers. Lesions are rarely pruritic, but furuncles may be painful. Facial furunculosis is usually seen in cold, wet winter/spring, when animals are bumping heads and fighting at feeding troughs; the first indication of disease may be

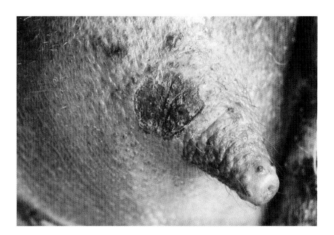

Figure 3.1-1 Impetigo. Annular erosion and crusts near base of teat.

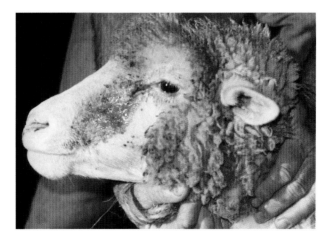

Figure 3.1-2 Staphylococcal Furunculosis. Ulceration and draining tracts on face.

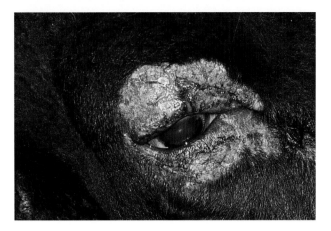

Figure 3.1-3 Staphylococcal Furunculosis. Crusts, ulceration, and fissuring (courtesy M. Smith).

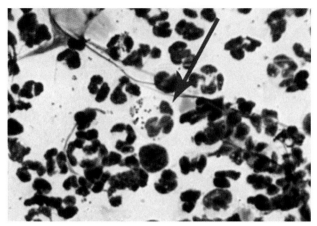

Figure 3.1-5 Staphylococcal Folliculitis. Direct smear (Diff-Quik stain). Suppurative inflammation with degenerate neutrophils, nuclear streaming, and phagocytosed cocci (arrow).

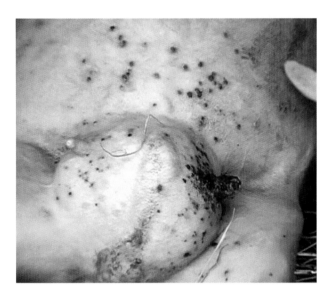

Figure 3.1-4 Staphylococcal Folliculitis. Erythematous papules and crusts on abdomen and medial thighs (courtesy J. Gourreau).

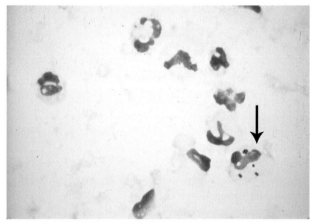

Figure 3.1-6 Staphylococcal Folliculitis. Direct smear (Gram stain). Degenerate neutrophils and phagocytosed Gram-positive cocci (arrow).

blood smeared on the face. Affected animals are usually otherwise healthy. Pending the inciting cause(s), single or multiple animals may be affected.

Staphylococcal dermatitis and folliculitis has been described in neonatal lambs. Lesions occur on the lips, perineum, ventral tail, abdomen, groin, and axillae. *S. aureus* or *S. xylosus* were isolated in culture.

Differential Diagnosis

Dermatophilosis, dermatophytosis, demodicosis, and contagious viral pustular dermatitis ("orf").

Diagnosis

1. Microscopy (direct smears)—Degenerate neutrophils, nuclear streaming, and phagocytosed cocci (Gram-positive; about 1 μm diameter) with folliculitis (Figs. 3.1-5 and 3.1-6). Furunculosis characterized by numerous macrophages, lympho-

cytes, eosinophils, and plasma cells in addition to the findings described for folliculitis (Fig 3.1-7).
2. Culture (aerobic).
3. Dermatohistopathology—Suppurative luminal folliculitis with intracellular cocci; pyogranulomatous furunculosis.

DERMATOPHILOSIS

Features

Dermatophilosis ("lumpy wool," "mycotic dermatitis") is a common, cosmopolitan skin disease. *Dermatophilus congolensis* proliferates under the influence of moisture (especially rain) and skin damage (especially ticks, insects, prickly vegetation). The disease is more common and more severe in tropical and subtropical climates and outdoor animals. There are no apparent sex or age predilections, and fine-wooled breeds (e.g., Suffolk, Romney) are more susceptible.

Lesions may occur anywhere. Common distributions include: face and pinnae; dorsum and flanks ("lumpy wool"); distal limbs (coronet to carpi/tarsi); scrotum (Figs. 3.1-8 to 3.1-12). An early serous to greasy exudate accumulates at the base of wool fibers,

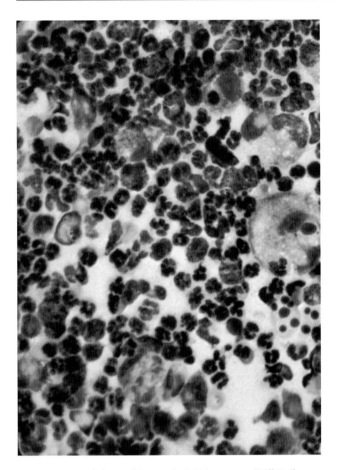

Figure 3.1-7 Staphylococcal Furunculosis. Direct smear (Diff-Quik stain). Pyogranulomatous inflammation with degenerate and nondegenerate neutrophils, macrophages, lymphocytes, and plasma cells.

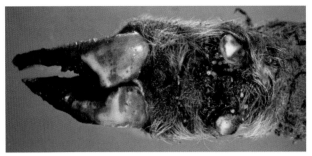

Figure 3.1-9 Dermatophilosis. Crusts and secondary myiasis ("maggots") on caudal pastern.

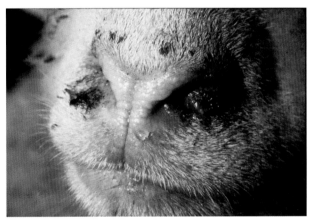

Figure 3.1-10 Dermatophilosis. Thick crusts on muzzle.

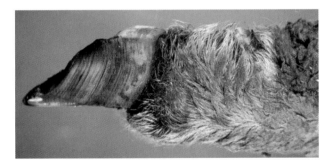

Figure 3.1-8 Dermatophilosis. Crusts on distal leg.

leading to matting of fibers. Later, hard, thick, dry crusts are formed ("lumpy wool"). As the wool grows out, the crusts persist as "pegs" or "pyramids" in the staple. In haired areas of skin, tufted papules and pustules coalesce and become exudative, which results in matted hairs within thick crusts. Erosions, ulcers, and thick, creamy, yellowish to greenish pus underlie the crusts. On the distal legs, bleeding, proliferative, fleshy masses ("mashed strawberries") underlie the crusts ("strawberry footrot"), and are believed to be a combination of dermatophilosis and contagious viral pustular dermatitis ("orf"). Acute lesions are painful, but not pruritic. Chronic lesions consist of dry crusts, scale, and alopecia. Typically, multiple animals are affected.

Dermatophilosis can cause major financial losses, especially through hide and wool damage; hide thickening ("coarse grain"); unevenness of hide ("spread cockle"); permanent enlargement of wool follicles ("pinhole"); secretory staining of wool ("yellow wool"). Dermatophilosis is a major predisposing factor for myiasis (fly-strike).

Dermatophilosis is a zoonosis. Human skin infections are uncommon and characterized by pruritic or painful pustular lesions in contact areas (Fig. 3.1-13).

Differential Diagnosis

Staphylococcal folliculitis and furunculosis, dermatophytosis, demodicosis, and zinc-responsive dermatitis.

Diagnosis

1. Microscopy (direct smears)—Degenerate neutrophils, nuclear streaming, and Gram-positive cocci in two-to-eight parallel rows forming branching filaments ("railroad tracks") (Fig. 3.1-14).
2. Culture (aerobic).
3. Dermatohistopathology—Suppurative luminal folliculitis and epidermitis with palisading crusts containing Gram-positive cocci in branching filaments.

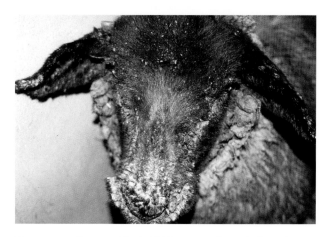

Figure 3.1-11 Dermatophilosis. Thick crusts on face and pinnae (courtesy P. Hill).

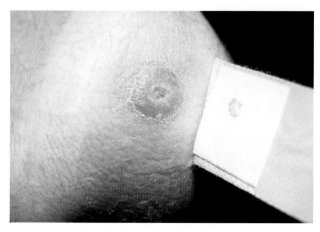

Figure 3.1-13 Dermatophilosis in a Human. Ruptured pustule and surrounding erythema on the elbow.

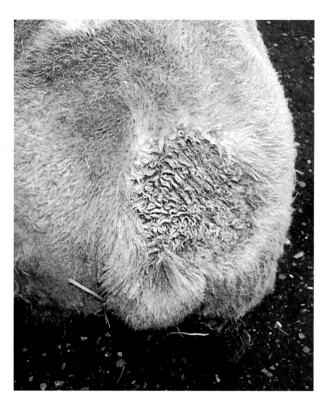

Figure 3.1-12 Dermatophilosis. Crusts on rump ("lumpy wool") (courtesy P. Scott).

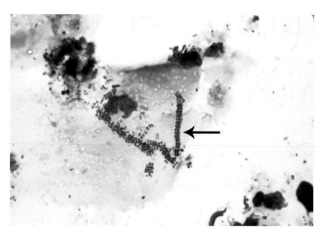

Figure 3.1-14 Dermatophilosis. Direct smear (Diff-Quik stain). Branching filaments composed of cocci ("railroad tracks").

MISCELLANEOUS BACTERIAL DISEASES

Table 3.1-1 Miscellaneous Bacterial Diseases

Abscess (Fig. 3.1-15)	Common and cosmopolitan; anywhere; fluctuant, often painful, subcutaneous, especially *Arcanobacterium pyogenes* and *Corynebacterium pseudotuberculosis*; rarely *Serratia marcescens* and *Burkholderia cepacia*; culture
Actinobacillosis ("leathery lips," "cruels") (Fig. 3.1-16)	Rare and cosmopolitan; cheek, lip, nose, neck; abscess, granuloma; thick green-yellow discharge; *Actinobacillus lignieresii*; culture and dermatohistopathology
Clostridial cellulitis (black leg; malignant edema, big head) (Fig. 3.1-17)	Uncommon and cosmopolitan; leg, perineum, abdomen ("black leg"; *Clostridium chauvoei*); anywhere ("malignant edema"; *C. septicum, C. sordelli, C. perfringens*); head and neck ("big head"; *C. novyi*); edema, exudation, variable necrosis and crepitus; systemic signs; culture and necropsy
Anthrax (Greek: coal, black eschar)	Uncommon and cosmopolitan; neck, brisket, flanks, abdomen, perineum; massive edema; *Bacillus anthracis*; systemic signs; zoonosis (cutaneous, respiratory, intestinal); culture and necropsy
Pseudomonas aeruginosa infection	Rare and cosmopolitan; wool-free areas (legs, scrotum); ulcer, crust, greenish exudates, foul odor; culture
"Staphylococcal scalded skin syndrome"	Very rare and undocumented; widespread exfoliative dermatitis, exudation, ulceration in two lambs; culture *S. aureus*; dermatohistopathology **not** confirmatory

Note: The participation of *Pseudomonas* spp. in fleece rot, *Bacillus* spp. in "pink rot," and of *Corynebacterium* spp. in "Bolo disease" is discussed in Chapter 3.7.

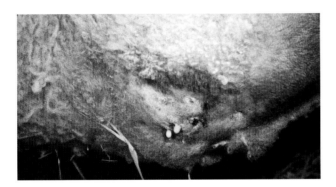

Figure 3.1-15 *Corynebacterium pseudotuberculosis* Abscess. Large swelling on sternum.

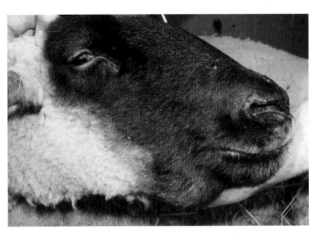

Figure 3.1-16 Actinobacillosis. Firm, movable swelling over mandible.

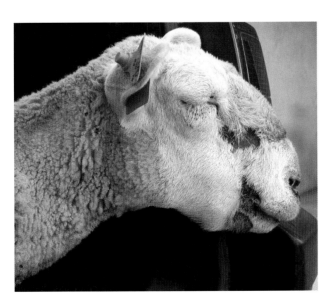

Figure 3.1-17 Clostridial Cellulitis. Cellulitis of head (courtesy R. Braque, coll J. Gourreau, AFSSA).

REFERENCES

Al Dughaym AM. 2004. Isolation of *Serratia, Arcanobacterium* and *Burkholderia* Species from Visceral and Cutaneous Abscesses in Four Emaciated Ewes. *Vet Rec* 155: 425.

Baird G. 2000. Differential Diagnosis of Non-Parasitic Skin Conditions in Sheep. *In Practice* 22: 72.

Gourreau JM, et al. 1994. Dermatite Staphylococcique du Mouton: Rôle de *Staphylococcus Xylosus. Point Vét* 26: 271.

Howard JL, Smith RA. 1999. Current Veterinary Therapy, Food Animal Practice. Ed 4. WB Saunders, Philadelphia, PA.

Martin WB, Aitken ID. 2000. Diseases of Sheep. Ed 3. Blackwell Science, Oxford, United Kingdom.

Radostits OM, et al. 2000. Veterinary Medicine. A Textbook of the Diseases of Cattle, Sheep, Pigs, Goats and Horses. Ed 9. WB Saunders, Philadelphia, PA.

Scott DW. 1988. Large Animal Dermatology. WB Saunders, Philadelphia, PA.

Yeruham I, et al. 1999. A Generalized Staphylococcal Scalded Skin-like Disease in Lambs. *J Vet Med B* 46: 635.

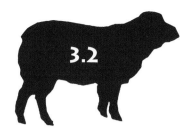

FUNGAL SKIN DISEASES

Dermatophytosis
Miscellaneous Fungal Diseases
    Pythiosis

DERMATOPHYTOSIS

Features

Dermatophytosis is an uncommon, cosmopolitan disease. It is most commonly caused by *Trichophyton verrucosum*, and less frequently by *T. mentagrophytes*, *Microsporum canis*, and *M. gypseum*. In temperate climates the disease is most common in fall and winter, especially in confined animals. There are no apparent breed or sex predilections, and young animals are most commonly affected.

Lesions can occur anywhere. *T. verrucosum* infections typically produce annular thick grayish to brownish crusts, especially on the head, face, and pinnae (Figs. 3.2-1 and 3.2-2). Wooled areas are less commonly involved, wherein hard, thick, crusted plaques are initially best detected by palpation. When matted wool and crust are removed, inflamed bleeding skin is revealed.

M. canis infections most commonly involve wooled areas—especially trunk, flank, rump—and produce clumps of wool matted with brownish exudates and dry crusts.

M. gypseum infections produce one to multiple lesions in show lambs. Lesions include annular areas of matted, discolored, easily epilated wool and erythema, erosion, and exudation.

Ovine dermatophytosis is typically nonpruritic. Affected animals are otherwise healthy. Typically multiple animals are affected.

Ovine dermatophytosis is a zoonosis. *T. verrucosum* infection in humans causes typical ringworm lesions or lesions in contact areas, especially hands, arms, neck, face, and scalp (Fig. 3.2-3).

Differential Diagnosis

Dermatophilosis, staphylococcal folliculitis, contagious viral pustular dermatitis (orf), and zinc-responsive dermatitis.

Diagnosis

1. Microscopy (trichography)—Plucked hairs placed in mineral oil or potassium hydroxide contain hyphae and arthroconidia (spores)(Figs. 3.2-4 and 3.2-5).
2. Culture.
3. Dermatohistopathology—Suppurative luminal folliculitis with fungal hyphae and arthroconidia in hairs.

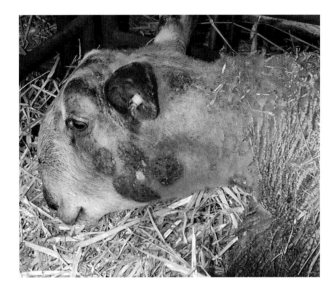

Figure 3.2-1 Dermatophytosis. Annular crusts on side of face (courtesy P. Scott).

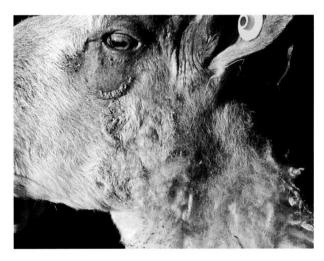

Figure 3.2-2 Dermatophytosis. Annular crusts on face (courtesy P. Scott).

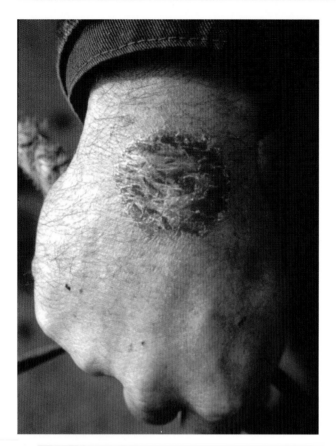

Figure 3.2-3 Dermatophytosis. Severely inflamed lesions on the hand caused by *Trichophyton verrucosum*.

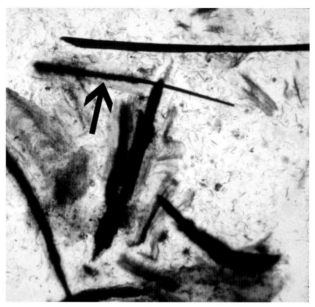

Figure 3.2-4 Dermatophytosis. Plucked hairs in mineral oil. Note thickened, irregular appearance of infected hair (arrow).

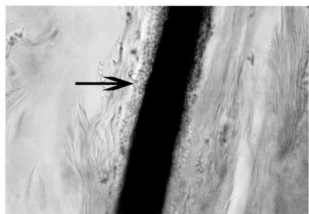

Figure 3.2-5 Dermatophytosis. Numerous arthroconidia (arrow) on surface of infected hair.

MISCELLANEOUS FUNGAL DISEASES

Table 3.2-1 Miscellaneous Fungal Diseases	
Pythiosis	Rare; South America; prolonged exposure to water; *Pythium insidiosum*; One or multiple ulcerated nodules and plaques (2.5 to 24 cm in diameter); especially legs and ventrum, dermatohistopathology, immunohistochemistry, culture

REFERENCES

Baird G. 2000. Differential Diagnosis of Non-Parasitic Conditions in Sheep. *In Practice* 22: 72.

Howard JL, Smith RA. 1999. Current Veterinary Therapy. Food Animal Practice. Ed 4. WB Saunders, Philadelphia, PA.

Hulliger GA, et al. 1999. Dermatophytosis in Show Lambs in the United States. *Vet Dermatol* 10: 73.

Jackson RB, et al. 1991. Endemic *Microsporum canis* Infection in a Sheep Flock. *Aust Vet J* 68: 122.

Lindemann D, Böhm KH. 1994. Ausbreitung einer *Microsporum-canis*-Infektion in einem Landwirtschaftlichen Betriet (Fallbeschreibung). *Berl Münch Tierärztl Wochen* 107: 413.

Martin WB, Aitken ID. 2000. Diseases of Sheep. Ed 3. Blackwell Science, Oxford, United Kingdom.

McKellar Q, et al. 1987. Ringworm Outbreak in Housed Sheep. *Vet Rec* 121: 168.

Power SB, Malone A. 1987. An Outbreak of Ringworm in Sheep in Ireland caused by *Trichophyton verrucosum*. *Vet Rec* 121: 218.

Radostits OM, et al. 2000. A Textbook of the Diseases of Cattle, Sheep, Pigs, Goats, and Horses. Ed 9. WB Saunders, Philadelphia, PA.

Sargison ND, et al. 2002. Ringworm caused by *Trichophyton verrucosum*—an Emerging Problem in Sheep Flocks. *Vet Rec* 150: 755.

Tabosa IM, et al. 2004. Outbreaks of Pythiosis in Two Flocks of Sheep in Northeastern Brazil. *Vet Pathol* 41: 412.

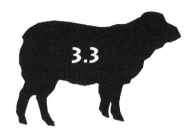

PARASITIC SKIN DISEASES

CHORIOPTIC MANGE

Features

Chorioptic mange ("foot mange," "scrotal mange") is uncommon in most parts of the world. It is caused by the mite *Chorioptes ovis*. There are no apparent breed, age, or sex predilections. Mite populations are usually much larger during cold weather. Thus, clinical signs are usually seen, or are more severe, in winter. Transmission occurs by direct and indirect contact.

Lesions are most commonly seen on the nonwooled areas, especially the lower hind legs and scrotum, but may also be present on the front legs, udder and teats, and rump (Figs. 3.3-1 through 3.3-4). Erythema and papules progress to scaling, oozing, crusts, and alopecia. Pruritus is usually intense. Scrotal lesions can cause infertility in rams. Severe infestations can reduce growth rates, as well as milk and meat yields. Typically, multiple animals are affected. Humans are not affected.

Differential Diagnosis

Sarcoptic mange, psoroptic mange, pediculosis, zinc-responsive dermatitis, insect hypersensitivity, and atopic dermatitis.

Diagnosis

1. Microscopy (Skin Scrapings in Mineral Oil)—Psoroptid mites, 0.3 to 0.5 mm in length (Figs 3.3-5 and 3.3-6).

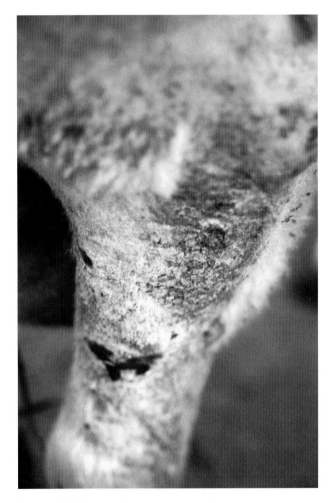

Figure 3.3-1 Chorioptic Mange. Alopecia, erythema, crusts, and excoriations on hind leg (courtesy J. Poncelet, coll. J. Gourreau, AFSSA).

2. Dermatohistopathology—Hyperplastic eosinophilic perivascular-to-interstitial dermatitis with eosinophilic epidermal microabscesses and parakeratotic hyperkeratosis (mites rarely seen).

PSOROPTIC MANGE

Features

Psoroptic mange ("sheep scab") is common to uncommon in most parts of the world. It is caused by the mite *Psoroptes ovis*. Differences in the pathogenicity or virulence of mite populations have been recognized and attributed to the existence of distinct "strains." In addition, *P. cuniculi* is an occasional cause of "ear

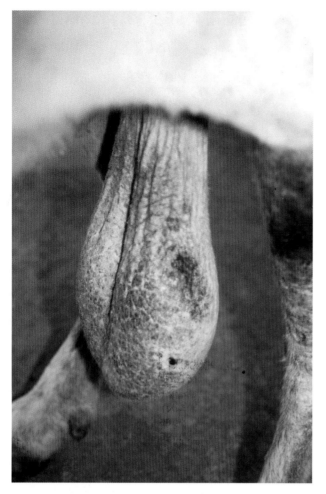

Figure 3.3-2 Chorioptic Mange. Crusts and erythema on scrotum (courtesy J. Poncelet, coll. J. Gourreau, AFSSA).

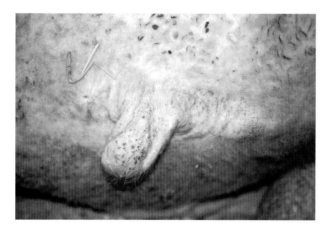

Figure 3.3-3 Chorioptic Mange. Erythema and crusts on udder (courtesy J. Poncelet, coll. J. Gourreau, AFSSA).

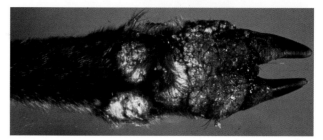

Figure 3.3-4 Chorioptic Mange. Severe crusting of foot (courtesy J. King).

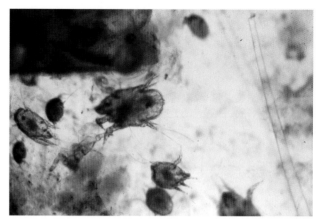

Figure 3.3-5 Chorioptic Mange. Multiple mites in a skin scraping.

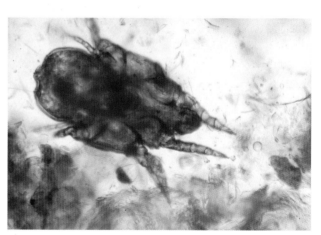

Figure 3.3-6 Chorioptic Mange. Adult mite in a skin scraping.

mites" in sheep. *P. ovis* allergens provoke an IgE-dependent immediate and late-phase response as well as a cell-mediated delayed-type hypersensitivity. There are no apparent breed, age, or sex predilections. Transmission occurs by direct and indirect contact. Mite populations are usually much larger during cold weather. Thus, clinical signs are usually seen, or are more severe, in winter.

The typical early signs of sheep scab are restlessness, head tossing, rubbing/chewing/scratching, and soiled/stained wool (especially over the shoulders). Early involvement of the shoulders, topline, and rump can progress to the entire body (Figs. 3.3-7 through 3.3-9). Vesicles and yellow to yellow-green pustules rupture, ooze, and develop into exuberant yellowish crusts. Typically the crust is surrounded by a moist yellow or faintly green zone of exudation with an outer ring of inflammation. Fleece overlying affected skin becomes increasingly stained, moist, soiled, and

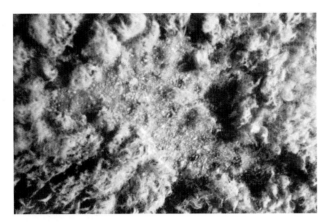

Figure 3.3-7 Psoroptic Mange. Alopecia, erythema, crusts, and excoriations over thorax (courtesy F. Personne, coll. J. Gourreau, AFSSA).

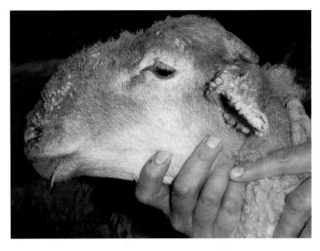

Figure 3.3-9 Psoroptic Mange. Thick crusts on pinna and bridge of nose (courtesy J. Natorp, coll. J. Gourreau, AFSSA).

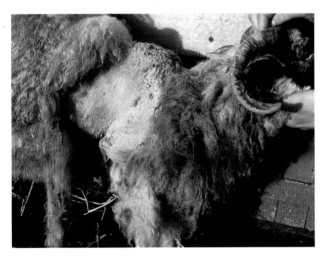

Figure 3.3-8 Psoroptic Mange. Alopecia, erythema, and thick yellow crusts over thorax (courtesy P. Scott).

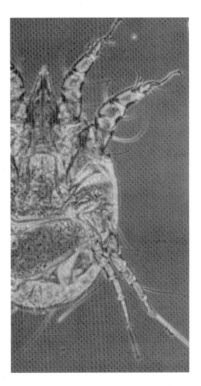

Figure 3.3-10 Psoroptic Mange. Adult *Psoroptes* mite (courtesy J. Georgi).

matted. Tufts and clumps of wool may be shed or pulled out, and self-trauma of exposed skin results in excoriations, ulcers, and secondary bacterial infection. Tags of loose wool are seen hanging from the fleece. Affected animals may be hyperesthetic and when stimulated by rubbing or scratching may exhibit a pronounced nibble reflex with protrusion of the tongue and lip smacking. Some animals will have seizures. Typically multiple animals are affected. Humans are not affected.

In some *P. ovis* outbreaks, clinical signs are limited to the ears. Head shaking and rubbing and scratching result in excoriation of the pinnae and base of the ears. Aural hematomas and resultant scarred and deformed ("cauliflower") pinnae may occur. As these animals typically have only ear involvement, the *P. ovis* populations involved may represent variant "strains" adapted to the otic environment. Occasionally, a similar syndrome may be produced by *P. cuniculi*.

In some animals, *P. ovis* mites persist in cryptic sites such as the groin, infraorbital fossa, perineum, and external auditory meatus.

Sheep scab can have devastating effects on sheep productivity: weight loss, reduced milk and meat productivity, downgrading of wool and hide, low birth weights of lambs and increased perina-

tal mortality, secondary bacterial infections, malnutrition, hypothermia, exhaustion, and death.

Differential Diagnosis

Sarcoptic mange, chorioptic mange, psorergatic mange, pediculosis, insect hypersensitivity, and atopic dermatitis.

Diagnosis

1. Microscopy (Skin Scrapings and/or Ear Swabs in Mineral Oil)—Psoroptid mites, 0.4 to 0.8 mm in length (Fig. 3.3-10). In sheep scab, mites tend to congregate at the margins of crusts.

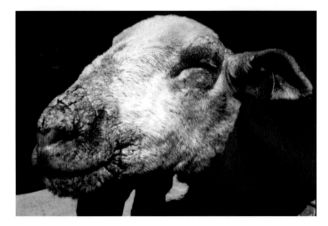

Figure 3.3-11 Sarcoptic Mange. Crusts on face and pinna (courtesy J. Poncelet, coll. J. Gourreau, AFSSA).

SARCOPTIC MANGE

Features

Sarcoptic mange (scabies, "head mange") is uncommon to rare in most parts of the world. It is caused by the mite *Sarcoptes scabiei var ovis*. There are no apparent breed, age, or sex predilections. Transmission occurs by direct and indirect contact.

Lesions are most commonly seen on the nonwooled areas such as the face, pinnae, and legs (Fig. 3.3-11). Erythema and papules progress to scaling, oozing, crusts, and alopecia. Pruritus is intense. Excoriation, lichenification, and hyperkeratosis are prominent in chronic cases. Peripheral lymphadenopathy is usually moderate to marked. Typically, multiple animals are affected. Weight loss, decreased milk production, hide damage, secondary bacterial (usually staphylococcal) pyoderma, and myiasis can occur due to the intense pruritus and irritation.

Sarcoptic mange is a potential zoonosis. Affected humans develop pruritic erythematous papules with crusts and excoriations on the arms, chest, abdomen, and legs (Fig. 3.3-12). In addition, although *Sarcoptes* mites tend to be species-specific, cross-infestation is possible, especially between sheep and goats.

Differential Diagnosis

Psoroptic mange, chorioptic mange, pediculosis, zinc-responsive dermatitis, insect hypersensitivity, and atopic dermatitis.

Diagnosis

1. Microscopy (Skin Scrapings in Mineral Oil)—Sarcoptic mites, 0.25 to 0.6 mm in length (Figs. 3.3-13 and 3.3-14). Ova (eggs) and scyballa (fecal pellets) may also be found (Fig. 3.3-15). Mites are often difficult to find, especially in chronic cases.
2. Dermatohistopathology—Hyperplastic eosinophilic perivascular-to-interstitial dermis with eosinophilic epidermal microabscesses and parakeratotic hyperkeratosis (mites rarely seen).

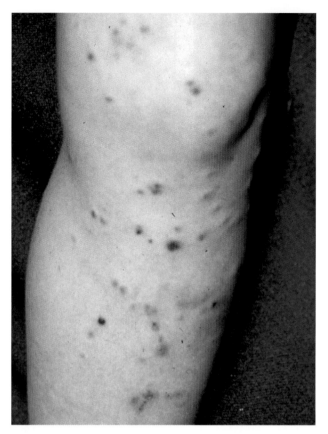

Figure 3.3-12 Sarcoptic Mange. Erythematous and crusted papules on the leg of a human with animal-origin scabies.

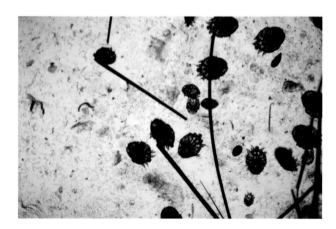

Figure 3.3-13 Sarcoptic Mange. Multiple mites in a skin scraping.

PEDICULOSIS

Features

Pediculosis (lice) is a common, cosmopolitan infestation caused by various lice. In the United States, recognized sheep lice include *Damalinia (Bovicola) ovis* (biting louse, "body louse," order Mallophaga) and *Linognathus ovillis* ("face louse") and *L. pedalis* ("foot louse") (sucking lice, order Anoplura). There are no apparent breed, age, or sex predilections. Louse populations are usually much larger during cold weather. Thus clinical signs are usually

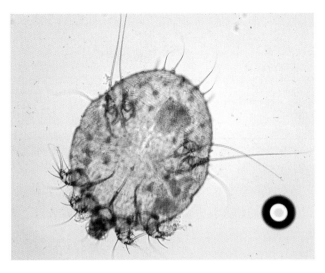

Figure 3.3-14 Sarcoptic Mange. Adult mite in a skin scraping.

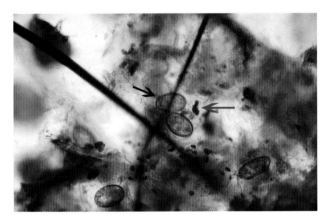

Figure 3.3-15 Sarcoptic Mange. Multiple eggs (black arrow) and fecal pellets (red arrow) in a skin scraping.

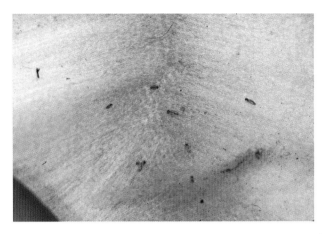

Figure 3.3-16 Pediculosis. Erythema, scaling, and numerous biting lice over back.

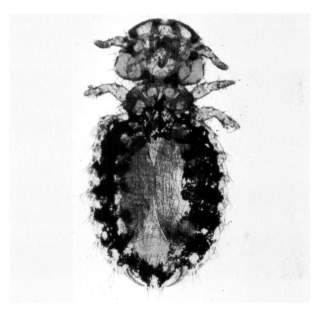

Figure 3.3-17 Pediculosis. Biting louse.

seen or are more severe in winter. Transmission occurs by direct and indirect contact.

D. ovis is most commonly seen over the dorsum, *L. ovillis* on the face, and *L. pedalis* on the legs and scrotum. Some animals will show no clinical signs. Most animals will have variable combinations of scaling, crusting, erythema, excoriation, and hair or wool loss (Fig. 3.3-16). Pruritus is usually marked, with affected animals constantly rubbing, chewing, scratching, and/or stomping. Louse infestations can be heavy in debilitated animals. Large populations of lice can cause anemia, especially in lambs. Heavy infestations can cause unthriftiness, decreased growth, and damage to wool and hides. Typically multiple animals are affected. Humans are not affected. *D. ovis* can be transmitted between sheep and goats.

Differential Diagnosis

Sarcoptic mange, chorioptic mange, psoroptic mange, psorergatic mange, and keds.

Diagnosis

1. History and Physical Examination—Sucking lice are bluish-gray in color. Biting lice are pale to brownish in color.
2. Microscopy (Lice and Hairs/Wool Fibers Placed in Mineral Oil)—Adult lice are large (3 to 6 mm in length) (Figs. 3.3-17 and 3.3-18). Ova (nits) are 1 to 2 mm in length and may be found attached to hair shafts/wool fibers (Fig. 3.3-19).

CALLIPHORINE MYIASIS

Features

Calliphorine myiasis (Greek: condition caused by flies) ("maggots," "flystrike") is common and cosmopolitan. *Lucilia* spp., *Phormia* spp., and *Calliphora* spp. flies are most important. Adult flies are attracted to decomposing organic matter (wounds, infections, soiled wool, etc.). Other predispositions include skin folds,

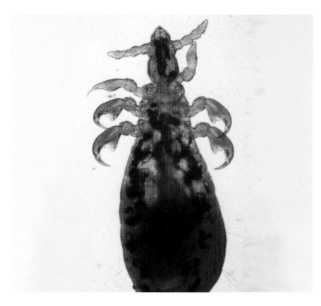

Figure 3.3-18 Pediculosis. Sucking louse.

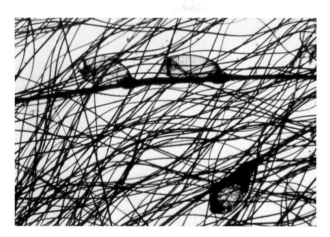

Figure 3.3-19 Pediculosis. Nits on hair shaft.

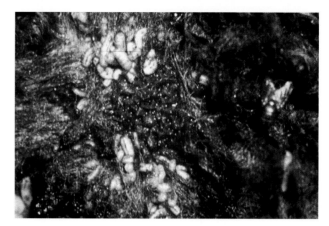

Figure 3.3-20 Calliphorine myiasis. Alopecia, ulceration, maggots, and flies (courtesy M. Smith).

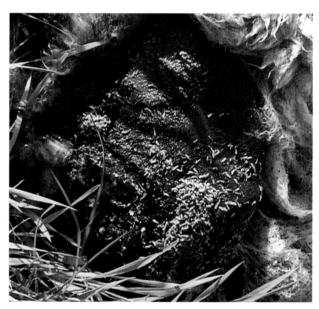

Figure 3.3-21 Calliphorine myiasis. Alopecia, ulceration, and numerous maggots (courtesy P. Scott).

long and/or fine wool, high temperature and humidity, and heavy rain. *Wohlfahrtia magnifica* is a sarcophagid fly, and the most important cause of traumatic myiasis in the Mediterranean Basin and parts of Europe. It especially affects the genitalia (breeding and lambing seasons), the heads of males (butting behavior), and shearing wounds. Calliphorine myiasis is most common in late spring, summer, and early fall.

Clinically, calliphorine myiasis is frequently classified in terms of the anatomic site attacked:

1. Wound strike
2. Breech strike
3. Tail strike
4. Head or poll strike
5. Pizzle (prepuce) strike
6. Foot strike
7. Body (usually dorsum) strike

Lesions are pruritic and painful, and animals shake, stomp, rub, scratch, and/or chew affected areas. Lesions consist of matted wool, alopecia, and foul-smelling ulcers, often with scalloped margins (Figs. 3.3-20 and 3.3-21). The ulcers often have a "honeycombed" appearance and are teeming with larvae ("maggots"). Animals are constantly agitated, and may die of toxemia and septicemia.

Diagnosis

1. History and physical examination.

MISCELLANEOUS PARASITIC DISEASES

Table 3.3-1 Miscellaneous Parasitic Diseases

Demodectic mange ("follicular mange") (Fig. 3.3-22)	Uncommon to rare; cosmopolitan; *Demodex ovis* (0.2 to 0.3 mm in length); no breed, age, sex predilections; asymptomatic papules and nodules; especially face, chin, and pinnae; widespread lesions and secondary bacterial (usually staphylococcal) infections usually seen in animals debilitated for other reasons; thick, caseous, whitish material expressed from incised lesion contains numerous mites (Fig. 3.3-23)
Psorergatic mange ("psorobic mange")	Uncommon and cosmopolitan; *Psorergates (Psorobia) ovis* (0.1 to 0.2 mm in length); especially winter and spring; especially Merinos; intense pruritus with rubbing, chewing, and kicking at fleece; matted, chewed, broken, and absent wool over lateral thorax, flanks, and thighs; scaling
Trombiculosis ("chiggers," "harvest mite")	Rare and cosmopolitan; late summer and fall; infested woods and fields; legs, face, pinnae, axillae, groin; papulocrustous dermatitis and variable pruritus; trombiculid larvae (0.2 to 0.4 mm in length, red to orange in color); e.g., *Trombicula (Eutrombicula) alfreddugesi, T. (Neotrombicula) autumnalis, T. sarcina*
Ticks	Common and cosmopolitan; most in spring and summer; especially ears, face, neck, axillae, groin, and legs; minimal lesions or papules and nodules centered around attached ticks; variable pain and pruritus; e.g., *Otobius megnini, Ixodes scapularis, I. cookei, I. pacificus, Rhipicephalus sanguineous, Dermacentor andersonii,* and *D. variabilis* in the United States; *D. reticulatus* reported to cause severe pruritus in the United Kingdom
Keds ("sheep ticks") (Fig. 3.3-24)	Uncommon and cosmopolitan; *Melophagus ovinus* (4 to 7 mm in length, red-brown in color); usually fall and winter; no breed, age, or sex predilections; especially long-wooled breeds; especially neck, sides, rump, and abdomen; intense pruritus results in broken wool, alopecia, and excoriations; heavy infestations can stain the wool (ked excrement) and cause anemia; keds transmit bluetongue virus
Fleas	Uncommon and cosmopolitan; *Ctenocephalides felis* ("cat flea"), 2 to 4 mm in length, brown in color; especially summer and fall; variable degrees of pruritus and papulocrustous dermatitis; especially legs and ventrum; some animals may develop hypersensitivity (allergy) to flea salivary antigens (see Chapter 3.5); heavy infestations in kids and debilitated animals may cause anemia and even death
Hydrotaea irritans flies ("head fly")	Common; Europe and Australia; especially summer; swarming flies initiate headshaking, rubbing, and scratching; excoriations progress to nonhealing ulcers and black crusts ("broken head," "black cap"); possible secondary bacterial infections and myiasis
Przhevalskiana silenus infestation	Uncommon, Asia and Europe; spring and early summer; subcutaneous nodules and cysts over back; lesions develop central pore in which third-stage larvae may be seen (10 to 12 mm in length)
Dermatobia hominis infestation	Uncommon; Central and South America; painful subcutaneous nodules with a central pore containing third-stage larvae (about 20 mm in length)
Screw-worm myiasis	Uncommon; Central and South America (*Callitroga hominivorax* and *C. macellaria*); Africa and Asia (*Chrysomyia bezziana* and *C. megacephala*); especially late spring, summer, and early fall; any wounded/damaged skin; foul-smelling ulcers with scalloped margins and a "honeycombed" appearance, teeming with larvae; painful and pruritic; humans are susceptible (e.g., skin, genitalia, ears, sinuses)
Elaeophoriasis ("sore head")	Uncommon; mountain ranges of western and southwestern United States; *Elaeophora schneideri* from mule deer (horse flies are intermediate hosts); no breed, age, or sex predilections; unilateral ulceration, hemorrhage, and pruritus of head, face, limbs, abdomen, and feet; dermatohistopathology
Strongyloidosis	Uncommon and cosmopolitan; no breed, age, and sex predilections; *Strongyloides papillosus*; pruritic dermatitis of feet, legs, and ventrum; fecal flotation
Pelodera dermatitis (rhabditic dermatitis)	Rare; mostly North America; no breed, age, or sex predilections; *Pelodera (Rhabditis) strongyloides* from filthy environment; pruritic dermatitis of feet, legs, and ventrum; skin scrapings (0.6 mm in length nematode larvae)
Hookworm dermatitis	Rare and cosmopolitan; no breed, age, or sex predilections; *Bunostomum trigonocephalum*; pruritic dermatitis of feet, legs, and ventrum; fecal flotation

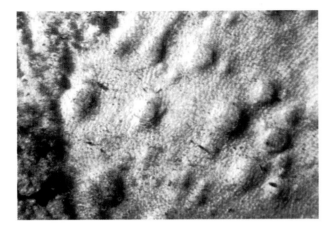

Figure 3.3-22 Demodectic Mange. Numerous nodules in clipped thoracic skin (courtesy C. Rees).

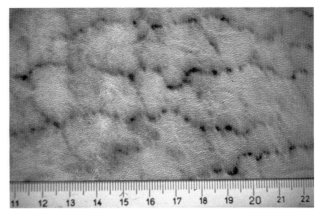

Figure 3.3-24 Keds. Numerous keds in wool over thorax (courtesy F. Personne, coll. J. Gourreau, AFSSA).

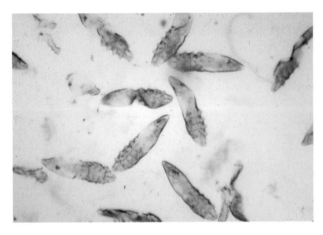

Figure 3.3-23 Demodectic Mange. Numerous mites from an incised and squeezed lesion.

REFERENCES

Abo-Shehada MN. 2005. Incidence of *Chrysomya bezziana* Screw-worm Myiasis in Saudi Arabia, 1999/2000. *Vet Rec* 156: 354.

Argüello MRH, et al. 2001. Effect of Moxidectin 1% Injectable Against Natural Infection of *Sarcoptes scabiei* in Sheep. *Vet Parasitol* 102: 143.

Bates PG. 1991. Ear Mites in Sheep. *Vet Rec* 128: 555.

Bates PG. 1996. Epidemiology of Subclinical Ovine Psoroptic Otoacariasis in Great Britain. *Vet Rec* 138: 388.

Ibrahim KEE, et al. 1987. Experimental Transmission of a Goat Strain of *Sarcoptes scabiei* to Desert Sheep and Its Treatment with Ivermectin. *Vet Parasitol* 26: 157.

Lee AJ, et al. 2002. Identification of an Antigen from the Sheep Scab Mite, *Psoroptes ovis*, Homologous with House Dust Mite Group I Allergens. *Parasite Immunol* 24: 413.

Lewis C. 1997. Update on Sheep Scab. *In Pract* 19: 558.

Martin WB, and Aitken ID. 2000. Diseases of Sheep. Ed. 3. Blackwell Science, Malden, MA.

Matthes HF, et al. 1996. Cross-Reacting Antibodies to *Sarcoptes suis*, *Chorioptes bovis*, and *Notoedres cati* and Anti-*P. ovis* IgE in Sera from Sheep Infested Naturally with *Psoroptes ovis*. *Int J Parasitol* 26: 437.

Meintjes T, et al. 2002. Host Preference of the Sheep Scab Mite, *Psoroptes ovis*. *J S Afr Vet Assoc* 73: 135.

Meintjes T, et al. 2002. On-Host Ecology and Off-Host Survival of the Sheep Scab Mite *Psoroptes ovis*. *Onderstepoort J Vet Res* 69: 273.

Meintjes T, et al. 2002. The Rate of Spread of Sheep Scab Within Small Groups of Merino and Dorper Sheep. *J S Afr Vet Assoc* 73: 137.

Morgan KL. 1991. Aural Haematomata, Cauliflower Ears, and *Psoroptes ovis* in Sheep. *Vet Rec* 128: 459.

Morgan KL. 1992. Parasitic Otitis in Sheep Associated with *Psoroptes* Infestation: A Clinical and Epidemiological Study. *Vet Rec* 130: 530.

O'Brien DJ, et al. 1994. Examination of Possible Transmission of Sheep Scab Mite *Psoroptes ovis* Between Host Species. *Vet Res Comm* 18: 113.

O'Brien DJ, et al. 1994. Survival and Retention of Infectivity of the Mite *Psoroptes ovis* Off the Host. *Vet Res Comm* 18: 27.

Radostits OM, et al. 2000. Veterinary Medicine. A Textbook of the Diseases of Cattle, Sheep, Pigs, Goats and Horses. Ed 9. WB Saunders, Philadelphia, PA.

Ramos JJ, et al. 1996. *Pelodera* Dermatitis in Sheep. *Vet Rec* 138: 474.

Scott DW. 1988. Large Animal Dermatology. WB Saunders, Philadelphia, PA.

Sinclair A. 1990. The Epidermal Location and Possible Feeding Site of *Psorergates ovis*, the Sheep Itch Mite. *Aust Vet J* 67: 59.

Small RW. 2005. A Review of *Melophagus ovinus* (L.), the Sheep Ked. *Vet Parasitol* 130: 141.

Sotiraki S, et al. 2005. Wohlfahrtiosis in Sheep and the Role of Dicyclanil in Its Prevention. *Vet Parasitol* 131: 107.

van den Broek AHM, et al. 2003. Cutaneous Hypersensitivity Reactions to *Psoroptes ovis* and Derp 1 in Sheep Previously Infested with *P. ovis*—the Sheep Scab Mite. *Vet Immunol Immunopathol* 91: 105.

van den Broek AH, Huntley JF. 2003. Sheep Scab: The Disease, Pathogenesis and Control. *J Comp Pathol* 128: 79.

VLA Surveillance Report. 2005. Sheep. *Vet Rec* 156: 161.

Winter AC. 1995. Wool Loss in Sheep. *Vet Annu* 35: 313.

Yeruham I, et al. 1986. Sheep Demodicosis (*Demodex ovis* Railliet, 1895) in Israel. *Rév Elev Méd Vét Pays Trop* 39: 363.

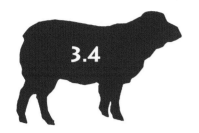

VIRAL AND PROTOZOAL SKIN DISEASES

3.4

Contagious Viral Pustular Dermatitis
Capripoxvirus Infection
Bluetongue
Foot-and-Mouth Disease
Miscellaneous Viral and Protozoal Diseases
    Border Disease
    Leishmaniosis
    Peste des Petits Ruminants
    Pseudorabies
    Rinderpest
    Scrapie
    Ulcerative Dermatosis

CONTAGIOUS VIRAL PUSTULAR DERMATITIS

Features

Contagious viral pustular dermatitis ("contagious ecthyma," "orf," "soremouth," "scabby mouth," "contagious pustular dermatitis," "thistle disease") is a common, cosmopolitan disease caused by *Parapoxvirus ovis*. Transmission occurs through contamination of skin abrasions. There are no apparent breed or sex predilections. Although all ages can be affected, the disease is primarily seen in 3 to 6 month old lambs. The disease tends to be seasonal, occurring most commonly in spring (lambing season) and toward the end of summer.

Lesions progress from papules to vesicles, and to pustules which become umbilicated and thickly crusted. Lesions are often painful, but not pruritic. Nonwooled areas of skin are primarily affected. In lambs, the lips, muzzle, nostrils, eyelids, and pinnae are most commonly affected (Figs. 3.4-1 through 3.4-3). The oral cavity, axillae, groin, coronets, interdigital spaces (Fig. 3.4-4), scrotum, teats, udder (Figs. 3.4-5 and 3.4-6), vulva, perineum, and distal legs are less commonly involved. Occasionally there is a generalized swelling of the head (*not* the pinnae) (Fig. 3.4-7). Oral lesions are raised, red-to-gray–to-yellowish papules and plaques with a surrounding zone of hyperemia, that become ulcerated (Fig. 3.4-8). Lesions may occur at the sites of various injuries such as tail-docking, ear-tagging, healing burns, and surgical sites. Generalized lesions may occur in animals debilitated for other reasons.

A so-called *papillomatous form* of the infection is seen, especially in rams, wherein large, persistent, proliferative "cauliflowerlike" and even pedunculated lesions up to 10 cm in diameter are seen on the head, pinnae, or distal legs (Figs. 3.4-9 through 3.4-11). So-called "strawberry foot rot" is seen on the coronets and distal legs, wherein fissured proliferative lesions expose raw, bleeding tissue which resembles "mashed strawberries." *Derma-*

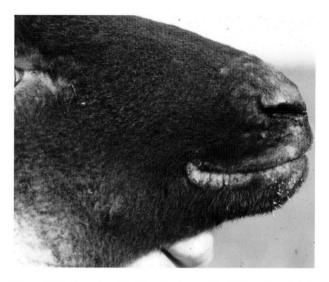

Figure 3.4-1 Contagious Viral Pustular Dermatitis. Mildly affected adult with crusts on the lips, muzzle, and nostrils.

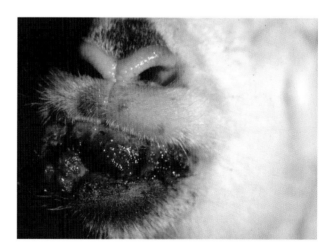

Figure 3.4-2 Contagious Viral Pustular Dermatitis. Proliferative crusts and ulcers on the lips of a lamb.

tophilus congolensis infection may complicate these lesions. In the so-called *venereal form*, small pustules and ulcers are seen on the mucocutaneous junction of the vulva (Fig. 3.4-12) and prepuce.

Occasionally, severe and persistent infections are seen. Extensive, proliferative, (sometimes "wart-like") and painful lesions occur (Fig. 3.4-13). Whether this involves different viral strains or genetic/immunologic susceptibility is not known.

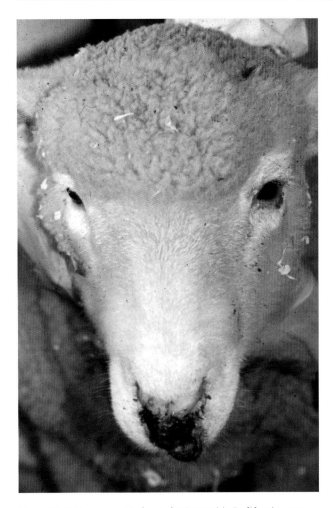

Figure 3.4-3 Contagious Viral Pustular Dermatitis. Proliferative crust and ulcer on the muzzle.

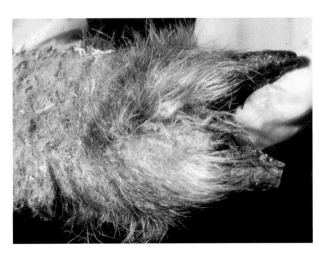

Figure 3.4-4 Contagious Viral Pustular Dermatitis. Proliferative ulcer and oozing of interdigital space.

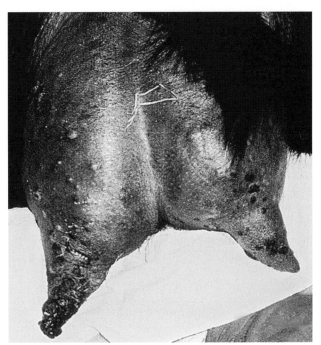

Figure 3.4-5 Contagious Viral Pustular Dermatitis. Multiple pustules and crusts on udder and teats (courtesy J. Gourreau).

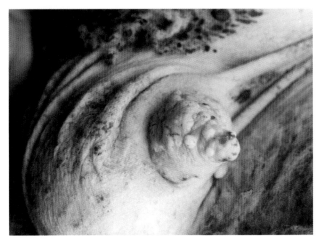

Figure 3.4-6 Contagious Viral Pustular Dermatitis. Pustules and crusts on teat and udder (courtesy R. Braque, coll. J. Gourreau, AFSSA).

Signs of systemic illness may include fever, depression, and decreased food consumption. Significant economic losses occur through loss of condition (failure to suck or eat), mastitis, abandonment, and secondary bacterial infections and myiasis. Morbidity in lambs usually approaches 100%, while mortality is usually around 1%, although it can be as high as 20%. Sheep are susceptible.

Contagious viral pustular dermatitis is a zoonosis. In humans, the condition is often called "ecthyma contagiosum," "orf," or "farmyard pox." Transmission can be direct, indirect, and even human-to-human. Lesions may be solitary or multiple, and occur most commonly on the fingers, arm, face, and leg (Figs. 3.4-14 and 3.4-15). Erythematous papules evolve into nodules with a red center, a white middle ring, and a red periphery. The lesions initially have a red, oozing surface, which then develops a dry crust through which black dots may be seen. Lastly, the lesions develop a papillomatous surface, a thick crust, and then regress. There is variable pain and pruritus.

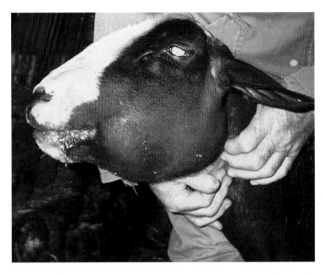

Figure 3.4-7 Contagious Viral Pustular Dermatitis. Extensive edema of head, but not pinnae (courtesy A. Quet, coll. J. Gourreau, AFSSA).

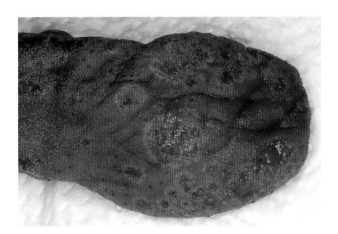

Figure 3.4-8 Contagious Viral Pustular Dermatitis. Ulcerated papules and plaque on tongue (courtesy J. Gourreau).

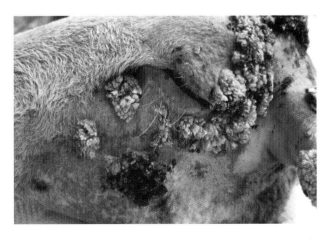

Figure 3.4-9 Contagious Viral Pustular Dermatitis. Multiple "wart-like" lesions in periocular region (courtesy of J. Gourreau).

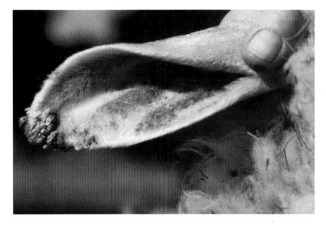

Figure 3.4-10 Contagious Viral Pustular Dermatitis. Wart-like lesions on tip of pinna (courtesy M. Maillet, coll. J. Gourreau, AFSSA).

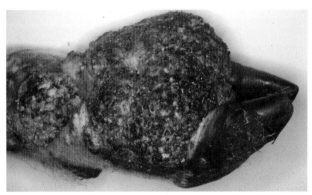

Figure 3.4-11 Contagious Viral Pustular Dermatitis. Wart-like lesions on distal leg (courtesy J. Gourreau).

Differential Diagnosis

Dermatophilosis, staphylococcal folliculitis, *Capripoxvirus* infection, ulcerative dermatosis, and zinc-responsive dermatitis.

Diagnosis

1. History and physical examination.
2. Dermatohistopathology and Electron Microscopy— Eosinophilic intracytoplasmic inclusion bodies in epithelial keratinocytes.
3. Viral isolation.
4. Viral antigen detection.

CAPRIPOXVIRUS INFECTION

Features

Capripoxvirus ("sheeppox") infections vary in severity, presumably because of differences in viral strains and/or host susceptibility. The disease occurs in the Middle East, Asia, Africa, and parts of Europe. Transmission occurs via contamination of skin abrasions, aerosol, or insect vectors. There are no apparent breed or sex predilections. Although all ages are susceptible, the disease is more severe in the young.

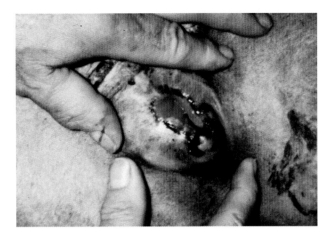

Figure 3.4-12 Contagious Viral Pustular Dermatitis. Ulcers and crusts at mucocutaneous junction of vulva (courtesy L. Rehby, coll. J. Gourreau, AFSSA).

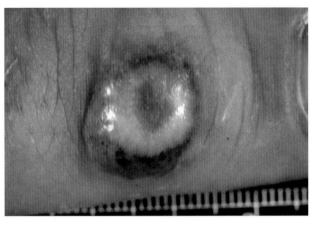

Figure 3.4-15 Contagious Viral Pustular Dermatitis. Solitary nodule (pustular, umbilicated, erythematous halo) on thumb of a human.

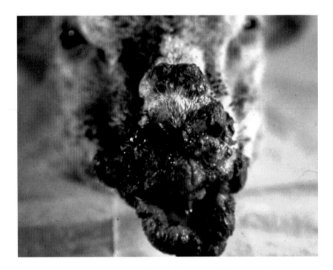

Figure 3.4-13 Contagious Viral Pustular Dermatitis. Extensive, severe proliferative crusts and ulcers (courtesy J. Asso, coll. J. Gourreau, AFSSA).

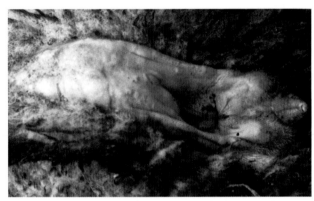

Figure 3.4-16 *Capripoxvirus* Infection. Multiple pustules on ventral tail and vulva. (courtesy J. Gourreau).

Initial pyrexia, depression, anorexia, rhinitis, and conjunctivitis are followed by skin lesions. Erythematous macules, papules, nodules, and pustules are seen. Vesicles are rarely observed. Pustules become umbilicated, ooze, and become crusted. Lesions often initially appear on hairless areas such as the ventral surface of the tail (Figs. 3.4-16 and 3.4-17), perineum, axillae, groin, and lateral (concave) surface of the pinnae. Lesions then commonly involve the lips, muzzle (Fig. 3.4-18), nostrils, eyelids, udder, teats, prepuce, and vulva. The entire body surface can be affected, as well as the oral mucosa. Oral lesions become ulcerated. Respiratory distress and facial edema are common. Mastitis may complicate teat lesions. A benign form occurs in adults, wherein only skin lesions are seen, especially on the ventral surface of the tail and perineal area.

Morbidity and mortality are usually 20% to 30%, but occasionally 70% to 80%. Economic losses include decreased meat, milk, and wool production, trade embargoes, and deaths. Presumably due to viral strain differences, goats may or may not be affected in a given outbreak.

Although a few literature reports indicate that ovine *Capripoxvirus* infections can be transmitted to humans (see contagious viral pustular dermatitis), current literature discounts this possibility.

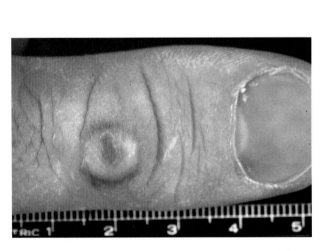

Figure 3.4-14 Contagious Viral Pustular Dermatitis. Solitary nodule (pustular, umbilicated, crusted, erythematous halo) on thumb of a human.

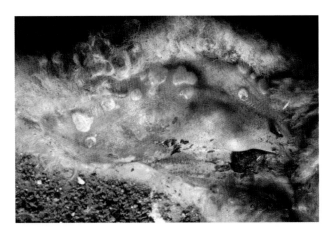

Figure 3.4-17 *Capripoxvirus* Infection. Many pustules—some of which are umbilicated—on ventral tail (courtesy J. Gourreau).

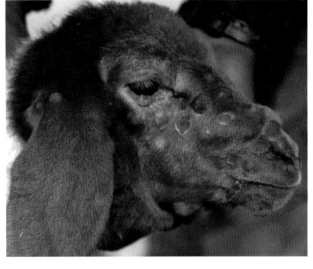

Figure 3.4-18 *Capripoxvirus* Infection. Multiple crusted nodules on face and pinna (courtesy J. Gourreau).

Differential Diagnosis

Contagious viral pustular dermatitis, staphylococcal folliculitis, dermatophilosis, bluetongue, peste des petits ruminants, and rinderpest.

Diagnosis

1. History and physical examination.
2. Dermatohistopathology and Electron Microscopy—Eosinophilic intracytoplasmic inclusion bodies in epithelial keratinocytes.
3. Necropsy examination.
4. Viral isolation.
5. Viral antigen detection.

BLUETONGUE

Features

Bluetongue ("soremouth," "sore muzzle," "ovine catarrhal fever") is an uncommon, cosmopolitan disease caused by an *Orbivirus*. Transmission occurs via *Culicoides* spp. gnats. There are no apparent breed, age, or sex predilections.

Fever, stiffness, lameness, and reluctance to move are often the first signs of infection. Affected animals often stand with an arched back, the head lowered, and the pinnae drooping due to edema. The lips, muzzle, coronets, feet, and less often the anus and vulva, are erythematous, edematous, and may develop ulcers and crusts (Figs. 3.4-19 and 3.4-20). The appearance of a dark red to purple band in the skin just above the coronet, when it occurs, is an important sign (Fig. 3.4-21). Cracking and separation of the hooves may be seen. The oral mucosa is hyperemic, and edematous, and the tongue is occasionally cyanotic ("blue tongue") (Fig. 3.4-22). Nasal discharge and hypersalivation are common. Anagen defluxion ("wool break") is common.

Morbidity may approach 50% to 75% and mortality varies from 0% to 50%. Economic losses include deaths, loss of meat and wool production, and trade embargoes.

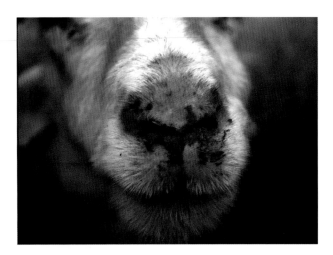

Figure 3.4-19 Bluetongue. Erythema, edema, and crusting of the muzzle (courtesy J. Gourreau).

Differential Diagnosis

Foot-and-mouth disease, *Capripoxvirus* infection, peste des petits ruminants, and rinderpest.

Diagnosis

1. History and physical examination.
2. Necropsy examination.
3. Viral isolation.
4. Viral antigen detection.

FOOT-AND-MOUTH DISEASE

Features

Foot-and-mouth disease ("aphthous fever"—Greek: painful vesicles and ulcers in mouth) is a highly contagious infectious disease of ruminants and swine caused by an *Aphthovirus* having seven

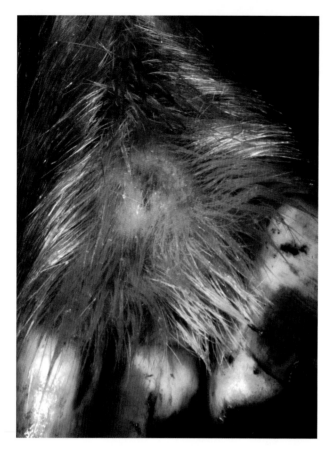

Figure 3.4-20 Bluetongue. Erythema and edema of the foot (courtesy J. Gourreau).

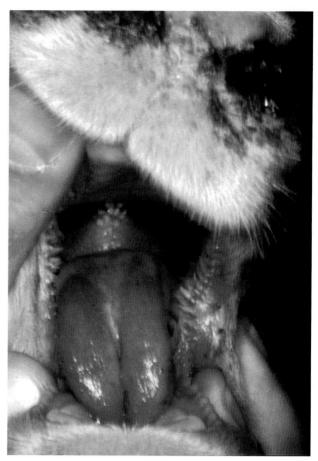

Figure 3.4-22 Bluetongue. Cyanotic ("blue") tongue (courtesy J. Gourreau).

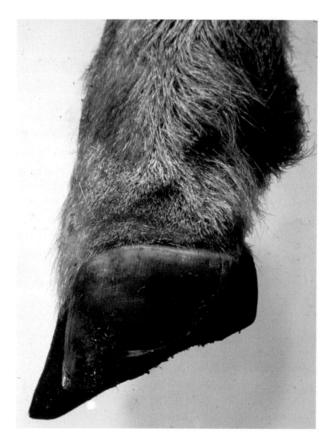

Figure 3.4-21 Bluetongue. Coronitis (courtesy J. King).

principal serotypes: A, O, C, South African Territories (SAT) 1, SAT 2, SAT 3, and Asia 1. The disease is endemic in Africa, Asia, and South America, and sporadic in Europe. Transmission occurs via aerosol, contact, insect vectors, and fomites. There are no breed, age, or sex predilections.

Lameness, fever, depression, and inappetence are usually the first signs of infection. Affected feet are hot and painful. Vesicles and bullae result in painful erosions and ulcers in the mouth, especially on the dental pad, and on the legs and occasionally the nostrils (Fig. 3.4-23). Lesions also occur on the coronets (Fig. 3.4-24), bulbs of the heels, the interdigital spaces, and occasionally the udder, teats, vulva, and prepuce.

Morbidity varies from 50% to 100% and mortality is usually low (less than 5%). Economic losses can be devastating: quarantine, slaughter, embargoes, and loss of trade. Foot-and-mouth disease is the number one foreign animal disease threat in the United States, and the most significant disease affecting free trade in animals and animal products internationally.

Humans may rarely develop vesicles on the hands (Fig. 3.4-25) and/or in the mouth.

Differential Diagnosis

Bluetongue, *Capripoxvirus* infection, peste des petits ruminants, and rinderpest.

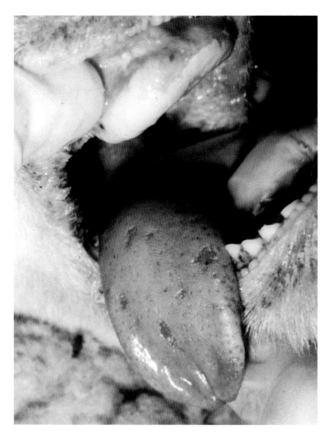

Figure 3.4-23 Foot-and-Mouth Disease. Multiple ulcers on tongue (courtesy S. Hammami, coll. J. Gourreau, AFSSA).

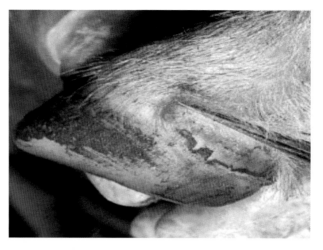

Figure 3.4-24 Foot-and-Mouth Disease. Ulceration of coronet (courtesy J. Gourreau).

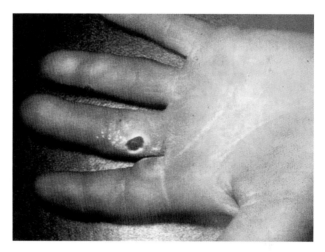

Figure 3.4-25 Foot-and-Mouth Disease. Ruptured vesicle on finger of a human (courtesy J. Gourreau).

Diagnosis

1. Virus Isolation—Vesicular fluid, epithelial lesions, heparinized blood.
2. Serology—Clotted blood.

MISCELLANEOUS VIRAL AND PROTOZOAL DISEASES

Table 3.4-1 Miscellaneous Viral and Protozoal Diseases

Border disease ("hairy shakers," "fuzzies," "hypomyelinogenesis congenita") (*Pestivirus*)	Uncommon to rare; cosmopolitan; neonatal neurological dysfunction (variable degrees of tremors to tonic-clonic skeletal muscle contractions involving the whole body ("shakers"); large, long primary hairs and wool fibers rise above the coat to form a halo over the dorsal neck, back, flanks, and rump ("hairy"); abnormal coat may also be abnormally pigmented; necropsy examination, viral isolation, viral antigen detection
Leishmaniosis	Very rare; South Africa; *Leishmania* sp.; crusts, alopecia, and edema; pinnae, nostrils, muzzle, lips, periocular region, face; dermatohistopathology
Peste des petits ruminants ("goat plague," "goat catarrhal fever," "Kata," "pseudorinderpest")(*Morbillivirus*)	Uncommon; Africa, Southeast Asia, and Middle East; ulcers on oral, nasal and ocular muscosae; ulcers and crusts of lips, eyelids, and nostrils; fever, ocular and nasal discharge, hypersalivation, and pneumonia; goats are susceptible; necropsy examination, viral isolation, viral antigen detection
Pseudorabies (Aujesky's disease, "mad itch") (Porcine *Herpesvirus 1*)	Very rare; cosmopolitan; intense, localized, unilateral pruritus with frenzied, violent licking, chewing, rubbing, and kicking at affected area; especially head, neck, thorax, flank, and perineum; fever, excitement, circling, convulsions, paralysis; cattle and goats are susceptible; viral antigen detection
Rinderpest ("cattle plague") (*Morbillivirus*)	Rare; Africa and Asia; ulcers on oral, nasal, and ocular mucosae; ulcers and crusts of lips, eyelids, and nostrils; fever, ocular and nasal discharge, hypersalivation, and diarrhea; cattle, swine, and goats are susceptible; necropsy examination, viral isolation, viral antigen detection
Scrapie (Fig. 3.4-26)	Uncommon; cosmopolitan; prion protein; 10% to 50% of flock; especially 2 to 5 years old; more or less bilaterally symmetrical intense pruritus results in wool loss; especially rump with cranial spread (Fig. 3.4-26); when lesional areas are rubbed, a characteristic nibbling response occurs ("the provocative scrapie test"); ataxia, incoordination, falling, muscle tremors, grinding of teeth (bruxism), trembling and spontaneous aggression:; brain histopathology, various immunohistochemical and Western blot procedures
Ulcerative dermatosis ("lip-and-leg ulcers," "ovine venereal disease") (unclassified *Poxvirus*) (Fig. 3.4-27)	Uncommon to rare; cosmopolitan; granulating ulcers (1 to 5 cm diameter) between lip and nostril (lip form) or interdigital spaces on craniolateral aspect of feet above coronet (leg form) or on prepucial orifice or vulva (venereal form); dermatohistopathology, viral isolation, viral antigen detection

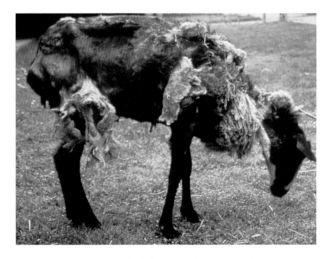

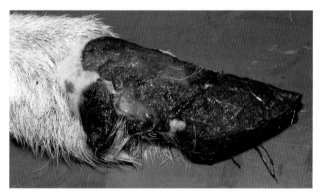

Figure 3.4-27 Ulcerative Dermatosis. Ulceration of leg above coronet (courtesy of P. Hill).

Figure 3.4-26 Scrapie. Marked alopecia and emaciation (courtesy J. Brugère-Picoux, coll. J. Gourreau, AFSSA).

REFERENCES

Buttner M, Rziha HJ. 2002. Parapoxviruses: From the Lesion to the Viral Genome. *J Vet Med B* 49: 7.

Cam Y, et al. 2005. Peste des Petits Ruminants in a Sheep and Goat Flock in Kayseri Province, Turkey. *Vet Rec* 157: 523.

Gavier-Widén D, et al. 2005. Diagnosis of Transmissible Spongiform Encephalopathies in Animals: A Review. *J Vet Diagn Invest* 17: 509.

Hajer I, et al. 1988. Capripox Virus in Sheep and Goats in Sudan. *Rev Elev Med Vet Pay Trop* 41: 125.

Hooser SB, et al. 1989. Atypical Contagious Ecthyma in a Sheep After Extensive Cutaneous Thermal Injury. *J Am Vet Med Assoc* 195: 1255.

Lewis C. 1996. Update on Orf. *In Pract* 18: 376.

Linnabarry RD, et al. 1991. Scrapie in Sheep. *Compend Cont Educ* 13: 511.

Martin WB, Aitken ID. 2000. Diseases of Sheep. Ed 3. Blackwell Science, Maulden, MA.

Radostits OM, et al. 2000. Veterinary Medicine. A Textbook of the Diseases of Cattle, Sheep, Pigs, Goats and Horses. Ed 9. WB Saunders, Philadelphia, PA

Scott DW. 1988. Large Animal Dermatology. WB Saunders Co, Philadelphia, PA.

Smith GW, et al. 2002. Atypical Parapoxvirus Infection in Sheep. *J Vet Intern Med* 16: 287.

Van Der Lugt JJ, et al. 1992. Cutaneous Leishmaniosis in a Sheep. *J S Afr Vet Assoc* 63: 74.

Wadhwa DR, et al. 2002. Occurrence of Peste des Petits Ruminants (PPR) Outbreak Among Migratory Goats and Sheep in Himachal Pradesh. *Indian J Vet Med* 22: 105.

Yeruham I, et al. 2000. Orf Infection in Four Sheep Flocks. *Vet J* 160: 74.

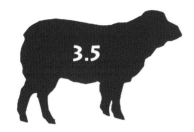

3.5

IMMUNOLOGICAL SKIN DISEASES

Insect Hypersensitivity
Flea Bite Hypersensitivity
Atopic Dermatitis

INSECT HYPERSENSITIVITY

Presumptive insect hypersensitivity has been reported. Hypersensitivity to *Culicoides* spp. and *Stomoxys calcitrans* salivary allergens is suspected. There are no apparent breed or sex predilections, and affected animals are usually 2 to 5 years old.

The syndrome is seasonal (spring to fall). In suspected *Culicoides* hypersensitivity, a pruritic, erythematous, crusted, excoriated, lichenified dermatitis is most commonly present on the ventral chest and abdomen, udder, and teats. The pinnae, periocular area, legs, and flanks are occasionally affected. Typically only one or a few animals in a flock are affected. In suspected *Stomoxys* hypersensitivity, the dermatitis is present on the rump, back, shoulders, and bridge of the nose, and up to 80% of a flock may be affected (Figs. 3.5-1 and 3.5-2).

FLEA BITE HYPERSENSITIVITY

Presumptive flea bite hypersensitivity has been reported. Hypersensitivity to *Ctenocephalides felis felis* (cat flea) salivary antigens is suspected. There are no apparent breed or sex predilections, and lambs and young adults are most commonly affected.

The syndrome is seasonal (summer to fall). A pruritic, crusted, excoriated dermatitis is most commonly present on the legs and ventrum. Flea excrement is present on the skin. Affected animals are usually otherwise healthy. Affected lambs may be anemic.

ATOPIC DERMATITIS

Presumptive atopic dermatitis (atopy) has been reported. Hypersensitivity to plants and molds was demonstrated by intradermal testing. No breed or sex predilections have been documented, and affected animals have been 2 to 5 years old.

The syndrome was seasonal (spring to fall) and pruritic. The dermatosis was more-or-less bilaterally symmetric, and involved the face, pinnae, axillae, ventral abdomen and thorax, udder, caudomedial thighs, and perineum (Figs. 3.5-3 to 3.5-6). Lesions included alopecia, erythema, lichenification, hyperpigmentation, and excoriation. Prescapular and prefemoral lymph nodes were enlarged, but affected animals were otherwise healthy. Hemograms and cytology of enlarged lymph nodes revealed eosinophilia.

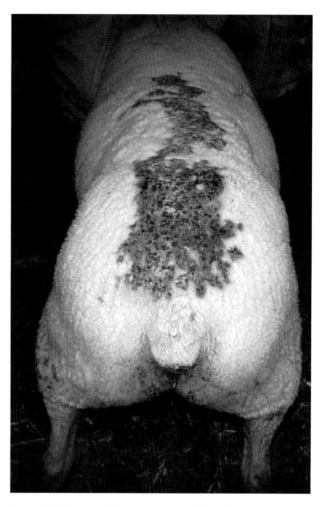

Figure 3.5-1 Suspected *Stomoxys* Hypersensitivity. Alopecia, erythema, and crusting over rump and back (courtesy J. Gourreau).

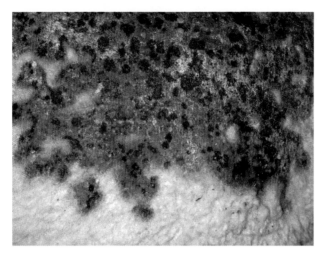

Figure 3.5-2 Close-up of Figure 3.5-1. Erythema, plaques, crusts, and alopecia over rump (courtesy J. Gourreau).

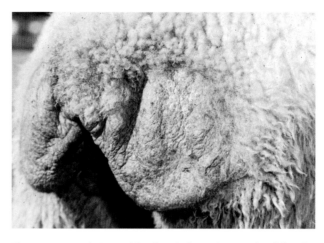

Figure 3.5-5 Atopic Dermatitis. Alopecia, hyperpigmentation, lichenification, and excoriation in perineum.

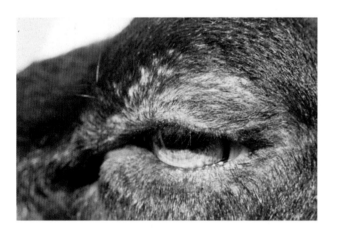

Figure 3.5-3 Atopic Dermatitis. Periocular scale, crust, and hypotrichosis.

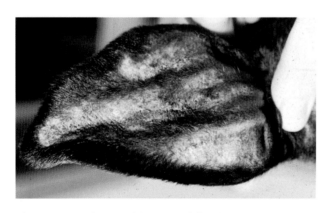

Figure 3.5-4 Atopic Dermatitis. Crust and alopecia on pinna.

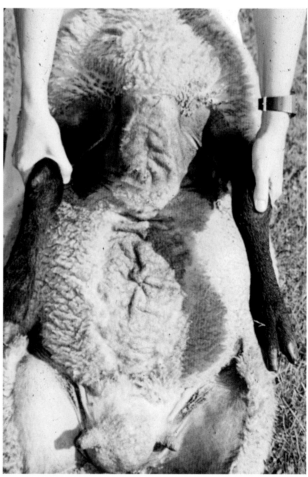

Figure 3.5-6 Atopic Dermatitis. Alopecia, hyperpigmentation, and lichenification of udder, ventral abdomen, ventral thorax, and axillae.

REFERENCES

Cannan RM, Lloyd S. 1988. Seasonal Allergic Dermatitis in Sheep. *Vet Rec* 123: 335.

Scott DW, Campbell SG. 1987. A Seasonal Pruritic Dermatitis Resembling Atopy in Sheep. *Agri-Pract* 8: 46.

Yeruham I, et al. 1993. Field Observations in Israel on Hypersensitivity in Cattle, Sheep and Donkeys Caused by *Culicoides*. *Aust Vet J* 70: 348.

Yeruham I, et al. 1997. An Apparent Flea-allergy Dermatitis in Kids and Lambs. *J Vet Med A* 44: 391.

Yeruham I, et al. 2000. Study of Apparent Hypersensitivity to *Culicoides* spp. in Sheep in Israel. *Vet Rec* 147: 360.

Yeruham I, et al. 2004. Seasonal Allergic Dermatitis in Sheep Associated with *Ctenocephalides* and *Culicoides* Bites. *Vet Dermatol* 15: 377.

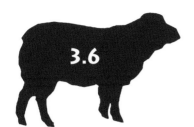

CONGENITAL AND HEREDITARY SKIN DISEASES

3.6

Hypotrichosis
Cutaneous Asthenia
Epidermolysis Bullosa
Miscellaneous Congenital and Hereditary Diseases
    Aplasia Cutis
    Congenital Goiter and Hypothyroidism
    Hereditary Photosensitivity and Hyperbilirubinemia
    Hypertrichosis

HYPOTRICHOSIS

Features

Hypotrichosis implies *clinically* a less than normal amount of hair that is hereditary and often congenital, and *histopathologically* a hypoplasia of hair follicles. These conditions are rare and cosmopolitan, and characterized by symmetrical hair and wool loss and skin that is initially normal in appearance. Exposed skin is susceptible to sunburn, infections, and contact dermatitis. Affected animals are intolerant to cold.

A viable hypotrichosis, autosomal recessive in nature, occurs in Polled Dorsets. The animals are hypotrichotic at birth, especially on the face and legs. Anecdotal reports indicate that ovine hypotrichosis occurs in other breeds as well (Fig. 3.6-1).

Diagnosis

1. History and physical examination.
2. Dermatohistopathology—Follicular hypoplasia.

CUTANEOUS ASTHENIA

Features

Cutaneous asthenia (dermatosparaxis, cutis hyperelastica, Ehlers-Danlos syndrome) is a group of inherited, congenital collagen dysplasias characterized by loose, hyperextensible, abnormally fragile skin that is easily torn by minor trauma. These disorders are rare and cosmopolitan. In most sheep, cutaneous asthenia is inherited as an autosomal recessive trait, and is associated with a deficiency in procollagen peptidase (aminopropeptidase, type I procollagen N-proteinase) activity. In Australian Border Leicester-Southdown crossbred lambs, the disorder was associated with an abnormality in the packing of collagen fibrils. An autosomal dominant form has been reported in New Zealand Romneys. Other breeds reported to have cutaneous asthenia include Norwegian Dala, Finnish crossbred Merino, White Dorper, and Romney.

From birth, affected sheep show variable degrees of cutaneous

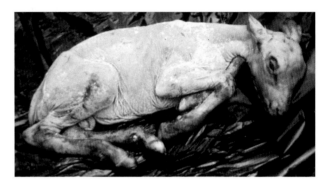

Figure 3.6-1 Hypotrichosis. Generalized alopecia in a lamb (courtesy J. Gourreau).

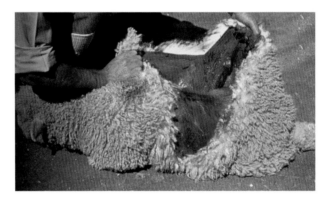

Figure 3.6-2 Cutaneous Asthenia. Huge tear in skin (courtesy J. King).

fragility and hyperextensibility (Figs. 3.6-2 through 3.6-4). The skin is often thin and easily torn, resulting in gaping ("fish mouth") wounds that heal with thin, papyraceous ("cigarette paper-like") scars. Wound healing may be delayed. Some lambs may have fragile internal organs and arteries. An autosomal dominant cutaneous asthenia in New Zealand Romney lambs was accompanied by osteogenesis imperfecta, marked joint laxity, moderate brachynathia inferior, small pink teeth, and subcutaneous edema.

Diagnosis

1. History and physical examination.
2. Dermatohistopathology—Collagen dysplasia, with small, fragmented, disorganized, loosely packed fibers.
3. Electron Microscopy—Abnormal structure and packing of collagen fibrils.

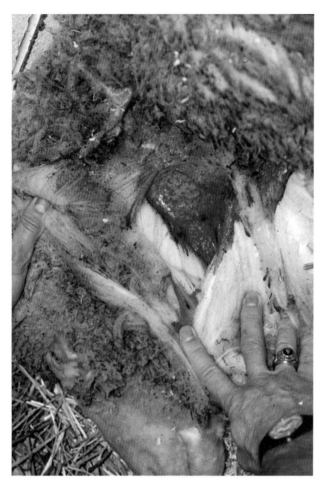

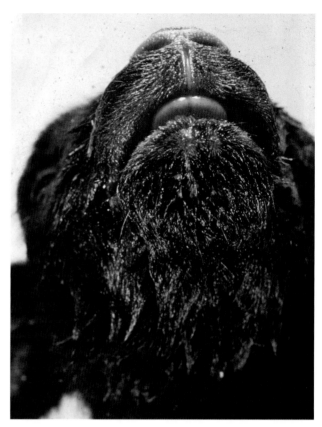

Figure 3.6-5 Epidermolysis Bullosa. Ulceration of muzzle and tongue (courtesy M. Alley).

Figure 3.6-3 Cutaneous Asthenia. Large tear in skin over thorax.

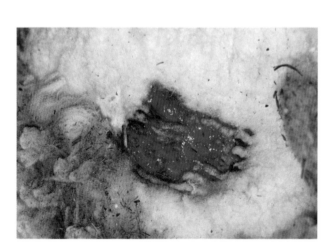

Figure 3.6-4 Same sheep as Figure 3.6-3. Skin tear over neck.

EPIDERMOLYSIS BULLOSA

Features

Epidermolysis bullosa is a group of hereditary mechanobullous diseases whose common primary feature is the formation of vesicles and bullae following trivial trauma. It is rare and cosmopolitan. In older veterinary literature, epidermolysis bullosa was mis-diagnosed as "aplasia cutis" or "epitheliogenesis imperfecta." The condition has been seen in numerous breeds, including Suffolk, Southdown, and Scottish Blackface.

Most reported cases of ovine epidermolysis bullosa resemble dystrophic epidermolysis bullosa, and are thought to be of autosomal recessive inheritance. A dystrophic epidermolysis bullosa was reported in Weisses Alpenschats in Switzerland. The condition was autosomal recessive, and associated with deficient collagen VII (anchoring fibrils).

Vesicobullous lesions and well-circumscribed ulcers are present at birth or within a few days after. Lesions are especially common in the oral cavity and on the distal limbs, pinnae, muzzle, and pressure points (Figs. 3.6-5 through 3.6-10). One or more hooves may be dysplastic or slough. Most animals die shortly after birth.

Diagnosis

1. History and physical examination.
2. Dermatohistopathology and Electron Microscopy—Subepidermal vesicular dermatitis with cleavage through the superficial dermis (dystrophic epidermolysis bullosa).

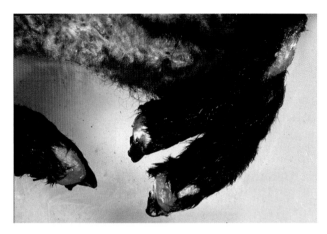

Figure 3.6-6 Epidermolysis Bullosa. Ulceration of legs and sloughing of hooves (courtesy M. Alley).

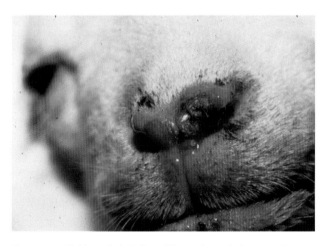

Figure 3.6-7 Epidermolysis Bullosa. Ulcerated muzzle (courtesy F. Ehrensperger, coll. J. Gourreau, AFSSA).

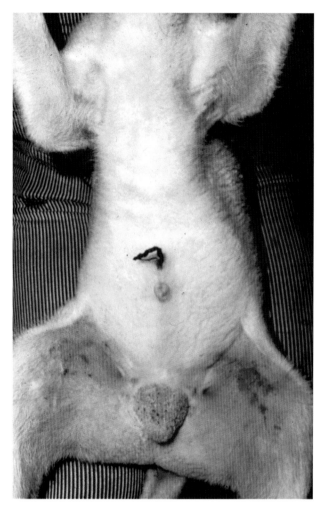

Figure 3.6-9 Epidermolysis Bullosa. Bullae and ulcers in axillae and groin (courtesy F. Ehrensperger, coll. J. Gourreau, AFSSA).

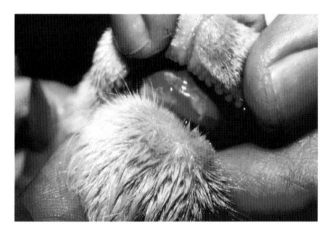

Figure 3.6-8 Epidermolysis Bullosa. Ulcerated lips and tongue (courtesy F. Ehrensperger, coll. J. Gourreau, AFSSA).

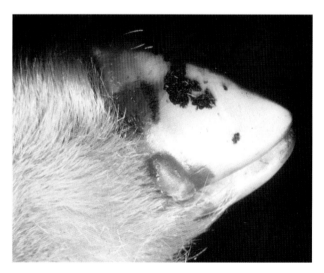

Figure 3.6-10 Epidermolysis Bullosa. Hemorrhagic bulla at coronary band (courtesy F. Ehrensperger, coll. J. Gourreau, AFSSA).

MISCELLANEOUS CONGENITAL AND HEREDITARY DISEASES

Table 3.6-1 Miscellaneous Congenital and Hereditary Diseases

Aplasia cutis	Very rare and cosmopolitan; solitary full-thickness ulcer at birth; especially leg
Congenital goiter and hypothyroidism	Rare and cosmopolitan; many breeds associated with maternal iodine deficiency; Merinos with presumed autosomal recessive defective thyroglobulin synthesis; born weak and die in hours or weeks; hair coat varies from short and fuzzy to completely absent; the skin is often thickened and puffy (myxedema)
Hereditary photosensitivity and hyperbilirubinemia	Very rare; Southdown (autosomal recessive); Corriedale (presumed hereditary); photodermatitis; abnormal liver function tests
Hypertrichosis	Maternal hyperthermia; Border disease (congenital *Pestivirus* infection) results in lambs born with a long, coarse birth coat and neurologic disorders)

REFERENCES

Arthur DG, et al. 1992. Lethal Osteogenesis Imperfecta and Skin Fragility in Newborn New Zealand Lambs. *N Z Vet J* 40: 112.

Bruckner-Tuderman L, et al. 1991. Animal Model for Dermolytic Mechanobullous Disease: Sheep with Recessive Dystrophic Epidermolysis Bullosa Lack Collagen VII. *J Invest Dermatol* 96: 452.

Martin WB, and Aitken ID. 2000. Diseases of Sheep. Ed 4. Blackwell Science, Malden, MA.

Radostits OM, et al. 2000. Veterinary Medicine. A Textbook of the Diseases of Cattle, Sheep, Pigs, Goats, and Horses. Ed 9. WB Saunders, Philadelphia, PA.

Scott DW. 1988. Large Animal Dermatology. WB Saunders, Philadelphia, PA.

Van Halderen A, and Green JR. 1988. Dermatosparaxis in White Dorper Sheep. *J S Afr Vet Assoc* 59: 45.

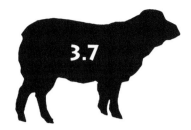

ENVIRONMENTAL SKIN DISEASES

BURNS

Features

Burns are occasionally seen and may be thermal (barn, forest, or brush fires; accidental spillage of hot solutions), electrical (electrocution; lightning strike), frictional (ropes; falls), chemical (improperly used topicals), or radiational (radiotherapy).

First-degree burns involve the superficial epidermis and are characterized by erythema, edema, heat, and pain. *Second-degree burns* affect the entire epidermis and are characterized by erythema, edema, heat, pain, and vesicles. *Third-degree burns* affect the entire epidermis, dermis, and appendages, and are characterized by necrosis, ulceration, anesthesia, and scarring. Burns are most commonly seen over the dorsum, face or udder and teats (Figs. 3.7-1 through 3.7-4).

Diagnosis

1. History and physical examination.

PRIMARY IRRITANT CONTACT DERMATITIS

Features

Primary irritant contact dermatitis is a common inflammatory skin reaction caused by direct contact with an offending substance. Moisture is an important predisposing factor, since it decreases the effectiveness of normal skin barriers and increases the intimacy of contact between the contactant and the skin. Substances known to cause contact dermatitis in sheep include: body excretions and secretions (feces, urine, wounds); caustics (acids, alkalis); crude oil, diesel fuel, and turpentine; improper

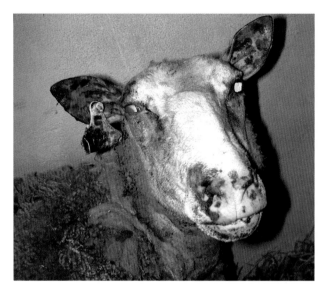

Figure 3.7-1 Burn. Edema, erythema, ulceration, and alopecia of face and ears due to barn fire (courtesy J. Gourreau).

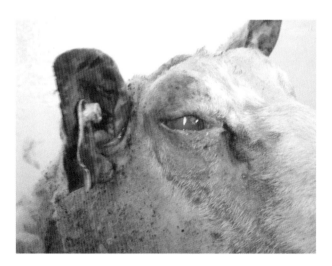

Figure 3.7-2 Same sheep as Figure 3.7-1. Note erythema and ulceration of pinna, facial swelling, and corneal edema (courtesy J. Gourreau).

use of sprays, rinses, and wipes; plants; wood preservatives; bedding; and filth.

The dermatitis varies in severity from erythema, edema, papules, and scale to vesicles, erosions, ulcers, necrosis, and crusts. Severe irritants, self-trauma, or secondary bacterial infections can result in alopecia, excoriation, lichenification, and scarring. Leukotrichia and leukoderma can be transient or perma-

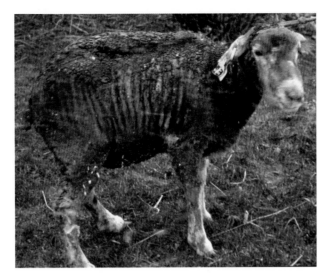

Figure 3.7-3 Burn. Swelling, erythema, and alopecia of face; charring of wool and skin due to barn fire.

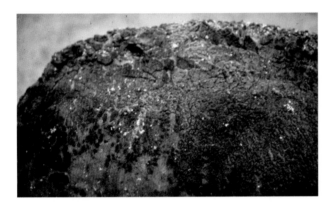

Figure 3.7-4 Same sheep as Figure 3.7-3. Charred wool and skin.

Table 3.7-1 Causes of Primary Photosensitization	
Source	**Photodynamic Agent**
Plants	
St. John's wort (*Hypericum perforatum*)	Hypericin
Buckwheat (*Fagopyrum esculentum*, *Polygonum fagopyrum*)	Fagopyrin, photofagopyrin
Bishop's weed (*Ammi majus*)	Furocoumarins
Dutchman's breeches (*Thamnosma texana*)	Furocoumarins
Wild carrot (*Daucus carota*), spring parsley (*Cymopterus watsonii*)	Furocoumarins
Cooperia pedunculata	Furocoumarins
Perennial ryegrass (*Lolium perenne*)	Perloline
Burr trefoil (*Medicago denticulata*)	Aphids
Alfalfa silage	?
Chemicals	
Phenothiazines, thiazides, acriflavines, rose bengal, methylene blue, sulfonamides, tetracyclines	

nent sequelae. In most instances, the nature of the contactant can be inferred from the distribution of the dermatitis: muzzle and distal legs (plants, environmental substances); face and dorsum (sprays, pour-ons, wipes); ventrum (bedding, filth); perineum and rear legs (urine, feces).

Diagnosis

1. History and physical examination.

PHOTODERMATITIS

Features

Photodermatitis (solar dermatitis, actinic dermatitis) is an inflammatory skin disease caused by exposure to ultraviolet light. *Phototoxicity* (sunburn) occurs on white skin, light skin, or damaged skin (e.g., depigmented or scarred) not sufficiently covered by hair. *Photosensitization* is classified according to the source of

the photodynamic agents (Tables 3.7-1 and 3.7-2): (1) primary photosensitization (a preformed or metabolically-derived photodynamic agent reaches the skin by ingestion, injection, or contact), (2) hepatogenous photosensitization (blood phylloerythrin levels are elevated in association with liver abnormalities), and (3) idiopathic photosensitization.

Skin lesions are usually restricted to light-skin, sparsely-haired areas but, in severe cases, can extend into the surrounding dark-skin areas too. Restlessness and discomfort often precede visible skin lesions. Typically there is rapid, painful, edematous swelling of the face and pinnae (Fig. 3.7-5). Erythema and edema may be followed by vesicles and bullae, ulceration, oozing, crusts, scales, and alopecia (Figs. 3.7-6 through 3.7-8). The skin may become dry and fissured, with the oozing of a yellowish transudate. In severe cases, pinnae, eyelids, tail, teats, and feet may slough. Secondary bacterial infections are common. Variable degrees of pruritus and pain are present. The muzzle, eyelids, lips, face, pinnae, back, perineum, distal legs, teats, and coronary bands are most commonly affected. Affected animals often attempt to protect themselves from sunlight.

Although photosensitized animals rarely die, resultant weight loss, damaged udders and teats, refusal to allow young to nurse, and secondary infections/flystrike all may lead to appreciable economic loss.

Diagnosis

1. History and physical examination.
2. Liver function testing should always be performed, whether or not clinical signs of liver disease are present.
3. Primary photodynamic agents can often be identified with various biological assay systems.

FLEECE ROT

Features

Fleece rot (wool rot, yolk rot, water rot, canary stain) is a common, cosmopolitan superficial dermatitis resulting from bacter-

Table 3.7-2 Causes of Hepatogenous Photosensitization

Source	Hepatotoxin
Plants	
Burning bush, fireweed (*Kochia scoparia*)	?
Ngaio tree (*Myoporum* spp.)	Ngaione
Lechuguilla (*Agave lechuguilla*)	Saponins
Rape, kale (*Brassica* spp.)	?
Coal oil brush, spineless horsebrush (*Tetradynia* spp.)	?
Moldy alfalfa hay	?
Sacahuiste (*Nolina texana*)	?
Salvation Jane (*Echium lycopsis*)	Pyrrolizidine alkaloids
Lantana (*Lantana camara*)	Triterpene
Heliotrope (*Heliotropium europaeum*)	Pyrrolizidine alkaloids
Tarweed, fiddle-neck (*Amsinckia* spp.)	Pyrrolizidine alkaloids
Crotalaria, rattleweed (*Crotalaria* spp.)	Pyrrolizidine alkaloids
Millet, panic grass (*Panicum* spp.)	?
Ganskweed (*Lasiospermum bipinnatum*)	?
Verrain (*Lippia rehmanni*)	Triterpenes
Bog asphodel (*Narthecium ossifragum*)	Saponins
Alecrim (*Holocalyx glaziovii*)	?
Vuusiektebossie (*Nidorella foetida*)	?
Anthanasia trifurcata	?
Asaemia axillaris	?
Fungi	
Pithomyces chartarum ("facial eczema")— on pasture, especially rye	Sporidesmin
Anacystis spp.—blue-green algae in water	Alkaloid
Periconia spp.—on Bermuda grass	?
Phomopsis leptostromiformis—on lupins	Phomopsin A
Infections	
Liver abscess	Bacteria/toxin
Rift Valley fever	Virus
Neoplasia	
Lymphoma	Malignant lymphocytes
Hepatic carcinoma	Malignant hepatocytes
Chemicals	
Copper	
Phosphorus	
Carbon tetrachloride	
Phenanthridium	

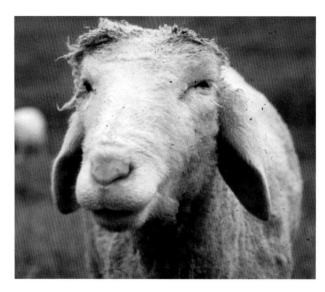

Figure 3.7-5 Photodermatitis. Swollen face and pinnae with early hepatic photosensitization.

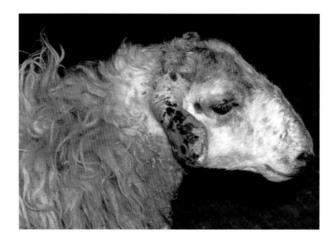

Figure 3.7-6 Photodermatitis. Facial swelling, erythema, crusting, and alopecia of pinnae and periocular area due to hepatic photosensitization (*Pithomyces chartarum*) (courtesy P. Bezille, coll. J. Gourreau, AFSSA).

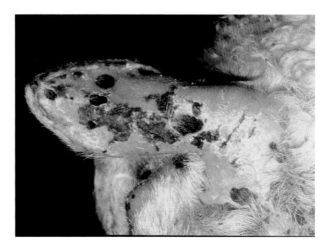

Figure 3.7-7 Same sheep as in Figure 3.7-6. Alopecia, erythema, and crusting of pinna (courtesy P. Bezille, coll. J. Gourreau, AFSSA).

ial proliferation induced by wetness and manifested by seropurulent exudation and matting of wool fibers. The condition has a seasonal incidence which coincides with months of maximum rainfall. Predisposing factors include increased wool staple length, less compact fleece, low wax content of fleece, and high suint content of fleece.

Subsequent to wetting (typically for 3 to 4 days), a marked proliferation of bacteria—almost exclusively *Pseudomonas* spp.—occurs on the skin and in the fleece. In mild cases, the fleece is discolored yellow, orange, green, blue (Fig. 3.7-9), brown, pink, or red—depending on the proliferating *Pseudomonas* spp. In more severe cases, the discoloration is accompanied by an exudative, superficial dermatitis which causes characteristic bands of matted fleece. Wool in affected areas is saturated and may epilate easily.

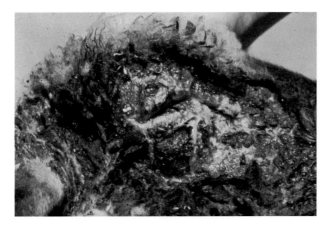

Figure 3.7-8 Photodermatitis. Severe necrosis, sloughing, and ulceration of face due to hepatic photosensitization.

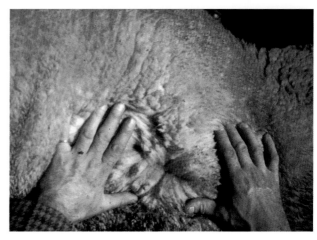

Figure 3.7-9 Fleece Rot. Early blue discoloration of the wool (courtesy M. Smith).

Some sheep rub and bite affected areas. Areas of fleece rot emanate putrid odors which attract flies. Lesions occur most commonly over the withers and along the back.

The prevalence of fleece rot within a flock varies from 14% to 92%. Economic losses from fleece damage and myiasis can be substantial.

Differential Diagnosis

Dermatophilosis (typically no crusts and ulcers seen with fleece rot), pink rot (Table 3.7-3), and bolo disease (Table 3.7-3).

Diagnosis

1. History and physical examination.
2. Culture.

MISCELLANEOUS DISEASES

Table 3.7-3 Miscellaneous Environmental Diseases

Bolo disease	*Corynebacterium* spp.; well-circumscribed areas of dark-grey to black patches or bands on or in the fleece; wool in areas shorter, fragile, less dense, with yellowish to grayish-white scale at base of staple; chalky-white deposits seen chronically; especially neck, shoulders and back
Foreign bodies	See Box 3.7-1
Frostbite	Rare and cosmopolitan; pinnae, tail tip, teats, scrotum, and feet; pale, hypoesthetic, cool skin that progresses to erythema, edema, scale, alopecia ± necrosis, dry gangrene, and slough
Hyalomma toxicosis (Fig. 3.7-10)	Uncommon; Africa; due to toxin of *Hyalomma truncatum* ticks; sudden onset fever, depression, hyperemic mucosae, hypersalivation, and nasal discharge; regionalized or generalized skin erythema, oozing, matted haircoat, pain, malodor; alopecia, ulceration; tips of pinnae and tail may slough
Iodism	Rare and cosmopolitan; excessive iodine-containing feeds or medicaments; nasal discharge, lacrimation, cough, variable appetite; severe skin scaling with or without partial alopecia, especially over dorsum neck, head, shoulders
Kaalsiekte	Rare; South Africa; nursing lambs ingest toxin in milk of ewes eating bitterkarro bush (*Chrysocana tenuifola*); diarrhea, haircoat shedding, pruritus when exposed to sunlight.
Mimosine toxicosis	Rare; humid and subhumid tropical lowlands; eating mimosine-containing plants (*Mimosa* and *Leucaena*); gradual loss of hair and variable hoof dysplasias
Pink rot	*Bacillus* spp.; follows prolonged wetting; bright pink discoloration of wool; fibers bound together in a creamy pink mass in the middle of the staple
Stachybotryotoxicosis	Rare; Europe; eating hay and straw contaminated by fungus *Stachybotrys atra* (macrocyclic trichothecenes); initial necrotic ulcers in mouth and on lips and nostrils; conjunctivitis, rhinitis, later fever, depression, anorexia, diarrhea, weakness, bleeding diathesis; isolate fungus and toxins from feed
Subcutaneous emphysema	Rare and cosmopolitan; sequel to tracheal perforation, esophageal rupture, pulmonary emphysema, penetrating wounds (external or internal; rib fracture); clostridial infections; soft, fluctuant, crepitant, subcutaneous swellings; usually nonpainful and not acutely ill (unless clostridial)

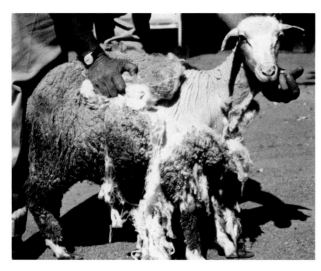

Figure 3.7-10 *Hyalomma* Toxicosis. Marked alopecia, easy epilation, and scaling with chronic disease (courtesy P. Bland).

Box 3.7-1 Draining tracts.

- A *fistula* is an abnormal passage or communication, usually between two internal organs or leading from an internal organ to the surface of the body.
- A *sinus* is an abnormal cavity or channel or fistula that permits the escape of pus to the surface of the body.
- *Draining tracts* are commonly associated with penetrating wounds that have left infectious agents and/or foreign material. Draining tracts may also result from infections of underlying tissues (e.g., bone, joint, lymph node) or previous injections.
- Foreign bodies include wood slivers, plant seeds and awns, cactus tines, fragments of wire, and suture material. Lesions include varying combinations of papules, nodules, abscesses, and draining tracts. Lesions occur most commonly on the legs, hips, muzzle, and ventrum.

REFERENCES

Howard JL, Smith RA. 1999. Current Veterinary Therapy. Food Animal Practice. Ed 4. W.B. Saunders, Philadelphia.

Martin WB, Aitken ID. 2000. Diseases of Sheep. Ed 3. Blackwell Science, Oxford, United Kingdom.

Radostits OM, et al. 2000. Veterinary Medicine. A Textbook of the Diseases of Cattle, Sheep, Pigs, Goats and Horses. Ed 9. WB Saunders, Philadelphia, PA.

Scott DW. 1988. Large Animal Dermatology. WB Saunders, Philadelphia, PA.

Suliman HB, et al. 1988. Zinc Deficiency in Sheep: Field Cases. *Trop Anim Hlth Prod* 20: 47.

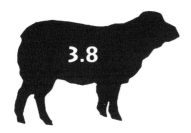

NUTRITIONAL SKIN DISEASES

3.8

Zinc-Responsive Dermatitis
Miscellaneous Nutritional Disorders
    Vitamin A Deficiency
    Cobalt Deficiency
    Copper Deficiency
    Iodine Deficiency
    Sulfur Deficiency

ZINC-RESPONSIVE DERMATITIS

Features

The characteristic dermatitis may be seen with true zinc deficiency or as an idiopathic zinc-responsive condition. Causes of deficiency include diets deficient in zinc; diets with excessive calcium, iron, phytates, and other chelating agents; and drinking water with excessive iron and other chelating agents. Zinc-responsive dermatoses are uncommon to rare. There are no apparent breed, sex, or age predilections.

More-or-less symmetrical erythema and scaling progress to crusting and alopecia. The face, pinnae, mucocutaneous junctions, pressure points, and distal legs are typically affected (Figs. 3.8-1 to 3.8-5). Some animals have a dull, rough, brittle haircoat. Pruritus may be intense or absent. Fleece/wool biting and eating may be seen. Secondary bacterial skin infections are common. Truly zinc-deficient animals have accompanying systemic signs, whereas animals with the idiopathic condition do not. With true zinc deficiency, multiple animals are often affected. With the idiopathic conditions, a single animal is typically affected.

Differential Diagnosis

Dermatophytosis, dermatophilosis, staphylococcal folliculitis, sarcoptic mange (when pruritic).

Diagnosis

1. Dermatohistopathology—Hyperplastic to spongiotic superficial perivascular-to-interstitial dermatitis with marked diffuse orthokeratotic to parakeratotic hyperkeratosis and a lymphoeosinophilic inflammatory infiltrate.
2. Analysis of diet.
3. Response to therapy.

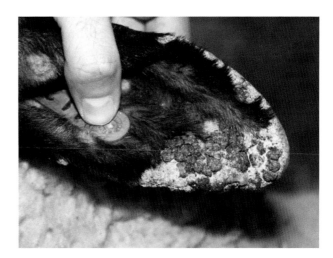

Figure 3.8-2 Zinc-Responsive Dermatitis. Alopecia and thick white-to-brown crusts on pinna.

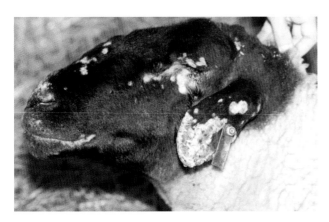

Figure 3.8-1 Zinc-Responsive Dermatitis. Alopecia and thick, whitish crusts on face and pinna.

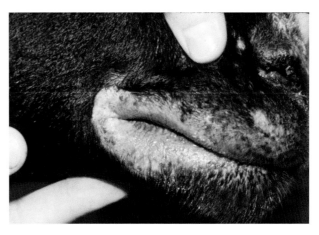

Figure 3.8-3 Zinc-Responsive Dermatitis. Alopecia and crusts on lips.

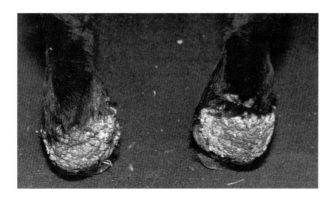

Figure 3.8-4 Zinc-Responsive Dermatitis. Thick crusts on caudal pasterns.

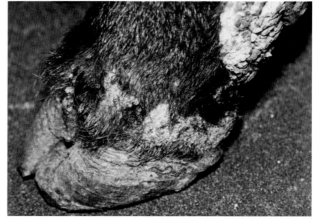

Figure 3.8-5 Zinc-Responsive Dermatitis. Thick crusts on distal leg.

MISCELLANEOUS NUTRITIONAL DISORDERS

Table 3.8-1 Miscellaneous Nutritional Disorders	
Vitamin A deficiency	Very rare; deficient diet; faded haircoat and generalized seborrhea; systemic signs; serum and liver concentrations of vitamin A, and vitamin A levels in diet
Cobalt deficiency	Very rare; deficient diet; rough , brittle, faded haircoat; systemic signs; serum and liver concentrations of cobalt and vitamin B_{12}
Copper deficiency	Rare; primary (deficient diet) or secondary (excess cadmium, molybdenum, or zinc in diet); rough, brittle, faded haircoat and loss of wool crimp; variable excessive licking; systemic signs; serum and liver concentrations of copper
Iodine deficiency	Very rare; maternal dietary deficiency; newborns, lambs; generalized alopecia and thick puffy skin (myxedema); systemic signs; serum concentrations of thyroid hormone and thyroid gland pathology
Sulfur deficiency	Rare; deficient diet; fleece-biting and alopecia, especially hips, abdomen, and shoulder; systemic signs; serum and liver concentrations of sulfur

REFERENCES

Howard JL, Smith RA. 1999. Current Veterinary Therapy. Food Animal Practice. Ed 4. W.B. Saunders, Philadelphia.

Martin WB, Aitken ID. 2000. Diseases of Sheep. Ed 3. Blackwell Science, Oxford, United Kingdom.

Radostits OM, et al. 2000. Veterinary Medicine. A Textbook of the Diseases of Cattle, Sheep, Pigs, Goats and Horses. Ed 9. WB Saunders, Philadelphia, PA.

Scott DW. 1988. Large Animal Dermatology. WB Saunders, Philadelphia, PA.

Suliman HB, et al. 1988. Zinc Deficiency in Sheep: Field Cases. *Trop Anim Hlth Prod* 20: 47.

Youde H. 2001. Preliminary Epidemiological and Clinical Observations on *Shimao zheng* (Fleece-Eating) in Goats and Sheep. *Vet Res Commun* 25: 585.

Youde H. 2002. An Experimental Study in the Treatment and Prevention of *Shimao Zheng* (Fleece-Eating) in Sheep and Goats in the Haizi Area of Akesai County in China. *Vet Res Commun* 26: 39.

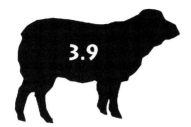

MISCELLANEOUS SKIN DISEASES

ANAGEN DEFLUXION

Features

Anagen defluxion ("anagen effluvium," "wool break," "wool slip") is uncommon and cosmopolitan. Various stressors (e.g., infectious diseases, metabolic disorders, mastitis, high fevers, winter shearing of housed sheep) result in temporary growth defects in hair shafts. Certain drugs (e.g., glucocorticoids, cyclophosphamide, epidermal growth factor) can also cause anagen defluxion. There are no apparent breed, sex, or age predilections.

Wool loss occurs suddenly, within days of the stressor. The wool loss may be regional, multifocal, or generalized, and is more-or-less bilaterally symmetric (Figs. 3.9-1 to 3.9-4). Skin in affected areas appears normal, unless secondarily inflamed by trauma, contact dermatitis, or photodermatitis. When fingers are rubbed over the surface of alopecic areas, wool stubble may be felt. Pruritus and pain are absent.

Differential Diagnosis

Hereditary hypotrichoses.

Diagnosis

1. Microscopy (pluck wool fibers in mineral oil)—Wool fiber diameter irregularly narrowed and deformed.
2. Dermatohistopathology—Apoptosis of wool matrix keratinocytes with or without dysplastic wool fibers.

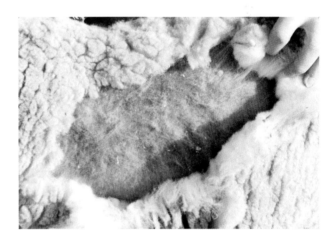

Figure 3.9-2 Close-up of Fig. 3.9-1. Wool can be easily epilated.

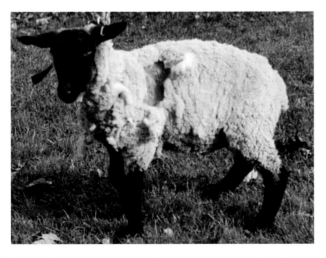

Figure 3.9-1 Anagen Defluxion. Alopecia occurring seven days after onset of fever and diarrhea.

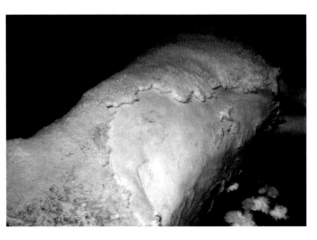

Figure 3.9-3 Anagen Defluxion. Widespread alopecia associated with severe systemic illness.

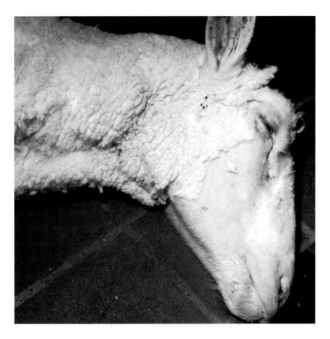

Figure 3.9-4 Same sheep as in Fig. 3.9-3. Facial alopecia.

REFERENCES

Gourreau JM, et al. 2003. Une Alopécie Quasiment Totale sur un Agneau en 12 à 18 Heures, Pourquoi. *Bull des GTV* 22: 6.

Howard JL, Smith RA. 1999. Current Veterinary Therapy. Ed 4. WB Saunders, Philadelphia, PA.

Scott DW. 1988. Large Animal Dermatology. WB Saunders, Philadelphia, PA.

Winter AC. 1995. Wool Loss in Sheep. *Vet Ann* 35: 313.

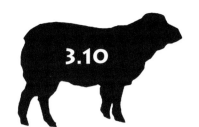

NEOPLASTIC AND NON-NEOPLASTIC GROWTHS

3.10

Papilloma
Squamous Cell Carcinoma
Miscellaneous Neoplastic and Non-Neoplastic Growths
    Basal Cell Tumor
    Fibroma
    Fibrosarcoma
    Neuroma
    Lipoma
    Lymphoma
    Melanoma
    Follicular Cyst
    Keratosis
        Actinic Keratosis
        Cutaneous Horn

PAPILLOMA

Features

Papillomas are uncommon cosmopolitan, benign neoplasms of keratinocytes. They are caused by papillomavirus. Infections follow direct or indirect contamination of various wounds. Given the various reported localizations for viral papillomas in sheep, it is probable that multiple types of ovine papillomavirus are involved. There are no apparent breed or sex predilections.

Filiform squamous papillomas occur in young sheep, especially on the fetlock area of the lower legs. Lesions are 15 to 25 mm in diameter and frondlike (Fig. 3.10-1). Similar lesions occur on the scrotum of rams. *Fibropapillomas* occur on the face, pinnae, legs, and teats of adult sheep (3 to 6 years old). Lesions are 0.5 to 1 cm in diameter, hyperkeratotic, and dome-shaped to pedunculated. Facial fibropapillomas can transform into squamous cell carcinomas. Papillomavirus DNA has been detected in perineal papillomas and squamous cell carcinomas.

Differential Diagnosis

Squamous cell carcinoma.

Diagnosis

1. Dermatohistopathology.

SQUAMOUS CELL CARCINOMA

Features

Squamous cell carcinoma is a common, cosmopolitan, malignant neoplasm of keratinocytes. They are especially common in sub-tropical and tropical climates, and at high altitudes. Ultraviolet light damage is important in the etiopathogenesis of this neoplasm, thus white-skin that is lightly haired or woolled is at risk. Facial fibropapillomas (viral) can transform into squamous cell carcinomas, and papillomavirus DNA has been detected in perineal squamous cell carcinomas (Figs. 3.10-2 to 3.10-4). Squamous cell carcinoma can rarely develop from the wall of follicular cysts. Adult to aged animals are most commonly affected, and Merinos may be at risk. There is no apparent sex predilection.

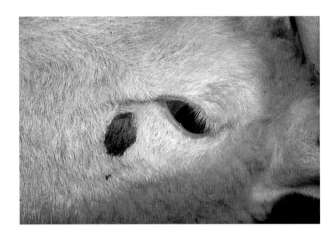

Figure 3.10-1 Papilloma. Hyperkeratotic mass below eye (courtesy M. Smith).

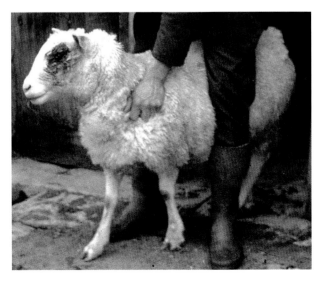

Figure 3.10-2 Squamous Cell Carcinoma. Ulcerated periocular lesion (courtesy G. Arnault, coll. J. Gourreau, AFSSA).

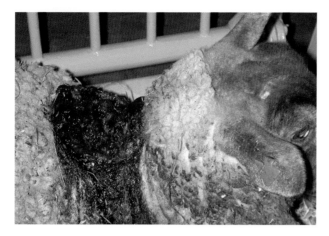

Figure 3.10-3 Squamous Cell Carcinoma. Ulcerated, proliferative lesion on withers (courtesy J. Gourreau).

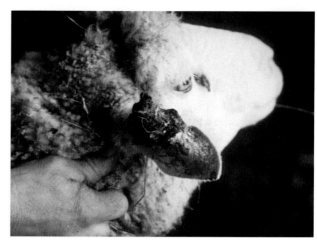

Figure 3.10-4 Squamous Cell Carcinoma. Crusted, proliferative lesion on pinna (courtesy R. Braque, coll. J. Gourreau, AFSSA).

Lesions may be single or multiple, and are most commonly seen on the muzzle, lips, eyelids, pinnae, perineum, and vulva. Early lesions are erythematous, scaly, crusty, and hyperkeratotic (actinic keratosis). Invasive squamous cell carcinomas may be proliferative (verrucous or cauliflower-like) or ulcerative (granulating and nonhealing).

Differential Diagnosis

Fibropapilloma, basal cell tumor (when ulcerated), various granulomas (infectious, foreign body).

Diagnosis

1. Microscopy (direct smears)—Keratinocytes showing various degrees of atypia.
2. Dermatohistopathology.

MISCELLANEOUS NEOPLASTIC AND NON-NEOPLASTIC GROWTHS

Table 3.10-1 Miscellaneous Neoplastic and Non-Neoplastic Growths

Basal Cell Tumor	Very rare; adult; solitary nodule, often ulcerated, head and neck; benign; direct smears and dermatohistopathology
Fibroma	Very rare; adult; solitary nodule, anywhere; benign; direct smear and dermatohistopathology
Fibrosarcoma	Very rare; adult; solitary nodule; anywhere; malignant; dermatohistopathology
Neuroma	Rare; young to adult; post-tail docking; painful nodule on end of tail; benign; dermatohistopathology
Lipoma	Very rare; adult; solitary subcutaneous nodule; trunk; benign; direct smears and dermatohistopathology
Lymphoma	Very rare; adult to aged; multiple subcutaneous nodules, 1 to 3 cm diameter, on thorax; malignant; direct smears and dermatohistopathology
Melanoma	Rare; adult to aged; Suffolks and Angoras may be predisposed; solitary or multiple melanotic nodules; anywhere; malignant; direct smears and dermatohistopathology
Follicular cyst (Fig. 3.10-5)	Uncommon; young to adult; may be hereditary in Merinos; solitary or multiple firm to fluctuant nodules; larger nodules can have firm, keratinous material protruding through a pore; anywhere; benign (squamous cell carcinoma may rarely develop in cyst wall); dermatohistopathology
Actinic keratosis	Common; adult to aged; ultraviolet light damaged white skin; solitary or multiple erythematous, scaly, crusty, hyperkeratotic plaques; premalignant; dermatohistopathology
Cutaneous horn	Rare; hornlike hyperkeratosis; usually overlying epithelial neoplasms (papilloma, squamous cell carcinoma, actinic keratosis, basal cell tumor); benign or malignant; dermatohistopathology

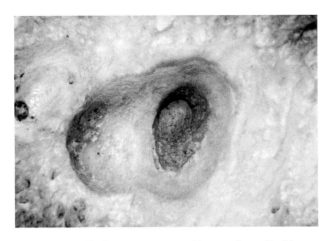

Figure 3.10-5 Follicular Cyst. Large cyst with protruding, yellowish, hard, keratinous material.

REFERENCES

French NP, Morgan KL. 1992. Neuromata in Docked Lambs' Tails. *Res Vet Sci* 52: 389.

Gorham SL, et al. 1990. Basal Cell Tumor in a Sheep. *Vet Pathol* 27: 466.

Green JR, et al. 1988. An Outbreak of Lymphosarcoma in Merino Sheep in the South Western Cape. *J So Afr Vet Assoc* 59: 27.

Hayward MLR, et al. 1993. Filiform Viral Squamous Papillomas in Sheep. *Vet Rec* 132: 86.

Head K. 1990. Tumours in Sheep. *In Pract* 12: 68.

Howard JO, and Smith RL. 1999. Current Veterinary Therapy. Food Animal Practice. Ed 4. WB Saunders, Philadelphia, PA.

Ramadan RO, et al. 1991. Squamous Cell Carcinoma in Sheep in Saudi Arabia. *Rev Elev Méd Vét Pays Trop* 44: 23.

Scott DW. 1988. Large Animal Dermatology. WB Saunders, Philadelphia, PA.

Tilbrook PA, et al. 1992. Detection of Papillomaviral-like DNA Sequences in Premalignant and Malignant Perineal Lesions of Sheep. *Vet Microbiol* 32: 327.

Trenfield K, et al. 1990. Detection of Papillomavirus DNA in Precancerous Lesions of the Ears of Sheep. *Vet Microbiol* 25: 103.

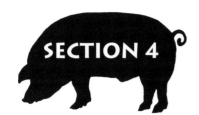

PORCINE

SECTION 4

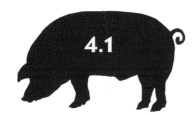

BACTERIAL SKIN DISEASES

4.1

Exudative Epidermitis
Staphylococcal Folliculitis
Spirochetosis
Erysipelas
Abscess
Actinomycosis
Septicemic Slough
Miscellaneous Bacterial Diseases
    Actinobacillosis
    Anthrax
    Clostridial Cellulitis
    Dermatophilosis
    Edema Disease
    Haemophilus parasuis Infection
    Necrobacillosis
    Streptococcal Infections
    Yersinia enterocolitica Infection

EXUDATIVE EPIDERMITIS

Features

Exudative epidermitis ("greasy pig disease") is typically an acute, exudative, vesicopustular disease. It is common and cosmopolitan, and caused by *Staphylococcus hyicus* subspecies *hyicus*—and rarely *S. chromogenes*—and predisposing factors include trauma, inadequate nutrition, other diseases, and stress. Virulent strains of *S. hyicus* produce an exfoliative toxin (exfoliatin) which produces widespread skin disease. The disease is common and primarily seen in suckling and recently weaned piglets. There are no apparent breed or sex predilections.

Clinically, exudative epidermitis has been divided into acute (peracute), subacute (acute), and chronic (subacute) forms. The acute and subacute forms are typically seen in suckling piglets, while the chronic form is usually seen in weaned piglets. However, the presentation can be highly variable. Morbidity varies from 10% to 90%, and mortality from 5% to 90% (average 20%).

In the *acute form*, a dark-brown, greasy exudate appears periocularly, followed by a vesicopustular eruption on the snout, lips, tongue, gums, and coronets (Figs. 4.1-1 through 4.1-6). Red-brown macules then appear behind the ears and on the ventral abdomen, groin, axilla, and medial thighs. The entire body is then covered by erythema, a moist greasy exudate, and thick brown crusts. Affected piglets show progressive depression, anorexia, and dehydration, and usually die within three to five days. Pruritus, pain, and pyrexia are usually absent.

The *subacute form* follows the general pattern of the acute form. The skin becomes thickened and wrinkled. The total body

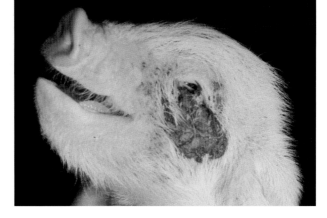

Figure 4.1-1 Exudative Epidermitis. Periocular brown waxy exudate.

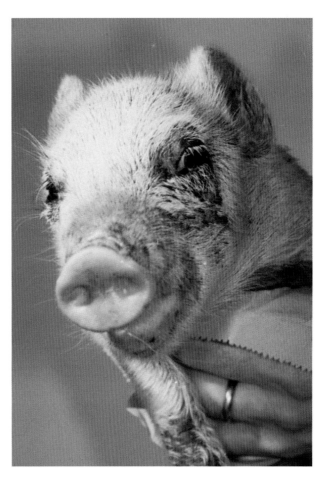

Figure 4.1-2 Exudative Epidermitis. Erythema, crusts, and brown waxy exudate on lips, bridge of nose, and periocular areas.

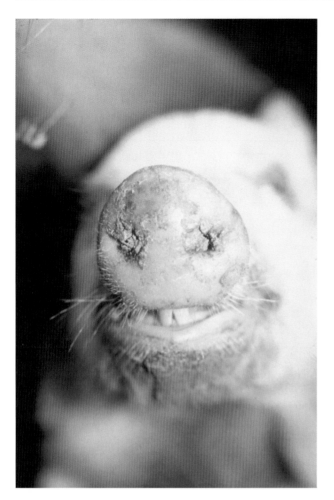

Figure 4.1-3 Exudative Epidermitis. Crusts and annular erosion on snout.

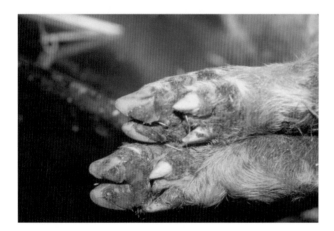

Figure 4.1-4 Exudative Epidermitis. Crusts and erosions on distal legs and coronets.

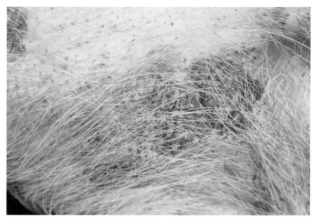

Figure 4.1-5 Exudative Epidermitis. Erythema and crust on ventral abdomen.

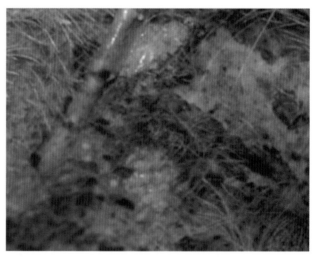

Figure 4.1-6 Exudative Epidermitis. Diffuse erythema, waxy brown crusts, and pustules on groin and medial thigh.

Other skin lesions that can be seen with exudative epidermitis include subcutaneous abscesses, and necrosis of the pinnae and tail.

Adults are uncommonly affected and have mild, localized lesions on the back or flanks.

Because of losses attributable to death, weight loss, stunting, and medical bills, exudative epidermitis can be a significant economic problem.

Differential Diagnosis

Parakeratosis, streptococcal pyoderma, biotin deficiency, and viral infections.

Diagnosis

1. Microscopy (direct smears)—Degenerate neutrophils, nuclear streaming, and phagocytosed cocci (Gram-positive, about 1 mm diameter) (see Fig. 4.1-12).
2. Culture (aerobic).

exudate becomes hardened and cracked. Parallel linear streaks of hair are matted together, revealing moist erythematous skin in-between ("furrows") (Figs. 4.1-7 and 4.1-8). Death often occurs within a week to 10 days.

The *chronic form* is characterized by erythema and waxy brown crusts confined to the ears and head (Fig. 4.1-9). The piglets are usually otherwise healthy.

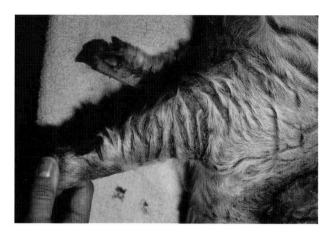

Figure 4.1-7 Exudative Epidermitis. Parallel rows of matted hair separated by areas of erythematous, waxy, alopecic skin ("furrows").

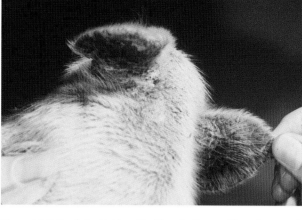

Figure 4.1-9 Exudative Epidermitis. Chronic disease with erythema and waxy brown crusts limited to the medial surface of the pinnae and the skin behind the ears.

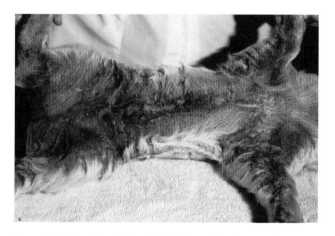

Figure 4.1-8 Exudative Epidermitis. Widespread erythema and waxy brown crusts.

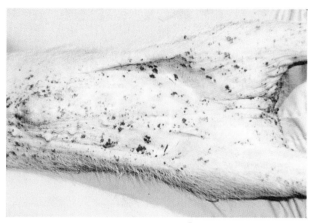

Figure 4.1-10 Staphylococcal Folliculitis. Widespread crusts and pustules.

3. Dermatohistopathology—Subcorneal to intragranular vesicular-to-pustular dermatitis with degenerate neutrophils and intracellular cocci.

FOLLICULITIS

Features

Folliculitis (hair follicle inflammation) is uncommon, cosmopolitan, and caused by an, as yet, uncharacterized, coagulase-positive *Staphylococcus* spp. There are no apparent breed or sex predilections, and the condition occurs most frequently in piglets less than eight weeks of age.

A pustular dermatitis covers much of the body, especially the ventral chest, abdomen, and hind quarters (Figs. 4.1-10 and 4.1-11). The white to yellowish pustules then rupture to form brown crusts. The condition is neither pruritic nor painful, and affected animals are otherwise healthy. One or multiple piglets may be affected.

Differential Diagnosis

None.

Diagnosis

1. Microscopy (direct smears)—Degenerate neutrophils, nuclear streaming, and phagocytosed cocci (Gram-positive, about 1 μm diameter)(Fig. 4.1-12).
2. Culture (aerobic).
3. Dermatohistopathology—Suppurative luminal folliculitis with degenerate neutrophils and intracellular cocci.

SPIROCHETOSIS

Features

Spirochetosis is an uncommon, cosmopolitan, poorly understood necrotic and ulcerative or granulomatous disease. It is thought to be caused by *Borrelia suis*, and predisposing factors include trauma and poor hygiene. Mixed infections (*Streptococcus* spp, *Arcanobacterium pyogenes, Staphylococcus hyicus*) are common. There are no apparent breed or sex predilections. Young animals (especially recently weaned) are most commonly affected, especially in large litters and disadvantaged, weaker piglets.

Lesions may occur anywhere, especially face (Figs. 4.1-13

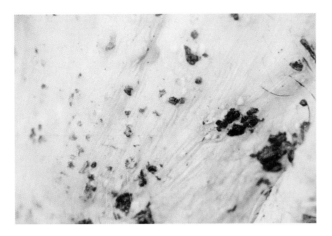

Figure 4.1-11 Close-up of Figure 4.1-10. Pustules and crusts.

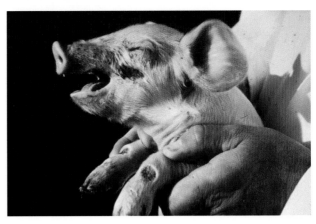

Figure 4.1-13 Spirochetosis. Necrosis and ulceration of the face (courtesy R. Cameron).

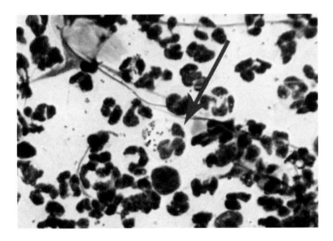

Figure 4.1-12 Staphylococcal Folliculitis. Direct smear (Diff-Quik stain). Suppurative inflammation with degenerate neutrophils, nuclear streaming, and phagocytosed cocci (arrow).

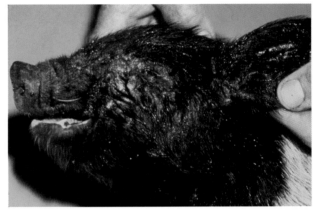

Figure 4.1-14 Spirochetosis. Necrosis and ulceration of the face.

through 4.1-15), head, pinnae, flank, and tail. Erythema and edema are followed by necrosis and ulceration. Granulomatous nodules ("ulcerative dermatitis," "granulomatous dermatitis")—often with central necrosis and slough—can occur, especially in pressure sores and calluses of older pigs. A gray-brown glutinous pus may be seen. Suckling piglets—especially those less than one week old—may develop bilateral necrotic ulcers, often covered by hard brown crusts, which can extend from the side of the face to the lower jaw. Large crusts can interfere with nursing. Bilateral ear lesions (necrotic and ulcerative) frequently begin at the base of the pinnae, extend distally, slough off, and leave a ragged bleeding margin (Fig. 4.1-16).

Differential Diagnosis

For necrotic and ulcerative lesions: streptococcal infection, necrobacillosis. For granulomatous lesions: other infections and foreign body granulomas.

Diagnosis

1. Microscopy (direct smears)—Suppurative or pyogranulomatous inflammation with spirochetes.

2. Dermatohistopathology—Necrotizing or pyogranulomatous dermatitis with spirochetes.

ERYSIPELAS

Features

Erysipelas (Greek: red skin) is an uncommon, cosmopolitan infectious disease caused by *Erysipelothrix (insidiosa) rhusiopathiae*. The organism is a Gram-positive pleomorphic rod (slender; about 0.3 μm × 1.7 μm). There are no apparent breed, or sex predilections, and pigs 3 months to 3 years old are most commonly affected.

Erysipelas occurs in acute, subacute, and chronic clinical forms. In the *acute form*, fever, depression, anorexia, and lameness are accompanied by bluish to purplish discoloration of the skin, especially in the abdomen, pinnae, and legs. Pinkish to red macules and papules may also be seen.

In the *subacute form*, erythematous papules and wheals enlarge to form square, rectangular, or rhomboidal plaques ("diamond skin disease"). The erythematous plaques often develop a purplish, necrotic center (Fig. 4.1-17).

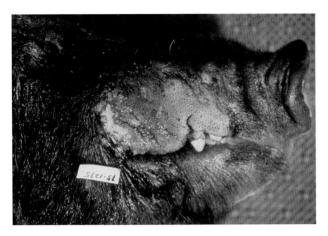

Figure 4.1-15 Spirochetosis. Necrotic plaque on face.

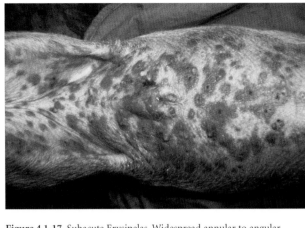

Figure 4.1-17 Subacute Erysipelas. Widespread annular to angular papules and plaques, some of which have central necrosis ("diamond skin disease") (courtesy R. Cameron).

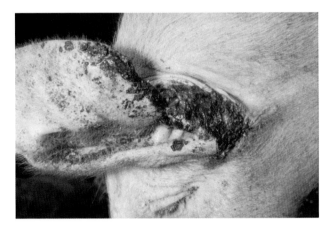

Figure 4.1-16 Spirochetosis. Necrosis and ulceration of the caudal pinnal margin (courtesy R. Cameron).

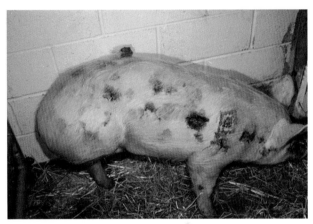

Figure 4.1-18 Chronic Erysipelas. Widespread angular to rectangular to square areas of necrosis.

The *chronic form* is characterized by necrosis and sloughing of the plaques, resulting in black, dry, firm areas of skin that peel away to reveal ulcers (Figs. 4.1-18 and 4.1-19). Occasionally, the pinnae, tail, and feet may slough as well (Figs. 4.1-20 through 4.1-22), and widespread alopecia may be seen.

Typically multiple animals are affected. Erysipelas is of great economic importance in swine operations.

Erysipelas is a zoonosis. Lesions are commonly seen on the hands and fingers, and consist of a painful, slowly progressive, discrete, purplish or erythematous cellulitis ("erysipeloid") (Fig. 4.1-23).

Differential Diagnosis

Actinobacillus suis infection.

Diagnosis

1. Culture (aerobic).
2. Necropsy—Skin lesions are characterized by neutrophilic vasculitis, suppurative hidradenitis, and necrotizing dermatitis.

ABSCESS

Features

Subcutaneous abscesses are a common, cosmopolitan problem. They usually follow contamination of skin wounds (accidents, fighting, surgery, infections, foreign bodies, ectoparasites). The most commonly involved bacteria are *Arocanobacterium pyogenes*, ß-hemolytic streptococci, *Staphylococcus aureus*, *S. hyicus*, and *Bacteroides* spp. There are no apparent breed, sex, or age predilections.

Subcutaneous abscesses may be single or multiple, and most commonly occur on the shoulder, neck, flank, pinnae, and tail (Figs. 4.1-24 and 4.1-25). Lesional heat and pain, and systemic signs are inconsistent. Typically a single, animal is affected.

Differential Diagnosis

Hematoma.

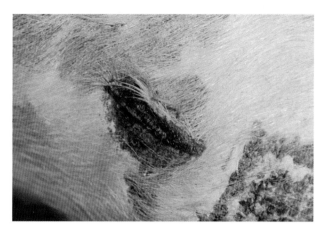

Figure 4.1-19 Close-up of Figure 4.1-18. Black areas of necrosis, and an ulcer created by partial sloughing of necrotic skin.

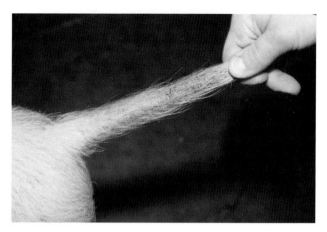

Figure 4.1-21 Chronic Erysipelas. Necrosis of distal tail.

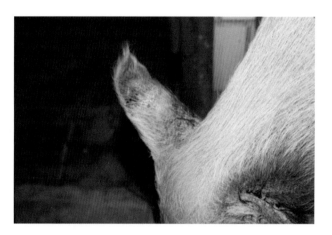

Figure 4.1-20 Chronic Erysipelas. Necrosis of distal pinnae.

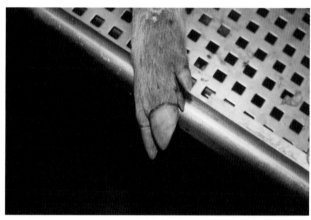

Figure 4.1-22 Chronic Erysipelas. Erythema and necrosis of distal leg.

Diagnosis

1. Microscopy (direct smears)—Suppurative inflammation with numerous intra- and extracellular cocci and/or rods.
2. Culture (aerobic and anaerobic).

ACTINOMYCOSIS

Features

Actinomycosis is a rare, cosmopolitan disease. *Actinomyces suis* contaminates various wounds. There are no breed or age predilections, and sows may be predisposed.

Lesions are most commonly seen affecting the udder, ventral abdomen, groin, and flank (Fig. 4.1-26). Firm nodules or tumors often develop draining tracts and discharge a yellowish pus containing yellowish-white granules ("sulfur granules") (Fig. 4.1-27). Affected animals are usually otherwise healthy. Typically a single animal is affected.

Differential Diagnosis

Other bacterial, fungal, or foreign body granulomas.

Diagnosis

1. Microscopy (direct smears)—Pyogranulomatous inflammation. Tissue granules contain Gram-positive, long filaments (less than 1 μm diameter).
2. Culture (anaerobic).
3. Dermatohistopathology—Nodular-to-diffuse pyogranulomatous dermatitis. Tissue granules are coated with Splendore-Hoeppli material and contain Gram-positive filaments.

SEPTICEMIC SLOUGH

Features

Septicemic slough is a rare, cosmopolitan, cutaneous reaction pattern. Septicemic salmonellosis—usually associated with *Salmonella choleraesuis* (Gram-negative rod) infection—is one recognized cause. There are no apparent breed or sex predilections, and young piglets are predisposed.

Lesions are most commonly seen on the pinnae, snout, feet, tail, and ventral abdomen (Figs. 4.1-28 through 4.1-30). Affected skin is initially bluish to purplish (cyanosis) due to intense dermal vascular dilatation and engorgement. This is a common

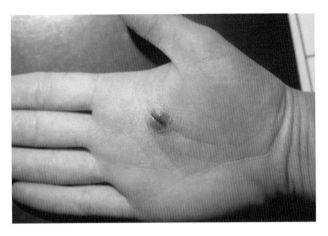

Figure 4.1-23 Erysipelas in a Human ("Erysipeloid"). Purple plaque on hand.

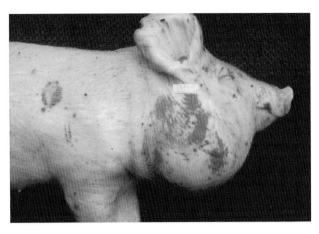

Figure 4.1-25 Huge subcutaneous abscess involving face and neck due to *Arcanobacterium pyogenes*.

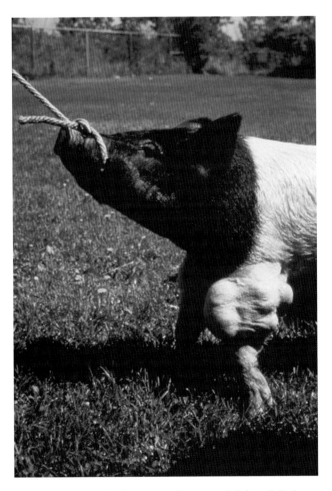

Figure 4.1-24 Multiple subcutaneous abscesses on left thoracic limb.

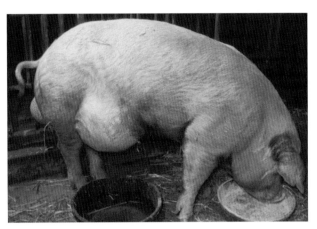

Figure 4.1-26 Actinomycosis. Firm tumor in flank.

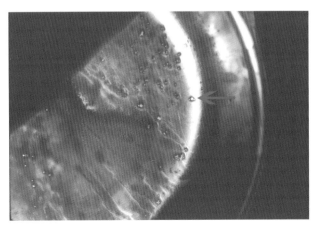

Figure 4.1-27 Actinomycosis. Seropurulent exudate containing "sulfur granules" (arrow) in a stainless steel bowl.

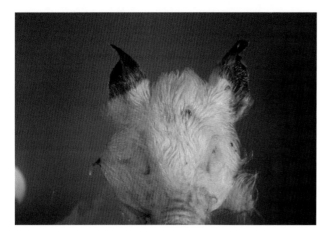

Figure 4.1-28 Septicemic Slough. Necrotic pinnae in a piglet with salmonellosis.

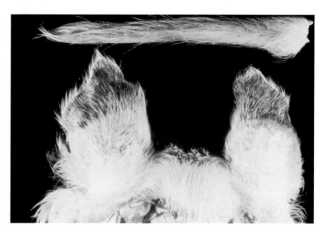

Figure 4.1-30 Septicemic Slough. Necrotic pinnae and sloughed tail in a piglet with salmonellosis.

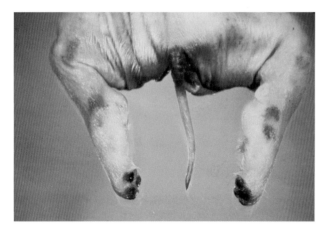

Figure 4.1-29 Septicemic Slough. Purpura and necrosis of tail, pelvic limbs, and feet in a piglet with salmonellosis.

Table 4.1-1 Differential Diagnosis for Symmetrical Cyanotic Extremities
Bacterial Infection
Actinobacillus pleuropneumoniae
Actinobacillus suis
Erysipelothrix rhusiopathiae (zoonosis: erysipeloid)
Escherichia coli (enterotoxigenic strains)
Haemophilus parasuis
Pasteurella multocida (zoonosis: skin infection)
Salmonella choleraesuis
Streptococcus suis (zoonosis: meningitis)
Rickettsial Infection
Eperythrozoon suis
Viral Infection
Iridovirus (African swine fever)
Pestivirus (classical swine fever)
Reproductive and respiratory syndrome virus

cutaneous reaction pattern in septicemic or toxemic pigs (Table 4.1-1). Some animals go on to develop thrombosis, which leads to necrosis and sloughing of affected skin, especially on the pinnae, tail, and feet. This is also a cutaneous reaction pattern in septicemic or toxemic pigs (Table 4.1-2). Typically animals are systemically ill, and one or more animals may be affected.

Differential Diagnosis

See Tables 4.1-1 and 4.1-2.

Diagnosis

1. Culture.
2. Necropsy.

Table 4.1-2 Differential Diagnosis for Symmetrical Sloughing of Extremities
Bacterial Infection
Actinobacillus suis
Erysipelothrix rhusiopathiae (zoonosis: erysipeloid)
Salmonella choleraesuis
Staphylococcus hyicus
Viral Infection
Pestivirus (classical swine fever)
Environmental
Frostbite

MISCELLANEOUS BACTERIAL DISEASES

Table 4.1-3 Miscellaneous Bacterial Diseases

Actinobacillosis	Uncommon and cosmopolitan; can produce cyanosis, sloughing of extremities or erysipelas-like disease; *Actinobacillus suis*; culture and necropsy
Anthrax (Greek: coal; black eschar)	Uncommon and cosmopolitan; face and neck; marked edema; *Bacillus anthracis*; systemic signs; *zoonosis* (cutaneous, respiratory, intestinal); culture and necropsy
Clostridial cellulitis (malignant edema; gas gangrene; blackleg)	Uncommon and cosmopolitan; groin, ventral abdomen, ventral neck, shoulder, head (*Clostridium septicum*); leg, face, neck (*C. chauvoei*); injection sites (*C. perfringens*); pitting edema, heat, pain, discoloration, variable crepitus; systemic signs; culture and necropsy
Dermatophilosis	Very rare and cosmopolitan; widespread exudation, crusting; *Dermatophilus congolensis*; *zoonosis* (cutaneous); direct smears, culture, dermatohistopathology
Edema disease	Uncommon and cosmopolitan; usually recently weaned pigs; edema and variable pruritus of eyelids, face, lips, pinnae, and neck; systemic signs; hemolytic, verotoxin-producing *Escherichia coli*; culture
Haemophilus parasuis infection (Fig. 4.1-31)	Uncommon and cosmopolitan; pinnal panniculitis (thickening of pinnae, especially concave surface); cutaneous cyanosis, meningitis; culture, dermatohistopathology, necropsy
Necrobacillosis (Figs. 4.1-32 and 4.1-33)	Uncommon and cosmopolitan; anywhere, especially lips, cheeks, legs, teats; *Fusobacterium necrophorum*; necrosis, ulceration, crusting, foul smell; variable systemic signs; culture
Streptococcal infections	Uncommon and cosmopolitan; B-hemolytic streptococci (*S. dysgalactia* group, serovars C and L) cause subcutaneous abscesses or pinnal necrosis (suckling piglets; unilateral or bilateral; especially tip and caudal edge); streptococci (especially Lancefield group C) cause contagious pustular dermatitis in suckling piglets (erythema, pustules, and crusts on groin, medial thighs, lips, periocular area, pinnae, rump, tail; premonitory systemic signs); culture
Yersinia enterocolitica infection	Uncommon and cosmopolitan; edema of eyelids, face, and abdomen; culture

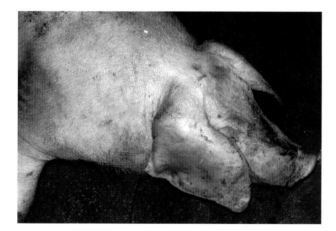

Figure 4.1-31 *Haemophilus parasuis* Infection. Swollen, erythematous pinnae due to panniculitis (courtesy R. Drolet).

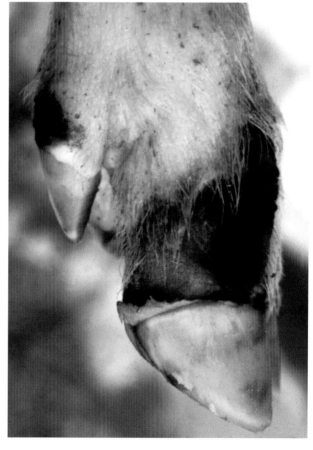

Figure 4.1-32 Necrobacillosis. Necrosis and ulceration of distal limb (courtesy J. Gourreau).

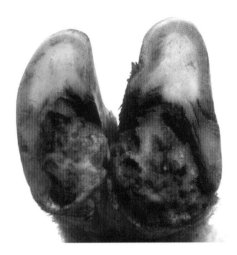

Figure 4.1-33 Necrobacillosis. Necrotic and proliferative lesions on foot (courtesy J. Gourreau).

REFERENCES

Aarestrup FM, Wegener HC. 1997. Association between production of fibrinolysin and virulence of *Staphylococcus hyicus* in relation to exudative epidermitis in pigs. *Acta Vet Scand* 38: 295.

Amass SF. 1999. Erysipelas: new disease or old problem revisited? *Comp Food Anim Med Manage* 21: 560.

Andersen LO, et al. 2005. Exudative Epidermitis in Pigs Caused by Toxigenic *Staphylococcus chromogenes. Vet Microbiol* 105: 291.

Drolet R, et al. 2000. Ear panniculitis associated with *Haemophilus parasuis* infection in growing-finishing pigs. *Int Pig Vet Soc Cong* 16: 528.

Hommerz J, et al. 1991. Characterization of 2 groups of Actinomyces-like bacteria isolated from purulent lesions in pigs. *J Vet Med B* 38: 575.

Howard JL, Smith RA. 1999. Current Veterinary Therapy. Food Animal Practice. Ed 4. WB Saunders, Philadelphia, PA.

Miniats OP, et al. 1989. *Actinobacillus suis* septicemia in mature swine: two outbreaks resembling erysipelas. *Can Vet J* 30: 943.

Radostits OM, et al. 2000. Veterinary Medicine. A Textbook of the Diseases of Cattle, Sheep, Pigs, Goats and Horses. Ed 9. WB Saunders, Philadelphia, PA.

Scott DW. 1988. Large Animal Dermatology. WB Saunders, Philadelphia, PA.

Straw BE, et al. 1999. Diseases of Swine. Ed 8. Iowa State Press, Ames.

Tanabe T, et al. 1996. Correlation between occurrence of exudative epidermitis and exfoliative toxin-producing ability of *Staphylococcus hyicus. Vet Microbiol* 48: 9.

White M. 1999. Skin lesions in pigs. *In Pract* 21: 20.

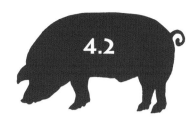

FUNGAL SKIN DISEASES

4.2

Dermatophytosis
Miscellaneous Fungal Diseases
    Aspergillosis
    Candidiasis
    Zygomycosis

DERMATOPHYTOSIS

Features

Dermatophytosis (ringworm) is a common cosmopolitan disease. It is most commonly caused by *Microsporum nanum*, and less frequently by *M. canis, Trichophyton mentagrophytes,* and *T. verrucosum*. There are no apparent breed, sex, or age predilections.

Lesions can occur anywhere, especially on the face, pinnae, and trunk (Figs. 4.2-1 and 4.2-2). Annular macular areas of erythema to brownish skin discoloration and dry brownish to orangish crusts are seen. Lesions may enlarge to several cm in diameter. Pustules may be seen at the periphery of lesions. Alopecia and pruritus are rare. Chronic infections—thick brown crusts—may be established behind the ears and spread onto the pinnae and the neck. Affected animals are otherwise healthy. Typically multiple animals are affected.

Porcine dermatophytosis is a zoonosis. *M. nanum* infection in humans causes typical ringworm lesions in contact areas, especially the face, scalp, and arms, and kerions on the scalp (Fig. 4.2-3).

Differential Diagnosis

Idiopathic recurrent dermatosis of sows.

Diagnosis

1. Culture.
2. Dermatohistopathology—Fungal hyphae and arthroconidia in surface and follicular keratin.

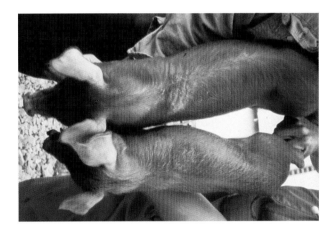

Figure 4.2-2 Dermatophytosis. Large annular area of crusting over trunk.

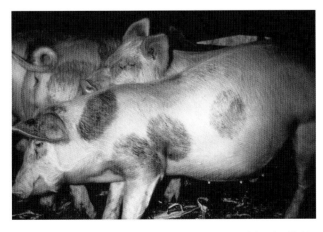

Figure 4.2-1 Dermatophytosis. Multiple annular areas of discolored skin and brown crusts (courtesy R. Cameron).

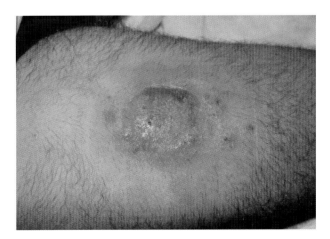

Figure 4.2-3 Dermatophytosis. Severely inflamed lesion with draining tracts (kerion) on the arm caused by *Microsporum nanum.*

MISCELLANEOUS FUNGAL DISEASES

Table 4.2-1 Miscellaneous Fungal Infections

Aspergillosis	Very rare; widespread papular dermatitis; *Aspergillus* spp.; culture and dermatohistopathology
Candidiasis	Rare and cosmopolitan; annular areas of moist erythema and gray surface exudate on ventral abdomen, medial thighs, and distal limbs; *Candida albicans*; culture and dermatohistopathology
Zygomycosis	Very rare; one or multiple subcutaneous nodules with draining tracts; *Rhizopus oryzae*; culture and dermatohistopathology

REFERENCES

Howard JL, Smith RA. 1999. Current Veterinary Therapy. Food Animal Practice. Ed 4. WB Saunders, Philadelphia, PA.

Radostits OM, et al. 2000. Veterinary Medicine. A Textbook of the Diseases of Cattle, Sheep, Pigs, Goats and Horses. Ed 9. WB Saunders, Philadelphia, PA.

Scott DW. 1988. Large Animal Dermatology. WB Saunders, Philadelphia, PA.

Straw BE, et al. 1999. Diseases of Swine. Ed 8. Iowa State Press, Ames.

White M. 1999. Skin lesions in pigs. *In Pract* 21: 20.

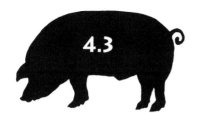

PARASITIC SKIN DISEASES

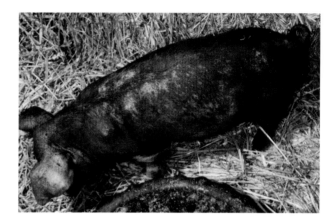

Figure 4.3-1 Sarcoptic Mange. Widespread crusts and alopecia, especially over pinnae, head, thorax, and rump.

SARCOPTIC MANGE

Features

Sarcoptic mange (scabies) is a common, cosmopolitan infestation caused by the mite *Sarcoptes scabiei var suis*. It is the most important skin disease of swine worldwide. Hypersensitivity (allergy) to mite antigens play an important role in the evolution of the dermatitis (type I and type IV hypersensitivity reactions involved). There are no apparent breed, age, or sex predilections. Transmission occurs by direct and indirect contact.

There are two clinical forms of sarcoptic mange. The most common form (the hypersensitive or allergic form) is seen most often in young growing pigs. Initial lesions include papules, crusts, and excoriations on and in the ears. Hematomas may develop on the lateral (inner) surface of the pinnae. A widespread, erythematous, maculopapular eruption then appears, especially over the rump, flanks, and abdomen (Figs. 4.3-1 and 4.3-2). In long-standing cases, the skin is thickened, lichenified, and crusted. Pruritus is intense.

The second, much less common form (the hyperkeratotic or chronic form) is seen most often in multiparous sows or in animals debilitated for other reasons. Thick, asbestos-like crusts develop in and on the ears (Fig. 4.3-3) and occasionally the head, neck, and distal legs (especially the hocks). Pruritus is moderate to intense.

Sarcoptic mange can be a cause of decreased weight gain, poor feed conversion efficiency, decreased milk production, decreased carcass value, decreased sow productivity, increased piglet mortality (due to crushing), and damage to facilities (constant rubbing). Multiple animals are affected, with a prevalence of 20% to 95% of the herd. Crusts in the ears of multiparous sows are the main reservoir of mites in a herd.

Sarcoptic mange is a potential zoonosis. Affected humans de-

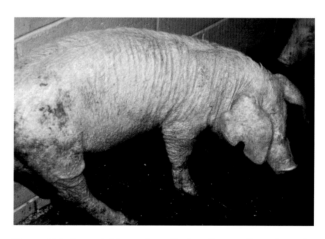

Figure 4.3-2 Sarcoptic Mange. Generalized erythema and papules, and multifocal crusts and excoriations (courtesy R. Cameron).

velop pruritic, erythematous papules with crusts and excoriations on the arms, chest, abdomen, and legs (Fig. 4.3-4).

Differential Diagnosis

Pediculosis, mosquitoes.

Diagnosis

1. History and physical examination.
2. Microscopy—Perhaps the most practical procedure is to make deep skin scrapings from the inner surface of the pinna and ear canal using melon ballers, bone curettes, or sharpened

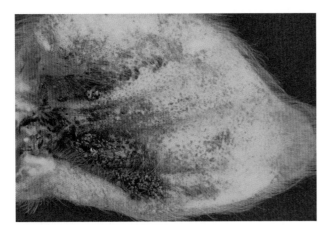

Figure 4.3-3 Sarcoptic Mange. Thick brownish crusts in ear canal and on inner surface of pinnae (courtesy T. Clark).

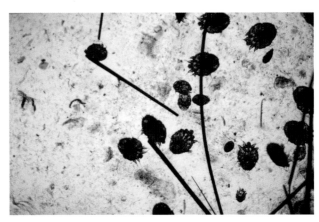

Figure 4.3-5 Sarcoptic Mange. Multiple mites in a skin scraping.

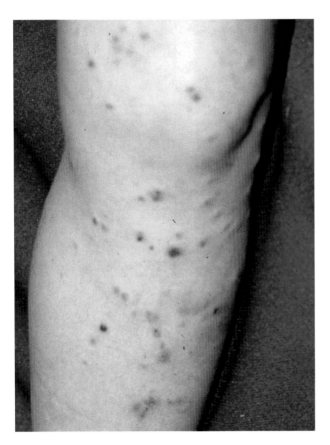

Figure 4.3-4 Sarcoptic Mange. Erythematous and crusted papules on the leg of a human with animal-origin scabies.

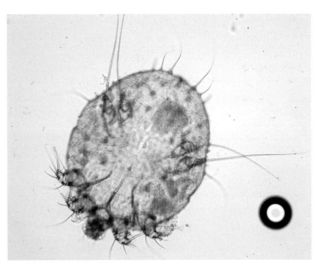

Figure 4.3-6 Sarcoptic Mange. Adult mite in a skin scraping.

3. Serodiagnosis—Various crude antigen preparations (*S. scabiei var suis, S. scabiei var vulpes*) have been used to detect circulating mite-specific antibodies by ELISA techniques. None are completely sensitive and specific. It is also important to realize that: (a) these tests should not be used in animals less than 10 weeks old; and (b) antibody titers remain positive for 9 to 12 months after the disease has been successfully treated.

PEDICULOSIS

Features

Pediculosis (lice) is a common, cosmopolitan infestation caused by the sucking louse, *Haematopinus suis.* There are no apparent breed, age, or sex predilections. Louse populations are usually much larger during cold weather. Thus, clinical signs are usually seen, or are more severe, in winter. Transmission occurs by direct and indirect contact.

Lice are most commonly seen on the ears, neck, axillae, groin, flanks, and medial surface of legs (Fig. 4.3-8). Pruritus is moderate to marked, and may be associated with erythema, papules, ex-

stainless steel teaspoons. The collected debris is placed in a petri dish, covered with mineral oil, and placed in an incubator overnight. The sample is examined with the aid of a 10× lens (dissecting scope or microscope), and mites (0.25 to 0.6 mm in length) are seen "swimming" in the oil (Figs. 4.3-5 and 4.3-6). Ova (eggs) and scyballa (fecal pellets) may also be found (Fig. 4.3-7). Unfortunately, skin scraping procedures have a low diagnostic sensitivity (about 33% in the hypersensitive form, and about 81% in the hyperkeratotic form).

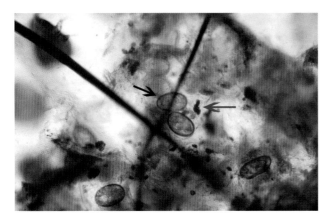

Figure 4.3-7 Sarcoptic Mange. Multiple eggs (black arrow) and fecal pellets (red arrow) in a skin scraping.

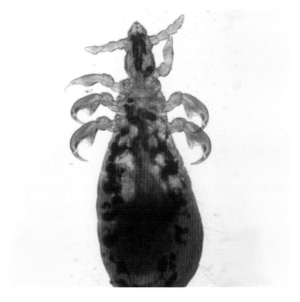

Figure 4.3-9 Pediculosis. Sucking louse.

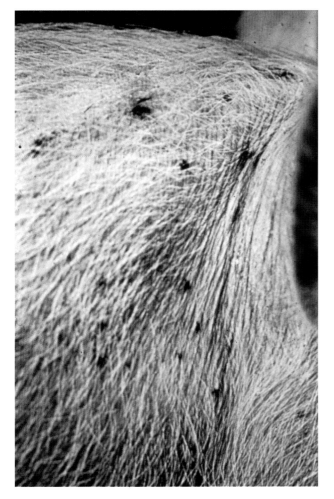

Figure 4.3-8 Pediculosis. Numerous lice on neck and shoulder.

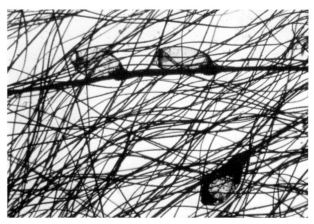

Figure 4.3-10 Pediculosis. Nits on hair shaft.

coriations, and crusts. Large populations of lice can cause anemia in young pigs, as well as decreased weight gain, decreased feed conversion efficiency and hide damage. Typically, multiple animals are affected. Lice are very host-specific, and humans would not be expected to be affected. Anecdotal reports indicate that *H. suis* can occasionally bite humans. Lice are involved in the transmission of swinepox.

Differential Diagnosis

Sarcoptic mange, mosquitoes.

Diagnosis

1. History and physical examination—*H. suis* is gray-brown in color.
2. Microscopy (Lice and Hairs Placed in Mineral Oil)—Adult lice are large (about 6 mm in length) (Fig. 4.3-9). Ova (nits) may be seen attached to hair shafts (Fig. 4.3-10).

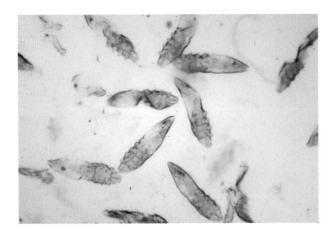

MISCELLANEOUS PARASITIC DISEASES

Table 4.3-1 Miscellaneous Parasitic Diseases

Demodectic mange ("follicular mange")	Uncommon and cosmopolitan; *Demodex phylloides* (about 0.25 mm in length), normal resident of hair follicles; associated with concurrent depressed immunity; skin-colored to erythematous papules on snout, eyelids, ventral neck/chest/abdomen, and medial thighs; neither painful nor pruritic; thick, caseous, whitish material expressed from incised lesion contains numerous mites (Fig. 4.3-11)
Ticks	Uncommon to rare; cosmopolitan; most in spring and summer; especially ears, face, neck, axillae, groin, and distal legs; minimal lesions or papules and nodules centered around attached ticks; variable pain and pruritus; e.g., *Dermacentor andersonii, D. nitens, D. variabilis, Amblyomma maculatum, Ixodes scapularis, Otobius megnini,* and *Ornithodoros turicata* in the United States
Fleas	Uncommon to rare; cosmopolitan; *Pulex irritans* ("human flea"), *Echidnophaga gallinacea* ("sticktight flea"), and *Ctenocephalides felis* ("cat flea"), 2 to 4 mm in length; *Tunga penetrans* ("chigger flea") in Africa; especially summer and fall; variable degrees of pruritus and papulocrustous dermatitis, especially trunk; transmit swinepox; *T. penetrans* affects feet, snout, scrotum, and teats (can produce agalactica)
Mosquitoes	Uncommon and cosmopolitan; especially *Aedes* spp.; spring, summer, fall; erythematous papules and wheals and moderate to severe pruritus; especially pinnae, abdomen, flanks, legs, and perineum
Biting flies	Uncommon and cosmopolitan; *Stomoxys calcitrans* ("stable fly"), *Simulium* spp. ("black fly"), and *Tabanus* spp. ("horse fly"); spring, summer, and fall; painful/pruritic papules and vesicles; especially legs, head, pinnae, and abdomen
Cuterebra spp. infestation	Rare; cosmopolitan; larvae of *Cuterebra* spp. flies; subcutaneous nodules and cysts with a central pore; especially the neck
Dermatobia hominis infestation	Uncommon; Central and South America; painful subcutaneous nodules with a central pore containing third-stage larvae (about 20 mm in length)
Calliphorine Myiasis ("maggots," "fly strike")	Common and cosmopolitan; especially *Lucilia* spp., *Calliphora* spp., and *Phormia* spp.; especially late spring, summer, and early fall; any wounded/damaged skin; foul-smelling ulcers with scalloped margins and a "honeycombed" appearance, teeming with larvae ("maggots"); usually painful and pruritic
Screw-worm myiasis	Uncommon; Central and South America (*Callitroga hominivorax* and *C. macellaria*); Africa and Asia (*Chrysomyia bezziana* and *C. megacephala*); especially late spring, summer, and early fall; any wounded/damaged skin; foul-smelling ulcers with scalloped margins and a "honeycombed" appearance, teeming with larvae; painful and pruritic; humans are also susceptible (e.g., skin, genitalia, ears, sinuses)
Suifilaria suis infestation	Rare; Africa; vesicular dermatitis, especially trunk; secondary bacterial infections cause abscesses; dermatohistopathology

Figure 4.3-11 Demodectic Mange. Numerous mites from an incised and squeezed lesion.

REFERENCES

Alexander JL. 2006. Screwworms. *J Am Vet Med Assoc* 228: 357.

Baker AS. 1999. Mites and Ticks of Domestic Animals. An Identification Guide and Information Source. The Stationary Office, London, UK.

Bornstein S, and Wallgren P. 1997. Serodiagnosis of Sarcoptic Mange in Pigs. *Vet Rec* 141: 8.

Bornstein S, and Zakrisson G. 1993. Clinical Picture and Antibody Response in Pigs Infected by *Sarcoptes scabiei var suis*. *Vet Dermatol* 4: 123.

Bowman DD. 1999. Georgis' Parasitology for Veterinarians. Ed. 7. WB Saunders, Philadelphia, PA.

Cole W. 1990. Suspected Hypersensitivity to Insect Bites in Market Pigs. *Can Vet J* 31: 845.

Davis DP, and Moon RD. 1990. Density of Itch Mite, *Sarcoptes scabiei* (Acari: Sarcoptidae) and Temporal Development of Cutaneous Hypersensitivity in Swine Mange. *Vet Parasitol* 36: 285.

Hogg A. 1989. The Control and Eradication of Sarcoptic Mange in Swine Herds. *Agri-Pract* 10: 8.

Jacobson M, et al. 1999. The Efficacy of Simplified Eradication Strategies Against Sarcoptic Mange Mite Infections in Swine Herds Monitored by an ELISA. *Vet Parasitol* 81: 249.

Melançon JJ. 1998. Sarcoptic Mange in Swine: Current Prevalence. *Comp Cont Educ* 20: 587.

Radostits OM, et al. 2000. Veterinary Medicine. A Textbook of the Diseases of Cattle, Sheep, Pigs, Goats, and Horses. Ed. 9. WB Saunders, Philadelphia, PA.

Scott DW. 1988. Large Animal Dermatology. WB Saunders, Philadelphia, PA.

Smets K, and Vercruysse J. 2000. Evaluation of Different Methods for the Diagnosis of Scabies in Swine. *Vet Parasitol* 90: 137.

Straw BE, et al. 1999. Diseases of Swine. Ed. 8. Iowa State University Press, Ames, IA.

van der Heijder HMJF, et al. 2000. Validation of ELISAs for the Detection of Antibodies to *Sarcoptes scabiei* in Pigs. *Vet Parasitol* 89: 95.

Wall R, et al. 2001. Veterinary Ectoparasites. Ed. 2. Blackwell Scientific, Oxford, UK.

Wooten-Saadi E., et al. 1988. Influence of Sarcoptic Mange and Cold and Ambient Temperature in Blastogenic Responses of Lymphocytes and Serum Cortisol Concentrations of Pigs. *Am J Vet Res* 49: 1555.

Zimmerman W, Kircher P. 1998. Serologische Bestandesuntersuchung und Sanierungsüberwachung der *Sarcoptes scabiei var suis* Infektion: Erste Vorläufige Resultate. *Schweiz Arch Tierheilk* 140: 369.

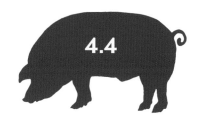

VIRAL AND PROTOZOAL SKIN DISEASES

4.4

Swinepox
Dermatitis and Nephropathy Syndrome
Foot-and-Mouth Disease
Miscellaneous Viral and Rickettsial Diseases
    Adenovirus Infection
    African Swine Fever
    Classical Swine Fever
    Eperythrozoonosis
    Parvovirus Vesicular Disease
    Porcine Reproductive and Respiratory Syndrome
    Rinderpest
    Swine Vesicular Disease
    Vesicular Exanthema
    Vesicular Stomatitis

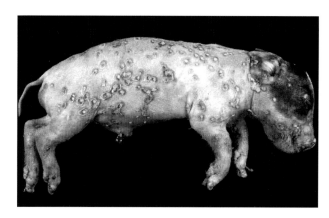

Figure 4.4-1 Swinepox. Generalized pustules and crusts in a piglet with congenital disease (*in utero* infection) (courtesy T. Clark).

SWINEPOX

Features

Swinepox is a cosmopolitan disease caused by *Suipoxvirus*. *Vaccinia* virus caused an identical syndrome. Hence, since the eradication of smallpox (variola) and the subsequent cessation of *Vaccinia* vaccination the prevalence of "swinepox" has decreased. The hog louse (*Haematopinus suis*) and various flies and mosquitoes are important in disease transmission. Transplacental infections result in neonatal disease (Fig. 4.4-1). There are no breed or sex predilections. All ages are affected, especially the young.

Lesions begin as erythematous macules which progress through papular, vesicular, and pustular phases. The vesicular phase is not often observed. Pustules become umbilicated (depressed center) and have a peripheral red, raised border (these lesions are the classic "pocks") (Figs. 4.4-2 through 4.4-5). The pustules then rupture, crust over, and heal (often with scars). Lesions occurring on the ventrolateral thorax and abdomen, medial thighs, and forelegs, udder, teats, and vulva are attributed to louse infestation. Lesions on the face, pinnae, and dorsum are attributed to fly and mosquito transmission. Very young animals can have generalized lesions. The lesions are neither painful nor pruritic. Systemic signs are rarely present.

Suipoxvirus does not cause lesions in humans (*Vaccinia* virus did).

Differential Diagnosis

Juvenile pustular psoriasiform dermatitis.

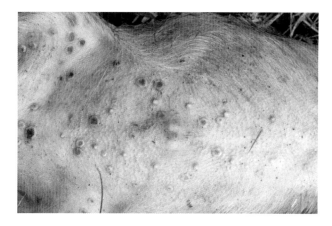

Figure 4.4-2 Swinepox. Numerous umbilicated and crusted pustules ("pocks") on the ventral thorax and abdomen.

Diagnosis

1. History and physical examination.
2. Dermatohistopathology—Eosinophilic intracytoplasmic inclusion bodies in epidermal keratinocytes.
3. Virus isolation.
4. Viral antigen detection.

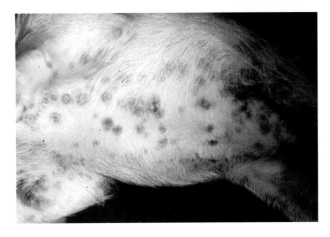

Figure 4.4-3 Swinepox. Numerous erythematous macules and plaques, crusts, and a few pustules on the ventral abdomen and thorax.

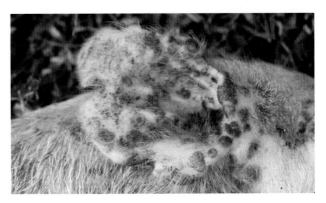

Figure 4.4-5 Swinepox. Numerous umbilicated and crusted pustules on pinnae.

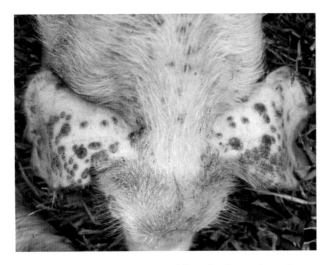

Figure 4.4-4 Swinepox. Numerous umbilicated and crusted pustules on the pinna.

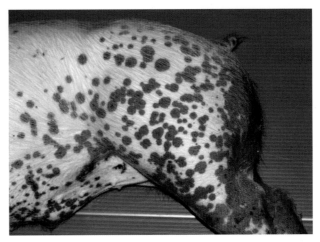

Figure 4.4-6 Dermatitis and Nephropathy Syndrome. Numerous deep red macules and plaques—many of which have a central black area (necrosis)—over thigh, flank, and abdomen (courtesy R. Drolet).

DERMATITIS AND NEPHROPATHY SYNDROME

Features

Dermatitis and nephropathy syndrome is a sporadic disease which is probably cosmopolitan. Porcine *Circovirus* type 2 and porcine reproductive and respiratory syndrome virus have been implicated as etiologic agents. Clinical signs are associated with an immune-complex, leukocytoclastic and necrotizing vasculitis. There are no apparent breed or sex predilections. Young animals, 6 to 16 weeks of age, are most commonly affected.

Erythematous to reddish-purple macules and papules evolve into patches and plaques. Larger papules and plaques often develop a central black area of necrosis and become covered with crusts (Figs. 4.4-6 and 4.4-7). Lesions are neither pruritic nor painful. Lesions occur most commonly on the hind quarters, perineum, legs, ventrolateral thorax and abdomen, and pinnae. Affected animals are depressed and inappetent. The morbidity is usually about 1%, but mortality can be high.

Differential Diagnosis

Erysipelas, actinobacillosis, adverse cutaneous drug reaction.

Diagnosis

1. History and physical examination.
2. Dermatohistopathology—Necrotizing, leukocytoclastic vasculitis.
3. Necropsy Examination—Lesions in kidneys and synovia. (vasculitis) and lungs (interstitial pneumonia).
4. Viral isolation from/viral antigen detection in affected tissues.

FOOT-AND-MOUTH DISEASE

Features

Foot-and-mouth disease ("aphthous fever"—Greek: painful vesicles and ulcers in mouth) is a highly contagious infectious disease of swine and ruminants caused by an Aphthovirus having 7 principal serotypes: A, O, C, South African Territories (SAT) 1, SAT 2, SAT 3, and Asia 1. The disease is endemic in Africa, Asia, and

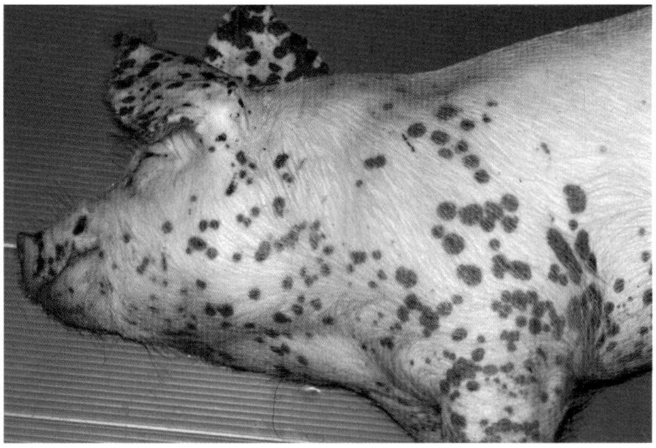

Figure 4.4-7 Dermatitis and Nephropathy Syndrome. Numerous deep red macules and plaques—many with central necrosis—over pinnae, face, neck, shoulder, and foreleg (courtesy R. Drolet).

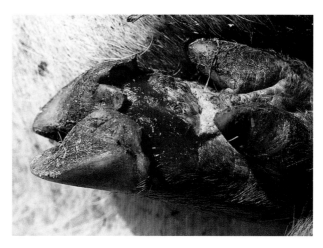

Figure 4.4-9 Foot-and-Mouth Disease. Ulceration of coronet and detachment of hoof (courtesy J. Gourreau).

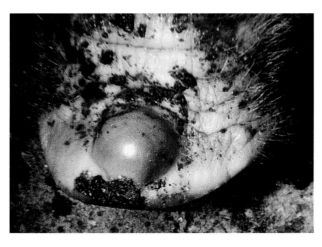

Figure 4.4-8 Foot-and-Mouth Disease. Intact bulla on snout (courtesy J. Gourreau).

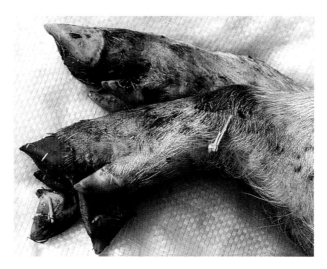

Figure 4.4-10 Foot-and-Mouth Disease. Sloughing of hooves (courtesy of J. Gourreau).

South America, and sporadic in Europe. Transmission occurs via aerosol, contact, insect vectors, and fomites. There are no breed, age, or sex predilections.

Lameness, fever, depression, and inappetence are usually the first signs of infection. Vesicles and bullae (up to 3 cm in diameter) develop into painful erosions and ulcers. Lesions are most commonly seen on the snout, nares, lips, tongue, hard and soft palates, coronets, and interdigital spaces and bulbs of the feet (Figs. 4.4-8 through 4.4-12). Nursing sows may have lesions on the teats and udder. In severe cases, the hooves may detach or severe laminitis may be followed by deformed hooves. Slobbering and chomping are common, and pregnant sows may abort.

Morbidity varies from 50% to 100%, and mortality is usually low (<5%), although occasional outbreaks are characterized by 50% mortality. Economic losses can be devastating: quarantine, slaughter, embargoes, and loss of trade. Foot-and-mouth disease is the number one foreign animal disease threat in the United States, and the most significant disease affecting free trade in animals and animal products internationally.

Humans may develop vesicles on the hands and/or in the mouth.

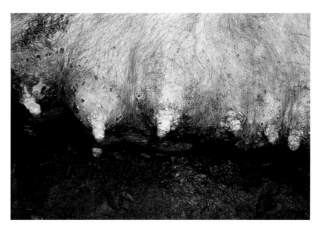

Figure 4.4-11 Foot-and-Mouth Disease. Pustules on teats. (courtesy J. Gourreau).

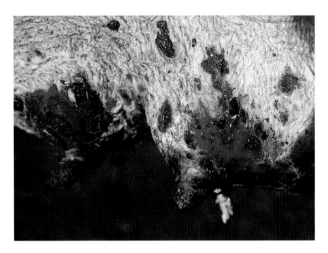

Figure 4.4-12 Foot-and-Mouth-Disease. Ulcers and crusts on teats and udder (courtesy J. Gourreau).

Differential Diagnosis

Swine vesicular disease, vesicular exanthema, and vesicular stomatitis are clinically identical to foot-and-mouth disease. Other differentials include ultraviolet light-induced vesiculobullous disease due to eating parsnip or celery, parvovirus vesicular disease, and chemical burns.

Diagnosis

1. Virus Isolation—Vesicular fluid, epithelial lesions, and heparinized blood.
2. Serology—Clotted blood.

MISCELLANEOUS VIRAL AND RICKETTSIAL DISEASES

Table 4.4-1 Miscellaneous Viral and Rickettsial Diseases

Adenovirus infection	Common; worldwide; skin cyanosis and subcutaneous edema in newborns; viral isolation and viral antigen detection
African swine fever (*Iridovirus*)	Common; Africa; red to red-blue to purplish discoloration of snout, pinnae, belly, flanks, legs, and rump; occasional skin necrosis; fever, anorexia, weakness, and incoordination; viral isolation and viral antigen detection
Classical swine fever ("hog cholera") (Fig. 4.4-13) (*Pestivirus*)	Uncommon; South America, Asia, Africa, parts of Europe; red to purplish discoloration of belly, medial thighs, snout, and pinnae; occasional necrotic areas on pinnae, tail, and vulva; fever, lethargy, conjunctivitis, diarrhea, vomiting, staggering; purplish blotching of pinnae and generalized hypotrichosis in chronic disease; congenital alopecia with *in utero* infection; viral isolation and viral detection
Eperythrozoonosis	Uncommon; cosmopolitan (especially North America and Europe); rickettsia *Eperythrozoon suis*; marbling (mottling) or red discoloration of pinnae (especially margins); occasional marked cyanosis of pinnae, tail, and distal legs; occasional necrosis of pinnal margins; occasional urticaria or macular purpuric eruption in chronic cases; fever, apathy, anemia; organism (0.2 to 2 μm diameter) adheres to erythrocytes; serology; rickettsial antigen detection
Parvovirus vesicular disease (Figs. 4.4-14 and 4.4-15)	Uncommon; cosmopolitan; vesicles and erosions on snout, coronet, interdigital spaces, and oral cavity; viral isolation and viral antigen detection
Porcine reproductive and respiratory syndrome (*Arterivirus*) (Fig. 4.4-16)	Uncommon; cosmopolitan; blotchy erythema and cyanosis of snout, pinnae, mammary gland, and vulva; anorexia, lethargy, fever, hyperpnea and dyspnea ("thumping"), and abortion; chemosis, diarrhea, and "thumping" in piglets; viral isolation and serology
Rinderpest (*Morbillivirus*)	Rare; Africa and Asia; erythema, papules, oozing, crusts, and alopecia over perineum, flanks, medial thighs, neck, scrotum, udder, and teats; cattle, sheep, and goats are susceptible; viral isolation and viral antigen detection
Swine vesicular disease (*Enterovirus*)	Uncommon; Asia and parts of Europe; vesicles, bullae, and erosions on snout, nares, lips, tongue, hard and soft palates, coronets, interdigital spaces, and occasionally teats; occasional sloughing of hooves; fever, slobbering, and chomping; possible abortion; viral isolation and viral antigen detection
Vesicular exanthema (*Calicivirus*) (Figs. 4.4-17 and 4.4-18)	Thought to be eradicated worldwide; vesicles, bullae, and erosions on snout, nares, lips, tongue, hard and soft palates, coronets, interdigital spaces, and occasionally teats; occasional sloughing of hooves; fever, slobbering, and chomping; possible abortion; viral isolation and viral antigen detection
Vesicular stomatitis (*Vesiculovirus*) (Fig. 4.4-19)	Uncommon; North, Central, and South America; especially summer and fall; vesicles, bullae, and erosions on snout, nares, lips, tongue, hard and soft palates, coronets, interdigital spaces, and occasionally teats; occasional sloughing of hooves; fever, slobbering, and chomping; possible abortion; cattle and goats are susceptible; viral isolation and viral antigen detection; influenza-like symptoms and occasional mucocutaneous vesicles and erosions in humans

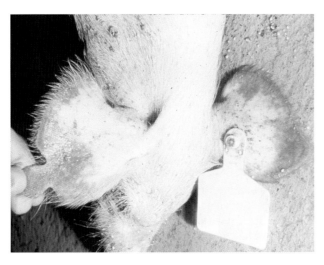

Figure 4.4-13 Classical Swine Fever (Hog Cholera). Blotchy, red-purple discoloration of pinnae (courtesy J. King).

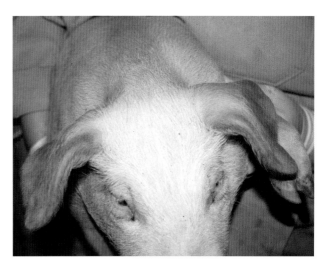

Figure 4.4-16 Porcine Reproductive and Respiratory Syndrome. Purple pinnae (courtesy R. Drolet).

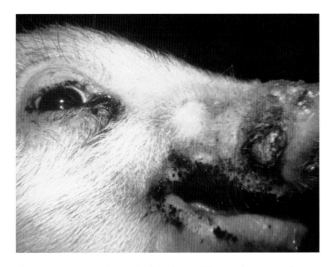

Figure 4.4-14 Parvovirus Vesicular Disease. Ulcers and crusts on face (courtesy H. Kresse, coll. J. Gourreau, AFSSA).

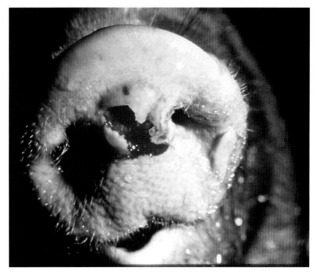

Figure 4.4-17 Vesicular Exanthema. Ulcers and crusts on snout (courtesy J. Gourreau).

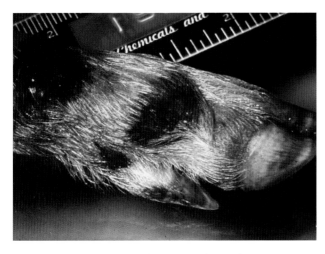

Figure 4.4-15 Parvovirus Vesicular Disease. Ulcers and crusts on coronet and distal leg (courtesy H. Kresse, coll. J. Gourreau, AFSSA).

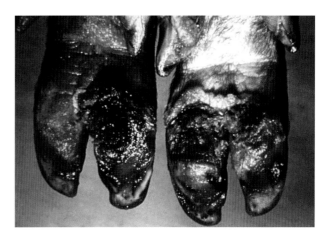

Figure 4.4-18 Vesicular Exanthema. Ulcers and crusts on coronets (courtesy J. Gourreau).

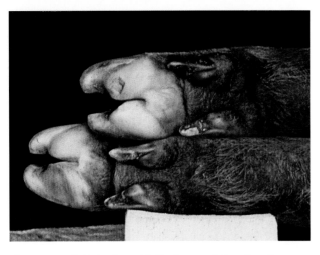

Figure 4.4-19 Vesicular Stomatitis. Erythema and ulceration of coronets and distal legs (courtesy J. Gourreau).

REFERENCES

Borst GHA, et al. 1990. Four Sporadic Cases of Congenital Swinepox. *Vet Rec* 127: 61.

Choi C, Chae C. 2001. Colocalization of Porcine Reproductive and Respiratory Syndrome Virus and Porcine Circovirus 2 in Porcine Dermatitis and Nephropathy Syndrome by Double-Labeling Technique. *Vet Pathol* 38: 436.

Grabarevi Z, et al. 2004. Pathological Observations on Pigs with Porcine Dermatitis and Nephropathy Syndrome in Croatia. *Vet Archiv* 74: 3.

Radostits OM, et al. 2000. Veterinary Medicine. A Textbook of the Diseases of Cattle, Sheep, Pigs, Goats and Horses. Ed. 9. WB Saunders, Philadelphia, PA.

Rosell C, et al. 2000. Identification of Porcine Circovirus in Tissues of Pigs with Porcine Dermatitis and Nephropathy Syndrome. *Vet Rec* 146: 40.

Scott DW. 1988. Large Animal Dermatology. WB Saunders, Philadelphia, PA.

Straw BE, et al. 1999. Diseases of Swine. Ed 8. Iowa State Press, Ames, IA.

Thibault S, et al. 1998. Cutaneous and Systemic Necrotizing Vasculitis in Swine. *Vet Pathol* 35: 108.

Van Halderen A, et al. 1995. Dermatitis/Nephropathy Syndrome in Pigs. *J So Afr Vet Assoc* 66: 108.

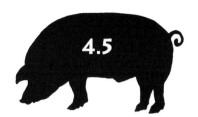

IMMUNOLOGICAL SKIN DISEASES

Urticaria
Bullous Pemphigoid

URTICARIA

Urticaria ("hives") is a rarely reported, cosmopolitan, variably pruritic, edematous skin disorder. It may be immunologic or nonimmunologic in nature. Incriminated causes include insects, arthropods, infections, topical agents, systemic medications, plants, and biologicals. There are no apparent age, breed, or sex predilections.

Urticarial reactions are characterized by the sudden onset of more-or-less bilaterally symmetric wheals, which may or may not be erythematous or pruritic. Lesions are typically flat-topped and steep-walled, of normal body temperature, and pit with digital pressure. Lesions may be annular, angular, arciform, or serpiginous. Individual lesions are typically evanescent, disappearing in 24 to 72 hours as new ones appear. They most commonly occur on the trunk and proximal limbs.

BULLOUS PEMPHIGOID

Bullous pemphigoid is a rare autoimmune disease described in adult Yucatan minipigs. Autoantibodies (IgG) target collagen XVII in the lamina lucida of the basement membrane zone.

Turgid, isolated or clustered vesicles occur especially over the dorsum. Vesicles occasionally evolve from erythematous and pruritic patches.

Diagnosis is confirmed by histopathology and immunodiagnostic testing.

REFERENCES

Luting X, et al. 2004. Molecular cloning of a cDNA encoding the porcine type XVII collagen noncollagenous 16A domain and localization of the domain to the upper part of porcine skin basement membrane zone. *Vet Dermatol* 15: 146.

Olivry T, et al. 2000. A spontaneously arising porcine model of bullous pemphigoid. *Arch Dermatol Res* 292: 37.

Scott DW. 1988. Large Animal Dermatology. WB Saunders, Philadelphia, PA

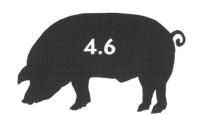

CONGENITAL AND HEREDITARY SKIN DISEASES

APLASIA CUTIS

Aplasia cutis ("epitheliogenesis imperfecta") is thought to be a simple autosomal recessive trait that produces a primary failure of embryonic ectodermal differentiation. It is rare and cosmopolitan.

Aplasia cutis has been seen in several breeds of swine with no sex predilection. The condition may be seen in individual piglets or with a familial incidence in litters. Affected piglets are born with typically one round or elliptical ulcer, 3 to 8 cm in diameter, especially over the back, loins, or leg (Fig. 4.6-1). Hydroureter, hydronephrosis, and skull and ear defects have occasionally been reported.

Diagnosis is based on history and physical examination.

DERMATOSIS VEGETANS

Features

Dermatosis vegetans is a hereditary and often congenital disorder characterized by a symmetrical erythematous maculopapular dermatitis, coronary band and hoof lesions, giant cell pneumonia, and a usually fatal course. It is rare and cosmopolitan. It occurs in Landrace pigs, as a simple autosomal recessive trait, with no sex predilection.

Skin and hoof lesions are often present at birth, but occasionally develop at 2 to 3 weeks of age. A symmetrical, erythematous maculopapular dermatitis develops on the ventral abdomen and medial thighs and spreads to the entire trunk. The skin lesions tend to expand peripherally, coalesce, and develop into dry, brownish-black, papillomatous, crusted plaques (Figs. 4.6-2 and 4.6-3). They are neither pruritic nor painful. The coronary bands become erythematous and edematous and are then covered with a yellowish-brown substance. The hooves become irregularly ridged and dysplastic (Fig. 4.6-4).

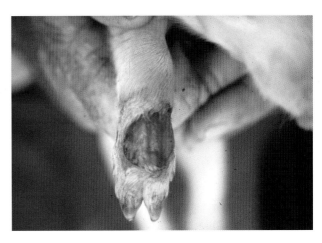

Figure 4.6-1 Aplasia Cutis. Congenital full-thickness ulcer over carpus (courtesy R. Cameron).

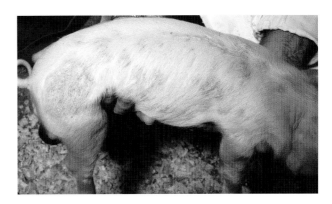

Figure 4.6-2 Dermatosis Vegetans. Multiple annular, heavily crusted plaques over trunk and hip (courtesy D. Percy).

The general condition of the piglets is initially good, but then a gradual deterioration and stunted growth is observed. Most piglets die at 5 to 6 weeks of age. Some piglets are febrile. Respiratory signs (acute or chronic interstitial or bronchopneumonia) precede death. Some piglets recover spontaneously but remain stunted.

Diagnosis

1. History and physical examination.
2. Dermatohistopathology—Intraepidermal pustular dermatitis (eosinophils and neutrophils), and multinucleated histiocytic giant cells in the dermis.

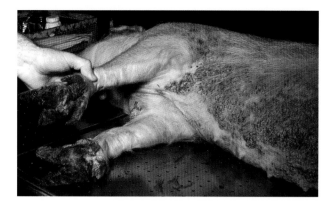

Figure 4.6-3 Dermatosis Vegetans. Coalescent crusted papules on ventrum and dysplastic hooves (courtesy D. Percy).

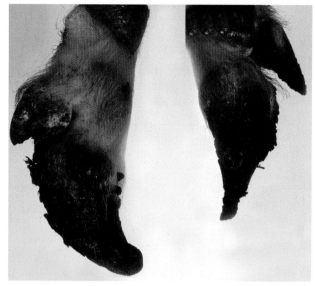

Figure 4.6-4 Dermatosis Vegetans. Dysplastic hooves (courtesy D. Percy).

MISCELLANEOUS CONGENITAL AND HEREDITARY SKIN DISEASES

Table 4.6-1 Miscellaneous Congenital and Hereditary Skin Diseases

Inherited congenital goiter and hairlessness	Very rare; Large Whites and Landrace crosses; probable autosomal recessive; newborn piglets; generalized alopecia and myxedema; goiter; serum concentrations of thyroxine and thyroid gland pathology
Cutaneous asthenia (Ehlers-Danlos Syndrome)	Very rare; Large White-Essex crossbred; born with few to numerous circular to oval, shallow depressions, 3 to 7 cm in diameter, especially over back, flanks, and thighs; affected skin very hyperextensible but not fragile
Focal cutaneous hypoplasia (congenital ectodermal defect)	Very rare; Essex and Large White, and crosses of these; born with 2 to 12 shallow skin depressions, 2 to 5 cm in diameter, irregular in shape, over the thorax and flank; affected skin alopecic and nonpigmented; dermatohistopathology (hypoplastic epidermis and collagen, absent hair follicles and sebaceous glands)
Hair whorls	Rare and cosmopolitan; whorls of hair on neck, rump, loin, and topline of newborn piglets; presumed autosomal recessive
Hypotrichosis	Rare; Mexican hairless and German swine (presumed autosomal dominant); other breeds (presumed autosomal recessive); widespread symmetrical hypotrichosis to alopecia; dermatohistopathology
Iodine deficiency	Very rare; maternal dietary deficiency; newborn piglets generalized alopecia and thick puffy skin (myxedema); systemic signs; serum concentrations of thyroid hormone and thyroid gland pathology
Progressive dermal collagenosis	Rare; Canada; post-puberal male miniature swine; symmetrical firm thickening (10X normal) of trunkal skin; occasionally raised, firm, papules to nodules on scrotum; dermatohistopathology (panniculus, deep dermis, and adnexae replaced by coarse, thick, interwoven collagen bundles)
Subcutaneous hypoplasia	Very rare; Large White; born with shallow depressions, 4 to 6 cm in diameter in skin over flanks and thighs; affected skin neither fragile nor hyperextensible; dermatohistopathology (hypoplasia of subcutis)
Wattles (tassels)	Uncommon and cosmopolitan; no breed or sex predilection; presumed autosomal dominant; congenital cylindrical, teat-like structures, 5 to 7 cm long, hanging from ventral mandibular area; dermatohistopathology

REFERENCES

Dunstan RW, Rosser EJ. 1986. Does a Condition Like Human Pityriasis Rosea Occur in Pigs? *Am J Dermatopathol* 8: 86.

Evensen O. 1993. An Immunohistochemical Study on the Cytogenetic Origin of Pulmonary Multinucleate Giant Cells in Porcine Dermatosis Vegetans. *Vet Pathol* 30: 162.

Evensen O, and Bratberg B. 1990. A Sequential Light Microscopic Study of the Pulmonary Lesions in Porcine Dermatosis Vegetans. *Res Vet Sci* 49: 50.

Howard JC, and Smith RA. 1999. Current Veterinary Therapy. Food Animal Practice. Ed. 4. WB Saunders, Philadelphia, PA.

McEwen BJE. 1993. Progressive Dermal Collagenosis of Male Miniature Swine. *Vet Dermatol* 3: 115.

Radostits OM, et al. 2000. Veterinary Medicine. A Textbook of the Diseases of Cattle, Sheep, Pigs, Goats and Horses. Ed. 9. WB Saunders, Philadelphia, PA.

Scott DW. 1988. Large Animal Dermatology. WB Saunders, Philadelphia, PA.

Straw BE, et al. 1999. Diseases of Swine. Ed 8. Iowa State Press, Ames IA.

Welchman DB, et al. 1994. An Inherited Congenital Goitre in Pigs. *Vet Rec* 135: 589.

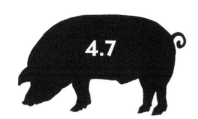

ENVIRONMENTAL SKIN DISEASES

Hematoma
Pressure Sore
Callus
Bites
Porcine Skin Necrosis
Photodermatitis
Miscellaneous Diseases
    Foreign Bodies
    Frostbite
    Polychlorinated Biphenyl Toxicosis
    Primary Irritant Contact Dermatitis
    Stachybotryotoxicosis
    Thallium Toxicosis

HEMATOMA

Features

A hematoma is a circumscribed area of hemorrhage into the tissue arising from vascular damage due to sudden, severe, blunt external trauma (e.g., a fall, a kick).

The lesions are usually acute in onset, subcutaneous, fluctuant, and may or may not be painful. The lesions are usually not warm to the touch. Hematomas are seen most commonly over the shoulder, flanks, and the hind quarters. Aural hematomas (Figs. 4.7-1 through 4.7-3) are most commonly seen in lop-eared breeds, and are associated with head shaking (scabies, pediculosis, meal in ears) or ear biting. Vulvar hematomas are seen in post-partum gilts and sows.

Differential Diagnosis

Abscess, neoplasm.

Diagnosis

1. History and physical examination.
2. Needle aspiration (blood).

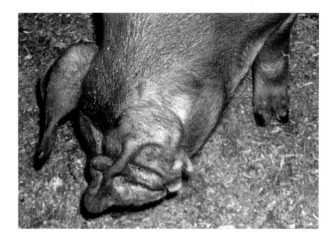

Figure 4.7-2 Cauliflower Ear. Firm, misshapen pinna post-hematoma (courtesy M. Smith).

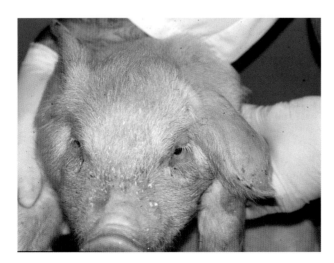

Figure 4.7-1 Hematoma. Left pinna is thickened, fluctuant, and mildly erythematous (courtesy R. Drolet).

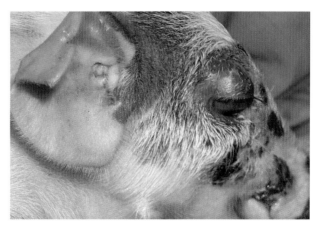

Figure 4.7-3 Hematoma. Right upper eyelid is thickened, fluctuant, and purplish (courtesy M. Smith).

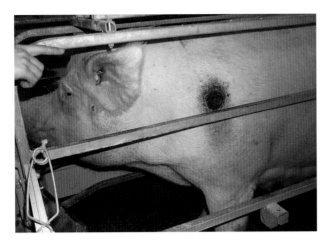

Figure 4.7-4 Pressure Sore. Annular crusted ulcer over left shoulder (courtesy M. Smith).

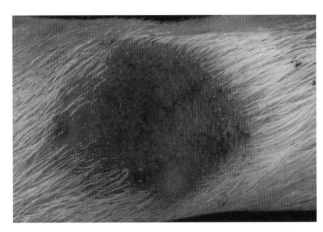

Figure 4.7-6 Callus. Oval, brownish, hyperkeratotic plaque on elbow (courtesy T. Clark).

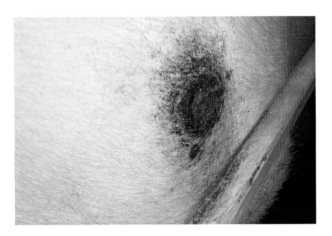

Figure 4.7-5 Close-up of pig in Figure 4.7-4. Annular crusted ulcer (courtesy M. Smith).

PRESSURE SORE

Features

Pressure sores (decubital ulcers) occur as a result of prolonged application of pressure which is concentrated in relatively small areas of the body, and is sufficient to compress the blood vasculature. Pressure sores are common and cosmopolitan. Risk factors include prolonged recumbency during parturition, reduced activity during early lactation, periparturient illness, rough concrete floors, thin body condition, and moist skin.

Pressure sores are most commonly seen in sows, especially on the scapula (Figs. 4.7-4 and 4.7-5), hip, mandible, hock, elbow, and carpus. Initial erythema to red-purple skin discoloration progresses to oozing, necrosis, and ulceration. Ulcers are usually deep and undermined at the edges. Secondary infections are common and healing is very slow.

Diagnosis

1. History and physical examination.

CALLUS

Features

A callus (Latin: hardened skin) is a localized area of epidermal hyperplasia and hyperkeratosis caused by intermittent pressure and friction, resulting in recurrent cutaneous ischemia and hyperplasia. Callosities are common and cosmopolitan and most commonly seen over bony prominences of swine housed on concrete floors with insufficient bedding.

Lesions appear as round or oval hyperkeratotic plaques. Secondary bacterial infection can produce callus pyoderma. Callosities are most commonly seen on the stifle, fetlock, elbow (Fig. 4.7-6), hock, and tuber ischii.

Diagnosis

1. History and physical examination.

BITES

Features

Vulva (Fig. 4.7-7) *and tail* (Fig. 4.7-8) *biting* are significantly associated with increased numbers of culled sows. Risk factors include once-a-day feeding, group size, number of sows per drinker, and providing water automatically.

Flank biting (Fig. 4.7-9) is most commonly seen in early weaned piglets (6 to 20 weeks old), and occasionally in fattening pigs. Erosions, ulcers, and edematous plaques with central necrosis are seen on the flanks, ribs, shoulders, and tuber ischii. Secondary bacterial infection (especially *Staphylococcus hyicus*) is common.

Ear biting (Fig. 4.7-10) may lead to secondary bacterial infection (*Staphylococcus hyicus*, streptococci, *Fusobacterium necrophorum*, spirochetes) and necrosis.

Diagnosis

1. History and physical examination.

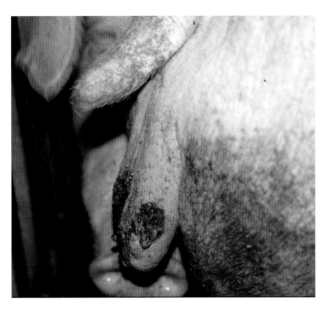

Figure 4.7-7 Vulva Biting. Annular crusted ulcers on vulva (courtesy R. Drolet).

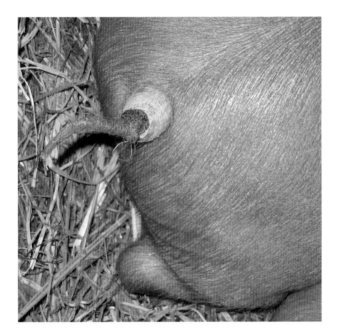

Figure 4.7-8 Tail Biting. Ulceration of tail base with necrosis of distal tail (courtesy M. Smith).

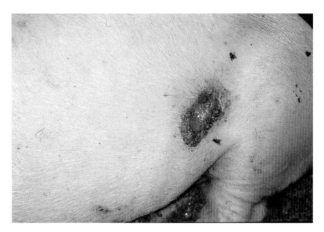

Figure 4.7-9 Flank Biting. Oval crusted ulcer in flank (courtesy R. Drolet).

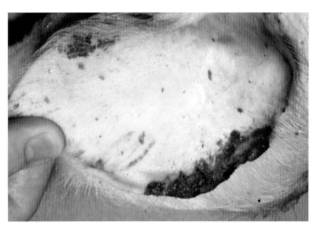

Figure 4.7-10 Ear Biting. Fresh ulcerated bite wounds and a section of necrotic, crusted pinnal margin.

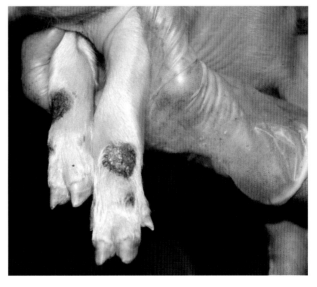

Figure 4.7-11 Skin Necrosis. Bilateral annular, crusted ulcers over carpi (courtesy R. Drolet).

PORCINE SKIN NECROSIS

Features

Porcine skin necrosis is common and cosmopolitan and seen in piglets within a few hours or days of birth. No breed predilection is apparent. The condition is seen most commonly with intensive husbandry systems with minimal bedding, rough concrete flooring, alkaline pH (alkali- and lime-washed pens), and contact dermatitis (caustic agents such as formalin and calcium hypochlorite).

Lesions are usually bilaterally symmetric over bony prominences, especially carpi (Fig. 4.7-11), hocks (Fig. 4.7-12), fetlocks,

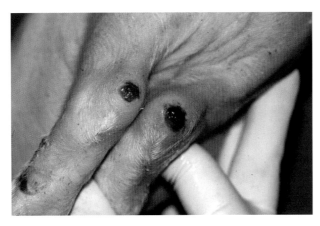

Figure 4.7-12 Skin Necrosis. Bilateral annular ulcers over hocks (courtesy R. Drolet).

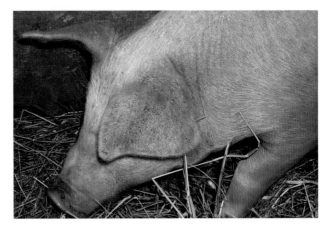

Figure 4.7-14 Photodermatitis. Diffuse erythema due to sunburn (courtesy M. Smith).

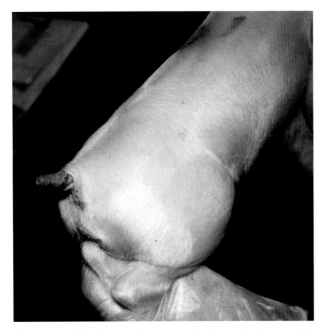

Figure 4.7-13 Skin Necrosis. Necrosis and sloughing of tail (courtesy R. Drolet).

Table 4.7-1 Causes of Primary Photosensitization

Source	Photodynamic Agent
Plants	
St. John's Wort (*Hypericum perforatum*)	Hypericin
Buckwheat (*Fagopyrum esculentum,* *Polygonum fagopyrum*)	Fagopyrin, photofagopyrin
Perennial ryegrass (*Lolium perenne*)	Perloline
Burr trefoil (*Medicago denticulata*)	Aphids
Alfalfa silage	?
Chemicals	
Phenothiazines	
Thiazides	
Acriflavines	
Rose Bengal	
Methylene blue	
Olaquindox	
Sulfonamides	
Tetracyclines	

elbows, teats, coronets, soles, and chin. Initial lesions are red-brown macules and patches which progress through necrosis, ulceration, and crusting.

Tail necrosis (Fig. 4.7-13) begins as erythema on the dorsal tail base. Scaling and fissures develop, and necrosis and ulceration encircle the entire tail root, resulting in sloughing of the tail.

Porcine skin necrosis may affect up to 75% of the litter and up to 50% of the litters. However, mortality and production losses are usually negligible.

Diagnosis

1. History and physical examination.

PHOTODERMATITIS

Features

Photodermatitis (solar dermatitis, actinic dermatitis) is an inflammatory skin disease caused by exposure to ultraviolet light. *Phototoxicity* (sunburn) occurs on white skin, light skin, or damaged skin (e.g., depigmented or scarred) not sufficiently covered by hair (Fig. 4.7-14). *Photosensitization* is classified according to the source of the photodynamic agents: (1) primary photosensitization (a preformed or metabolically-derived photodynamic agent reaches the skin by ingestion, injection, or contact) (Table 4.7-1); and (2) idiopathic photosensitization.

Skin lesions are usually restricted to light-skin, sparsely-haired areas but, in severe cases, can extend into the surrounding dark-skin areas too. Restlessness and discomfort often precede visible skin lesions. Erythema and edema may be followed by vesicles and bullae, ulceration, oozing, crusts, scales, and alopecia (Fig. 4.7-15). Secondary bacterial infections are common. In severe cases, necrosis and sloughing may occur. Variable degrees of pru-

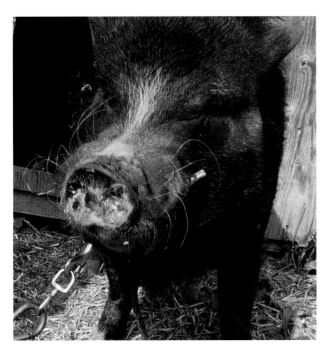

Figure 4.7-15 Photodermatitis. Erythema and ulceration of snout due to photosensitization (courtesy M. Smith).

ritus and pain are present. The muzzle, eyelids, lips, face, pinnae, back, perineum, distal legs, teats, and coronary bands are most commonly affected. In severe cases, pinnae, tail, and teats may slough. Affected animals often attempt to protect themselves from sunlight.

In New Zealand, an ultraviolet light-induced vesiculobullous disease is seen in white pigs eating parsnips or celery infected with the fungus *Sclerotinia sclerotiorum*. Vesicles, bullae, erosions, and ulcers occur on the snout and feet. Oral lesions and systemic signs are absent.

Although photosensitized animals rarely die, resultant weight loss, damaged udders and teats, refusal to allow young to nurse, and secondary infections/flystrike all may lead to appreciable economic loss.

Diagnosis

1. History and physical examination.
2. Primary photodynamic agents can often be identified with various biological assay systems.

MISCELLANEOUS DISEASES

Table 4.7-2 Miscellaneous Environmental Dermatoses

Foreign Bodies	See Box 4.7-1
Frostbite	Rare and cosmopolitan; pinnae, tail tip, teats, scrotum, and feet; pale, hypoesthetic, cool skin that progresses to erythema, edema, scale, alopecia ± necrosis, dry gangrene, and slough
Polychlorinated biphenyl (PCB) toxicosis	Very rare; industrialized areas; eating PCBs which have numerous industrial uses and serious environmental contamination potential; erythema of snout and anus, diarrhea, decreased growth; PCB levels in tissues (especially fat)
Primary irritant contact dermatitis	Uncommon and cosmopolitan; body excretions and secretions (feces, urine, wounds); caustics (acids, alkalis, salt, lime); crude oils and fuels; improper use of topicals; pentachlorophenol (waste motor oil, fungicides, wood preservatives, moth-proofers); bedding; filth; tiamulin (presumably due to tiamulin or a metabolite being passed in urine or feces); variable degrees of dermatitis where exposed to contactant
Stachybotryotoxicosis	Rare; Europe; eating hay and straw contaminated by the fungus *Stachybotrys atra* (macrocyclic trichothecenes); initial necrotic ulcers in mouth and on lips and nostrils; conjunctivitis and rhinitis; later fever, depression, anorexia, diarrhea, weakness, bleeding diathesis; isolate fungus and toxins from feed
Thallium toxicosis	Very rare and cosmopolitan; eating thallium in rodenticides; generalized alopecia and erythema, with necrosis around eyes and mouth; salivation, colic, diarrhea, dyspnea, weakness, emaciation; urine thallium concentration

Box 4.7-1 Draining tracts

- A *fistula* is an abnormal passage or communication, usually between two internal organs or leading from an internal organ to the surface of the body.
- A *sinus* is an abnormal cavity or channel or fistula that permits the escape of pus to the surface of the body.
- Draining tracts are commonly associated with penetrating wounds that have left infectious agents and/or foreign material. Draining tracts may also result from infections of underlying tissues (e.g., bone, joint, lymph node) or previous injections.
- Foreign bodies include wood slivers, plant seeds and awns, cactus tines, fragments of wire, and suture material. Lesions include varying combinations of papules, nodules, abscesses, and draining tracts. Lesions occur most commonly on the legs, hips, muzzle, and ventrum.

REFERENCES

Blowey RW. 1999. Piglet tail necrosis. *Vet Rec* 144: 55.

Davies PR, et al. 1999. Epidemiological study of decubital ulcers in sows. *J Am Vet Med Assoc* 208: 1058.

Howard JL, and Smith RL. 1999. Current Veterinary Therapy. Food Animal Practice. Ed 4. WB Saunders, Philadelphia, PA.

Mirt D. 1999. Lesions of so-called flank biting and necrotic ear syndrome in pigs. *Vet Rec* 144: 92.

Montgomery JF, et al. 1987. A vesiculobullous disease in pigs resembling foot and mouth disease I. Field Cases. *NZ Vet J* 35: 21.

Montgomery JF, et al. 1987. A vesiculobullous disease in pigs resembling foot and mouth disease II. Experimental reproduction of the lesion. *NZ Vet J* 35: 27.

Radostits OM, et al. 2000. Veterinary Medicine. A Textbook of the Diseases of Cattle, Sheep, Pigs, Goats and Horses. Ed 9. WB Saunders, Philadelphia, PA.

Rizvi S, et al. 1998. Risk factors for vulva biting in breeding sows in southwest England. *Vet Rec* 143: 654.

Scott DW. 1988. Large Animal Dermatology. WB Saunders, Philadelphia, PA.

Straw BF, et al. 1999. Diseases of Swine. Ed 8. Iowa State Press, Ames, IA.

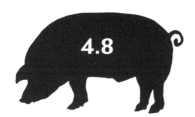

NUTRITIONAL SKIN DISEASES

PARAKERATOSIS

Features

Parakeratosis is an uncommon, cosmopolitan, nutrition-related metabolic disorder. Dietary zinc, essential fatty acids, calcium and other chelating agents, and other disease conditions play a role in the pathogenesis of the disorder. There are no apparent breed, or sex predilections, and the disorder typically occurs in housed feeder pigs between the ages of 7 and 20 weeks.

More-or-less symmetrical erythematous macules and papules appear on the ventral abdomen and medial thighs. The dermatitis then becomes widespread, especially the legs, ventrum, face, pinnae, and tail (Figs. 4.8-1 to 4.8-3). Hard, dry, brownish-to-blackish crusts develop. Pruritus and greasiness are absent. Secondary bacterial infections and subcutaneous abscesses are not uncommon. Systemic signs are frequently present. Multiple animals are typically affected.

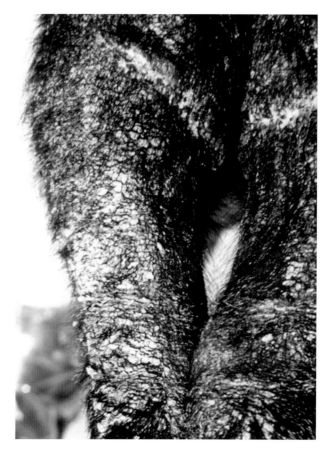

Figure 4.8-2 Parakeratosis. Thick crusts on legs.

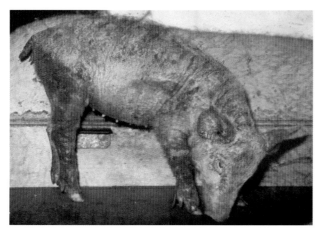

Figure 4.8-1 Parakeratosis. Widespread erythema and crusting.

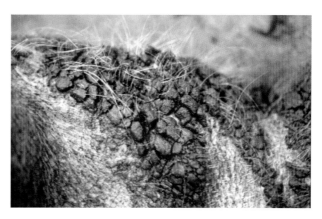

Figure 4.8-3 Parakeratosis. Thick, black, fissured crusts.

Differential Diagnosis

None.

Diagnosis

1. Dermatohistopathology—Hyperplastic to spongiotic superficial perivascular-to-interstitial dermatitis with marked diffuse parakeratotic hyperkeratosis and a lymphoeosinophilic inflammatory infiltrate.
2. Analysis of diet.
3. Response to therapy.

MISCELLANEOUS NUTRITIONAL DISORDERS

Table 4.8-1 Miscellaneous Nutritional Disorders

Essential fatty acid deficiency	Very rare; deficient diet; generalized scaling and alopecia; brownish exudate on ears, axillae, and flanks; increased susceptibility to skin infection; EFA levels in diet
Vitamin A deficiency	Very rare; deficient diet; rough, dry, faded haircoat and generalized seborrhea; systemic signs; serum and liver concentrations of vitamin A, and vitamin A levels in diet
Biotin deficiency	Very rare; deficient diet; generalized scaling, crusting, and alopecia; ulcers on thighs and abdomen; systemic signs; biotin levels in diet
Niacin deficiency	Very rare; deficient diet; generalized scaling and crusting; systemic signs; niacin levels in diet
Pantothenic acid deficiency	Very rare; deficient diet; patchy alopecia and periocular accumulation of brown exudate; systemic signs; pantothenic acid levels in diet
Riboflavin deficiency	Very rare; deficient diet; generalized scaling and focal ulcers; systemic signs; riboflavin deficiency in diet
Vitamin E deficiency	Very rare; deficient diet; newborn piglets; generalized scaly skin; systemic signs; plasma concentration of vitamin E, vitamin E levels in diet
Iodine deficiency	Very rare; maternal dietary deficiency; newborn piglets; generalized alopecia and thick puffy skin (myxedema); systemic signs; serum concentration of thyroid hormone and thyroid gland pathology

REFERENCES

Howard JL, Smith RA. 1999. Current Veterinary Therapy. Food Animal Practice. Ed 4. WB Saunders, Philadelphia, PA.

Radostits OM, et al. 2000. Veterinary Medicine. A Textbook of the Diseases of Cattle, Sheep, Pigs, Goats and Horses. Ed 9. WB Saunders, Philadelphia, PA.

Scott DW. 1988. Large Animal Dermatology. WB Saunders, Philadelphia, PA.

Straw BE. 1999. Diseases of Swine. Ed 8. Iowa State Press, Ames, IA.

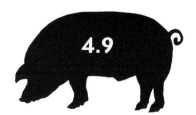

MISCELLANEOUS SKIN DISEASES

Juvenile Pustular Psoriasiform Dermatitis
Other Disorders
    Dermatosis Erythematosa
    Hyperkeratosis
    Porcine Ulcerative Dermatitis Syndrome
    Recurrent Dermatosis of Sows
    Vices

JUVENILE PUSTULAR PSORIASIFORM DERMATITIS

Features

Juvenile pustular psoriasiform dermatitis ("pityriasis rosea") is a common, cosmopolitan disorder. The cause and pathogenesis are unknown, but heredity appears to play a role. The condition occurs in 3–14 week old piglets of either sex, and white breeds—especially Landrace—seem to be more commonly affected.

A more-or-less symmetrical distribution of erythematous macules and papules begins on the ventral abdomen and medial thighs, and extends to involve most of the ventrum, and occasionally the lateral and dorsal aspects of the trunk (Figs. 4.9-1 to 4.9-4). Lesions enlarge peripherally, develop central craters, and become covered with bran-like scale. Evolution of lesions usually produces annular, arciform, serpiginous and polycyclic shapes. Pruritus is absent, and affected animals are usually otherwise healthy. One or multiple piglets in a litter may be affected.

Differential Diagnosis

Swinepox, dermatosis vegetans.

Diagnosis

1. Culture—Sterile.
2. Dermatohistopathology—Psoriasiform superficial perivascular-to-interstitial dermatitis with prominent parakeratotic hyperkeratosis and numerous eosinophils and neutrophils. Intraepidermal pustules containing eosinophils and neutrophils are prominent in early lesions.

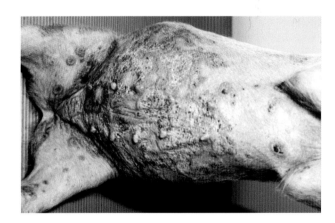

Figure 4.9-2 Juvenile Pustular Psoriasiform Dermatitis. Annular and coalescent erythematous plaques, many with central depressions covered with brownish scale.

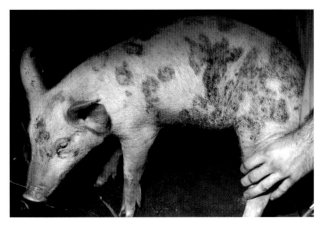

Figure 4.9-1 Juvenile Pustular Psoriasiform Dermatitis. Multiple annular to polycyclic areas of erythema and crusting.

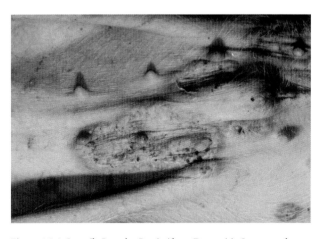

Figure 4.9-3 Juvenile Pustular Psoriasiform Dermatitis. Large, erythematous plaques with central healing and thin brownish scale.

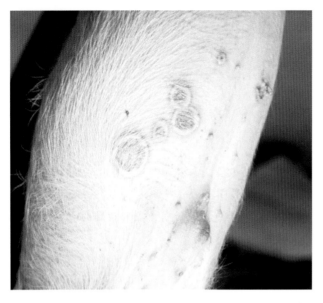

Figure 4.9-4 Juvenile Pustular Psoriasiform Dermatitis. Anular, pustular plaques with central depression and brownish scale.

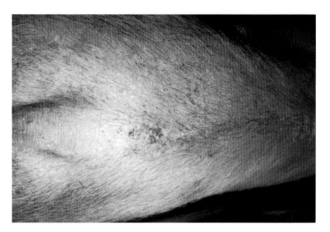

Figure 4.9-5 Hyperkeratosis. Waxy brown scale and crust over dorsum.

OTHER DISORDERS

Table 4.9-1 Miscellaneous Skin Disorders	
Dermatosis erythematosa	Common (?); idiopathic; adults; indoors or outdoors; acute erythema over large areas of body (especially pinnae, sides, abdomen); nonpruritic, nonpainful; otherwise healthy
Hyperkeratosis (Figs. 4.9-5 and 4.9-6)	Common; idiopathic; intensively-housed sows and boars; brownish, waxy material accumulates (normal skin underneath); localized to dorsal neck and shoulders, or entire dorsum and flanks; nonpruritic; healthy otherwise
Porcine ulcerative dermatitis syndrome (Figs. 4.9-7 and 4.9-8)	Uncommon and cosmopolitan; mostly adult sows; chronic ulcers with thickened margins and crusts; especially perineum, lateral thighs, mammae, lateral thorax, lateral abdomen, and convex surface of pinnae; lesions may resolve during lactation, but reappear after weaning; dermatohistopathology
Recurrent dermatosis of sows (Figs. 4.9-9 and 4.9-10)	Rare; idiopathic; sows; occurs/recurs in farrowing house, disappears after leaving farrowing house; erythematous macules and patches enlarge and become scaly; hairs in lesion become discolored brown; especially on trunk, and only in white skin; no pruritus; otherwise healthy
Vices	Common and cosmopolitan; stressors include increased competition for space, food, and water; *tail biting* (growing pigs) and *vulva biting* (especially late pregnancy)

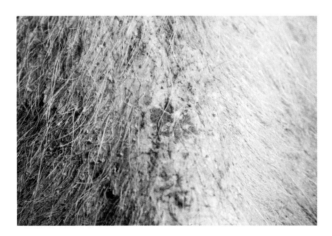

Figure 4.9-6 Close-up of Figure 4.9-5.

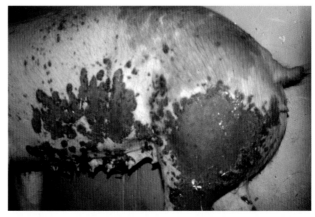

Figure 4.9-7 Porcine Ulcerative Dermatitis Syndrome. Ulcers with thickened, crusted margins on thigh, side, and mammae.

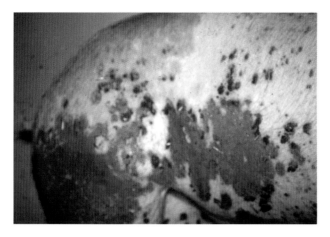

Figure 4.9-8 Same pig as in Figure 4.9-7. Ulcerative lesions on other side.

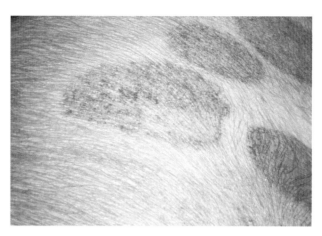

Figure 4.9-10 Close-up of Figure 4.9-9. Brownish discoloration of hairs.

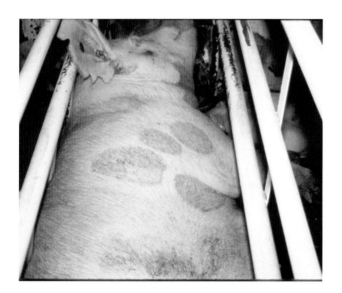

Figure 4.9-9 Recurrent Dermatosis of Sows. Annular areas of erythema.

REFERENCES

Dunstan RW, Rosser EJ. 1986. Does a condition like human pityriasis rosea occur in pigs? *Am J Dermatopathol* 8: 86.

Howard JL, Smith RA. 1999. Current Veterinary Therapy. Food Animal Practice. Ed 4. WB Saunders, Philadelphia, PA.

Schmoll F, et al. 2004. Clinical and pathological features of the porcine ulcerative dermatitis syndrome (PUDS). *J Vet Med A* 51: 15.

Scott DW. 1988. Large Animal Dermatology. WB Saunders, Philadelphia, PA.

Scott DW, et al. 1989. Clinicopathologic studies on a chronic, recurrent dermatosis of sows. *Agri-Pract* 10: 43.

White M. 1999. Skin lesions in pigs. *In Pract* 21: 20.

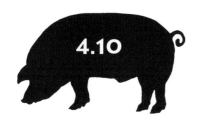

NEOPLASTIC AND NON-NEOPLASTIC GROWTHS

4.10

PAPILLOMA

Features

Papillomas are rare, cosmopolitan, benign neoplasms of keratinocytes. Viral etiology is suspected but not proved. No age, breed, or sex predilections are apparent. Congenital papillomas have been reported.

Lesions may be solitary or multiple, and commonly affect the face and external genitalia (Fig. 4.10-1). Lesions are dome-shaped to pedunculated, 3 to 15 cm in diameter, and cauliflower-like. The surface is hyperkeratotic and may have frond-like keratinous projections.

Differential Diagnosis

Scrotal hemangiomas.

Diagnosis

1. Dermatohistopathology.

HEMANGIOMA

Features

Hemangiomas are uncommon, cosmopolitan, benign neoplasms of endothelial cells. They occur most frequently in the scrotum of Yorkshire and Berkshire boars, and may be hereditary. Nonscrotal hemangiomas may occur anywhere on the body, may be congenital, and have no apparent age, breed, or sex predilections.

Scrotal hemangiomas begin as multiple, tiny reddish to purplish papules and become increasingly hyperkeratotic and verru-

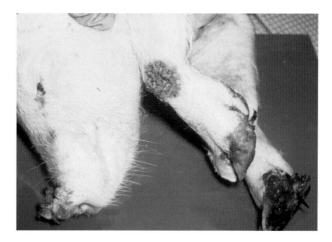

Figure 4.10-1 Papillomas. Multiple, clustered, hyperkeratotic, cauliflower-like lesions on snout and carpus.

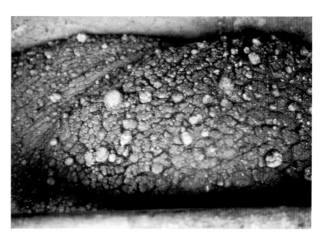

Figure 4.10-2 Hemangiomas. Multiple hyperkeratotic papules on scrotum.

cous in appearance (Fig. 4.10-2). Nonscrotal hemangiomas are typically solitary and can occur anywhere on the body. Solitary hemangiomas are typically reddish to bluish to blackish in color, fluctuant, and may bleed easily.

Differential Diagnosis

Papillomas (scrotal hemangiomas), hemangiosarcoma, melanocytic neoplasm.

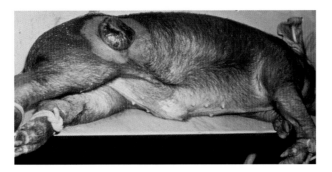

Figure 4.10-3 Melanoma. Large, firm, melanotic, ulcerated tumor in flank (area has been clipped and scrubbed with povidone-iodine).

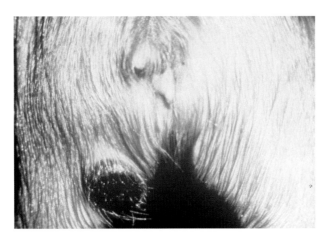

Figure 4.10-4 Melanocytoma. Firm, melanotic nodule on caudal thigh.

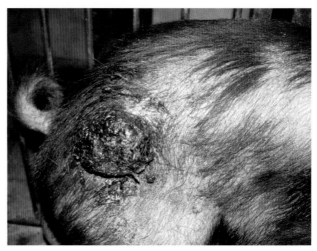

Figure 4.10-5 Melanoma. Ulcerated, melanotic tumor on hip (courtesy R. Drolet).

Diagnosis

1. Dermatohistopathology.

MELANOCYTIC NEOPLASMS

Features

Melanocytic neoplasms (benign or malignant proliferations of melanocytes) are generally rare and cosmopolitan in swine. However, melanocytic neoplasms occur frequently in certain breeds: Duroc, Sinclair miniature, Hormel, Hampshire, and Iberian. The predisposition is hereditary in the latter four breeds, and is an au-tosomal dominant trait in Durocs and Sinclair miniatures. In the predisposed breeds, melanocytic neoplasms may be congenital or appear early in life. There is no apparent sex predilection.

In the predilected breeds, the vast majority of neoplasms are melanocytomas (benign) as opposed to melanomas (malignant). Lesions may be solitary or multiple, and can occur anywhere on the body, especially the trunk (Figs. 4.10-3 to 4.10-5). Lesions vary from well-circumscribed, flat, and evenly pigmented, to ir-regular, nodular, variably pigmented, and ulcerated. Lesions vary from 0.3 to 25 cm diameter. Up to 95% of affected piglets undergo complete spontaneous remission by one year of age. Regression may be associated with the development of vitiligo and perilesional depigmentation. Up to 95% of the animals in affected herds can be affected.

Differential Diagnosis

Hemangioma and hemangiosarcoma (solitary lesions).

Diagnosis

1. Microscopy (direct smears)—Melanocytes showing variable degrees of melanization and atypia.
2. Dermatohistopathology.

MISCELLANEOUS NEOPLASTIC AND NON-NEOPLASTIC GROWTHS

Table 4.10-1 Miscellaneous Neoplastic and Non-Neoplastic Growths

Squamous cell carcinoma	Rare; adult to aged; solitary or multiple ulcerated plaques or nodules; white skin; malignant; direct smears and dermatohistopathology
Fibroma (fibrous polyp)	Rare; adult to aged; especially sows; solitary polyp or nodule; anywhere (especially pinna, neck, back); benign; direct smears and dermatohistopathology
Fibrosarcoma (Fig. 4.10-6)	Very rare; adult to aged; rarely congenital; solitary nodule, up to 15 cm diameter; anywhere (especially sternum); malignant; dermatohistopathology
Fibroleiomyoma	Very rare; adult; solitary crusted nodule, 2.5 cm diameter; pinna; benign; dermatohistopathology
Epitrichial (apocrine) adenoma	Very rare; adult; solitary nodule; anywhere; benign; direct smears and dermatohistopathology
Neurofibroma (neurofibromatosis) (Figs. 4.10-7 and 4.10-8)	Rare and geographically restricted; probably hereditary; 1% to 7% of piglets affected; one or multiple firm, dermal or subcutaneous nodules, up to 30 cm diameter; anywhere; benign; dermatohistopathology
Hemangiosarcoma	Very rare; adult; solitary nodule; anywhere; malignant; dermatohistopathology
Mast Cell Tumor	Very rare; adult; single or multiple, firm to fluctuant, dermal to subcutaneous papules and nodules (0.2 to 2 cm diameter); anywhere; benign or malignant; direct smears and dermatohistopathology
Histiocytosis	Very rare; congenital; generalized purpuric macules and papules; dermatohistopathology
Actinic Keratosis	Rare; adult to aged; ultraviolet light damaged white skin; solitary or multiple erythematous, scaly, crusty, hyperkeratotic plaques; pre-malignant; dermatohistopathology
Organoid Nevus (Fig. 4.10-9)	Very rare; congenital; solitary polyp on pinna; benign; dermatohistopathology

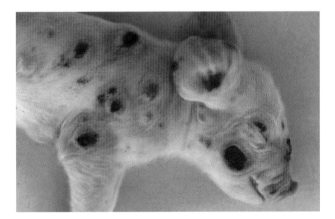

Figure 4.10-6 Congenital Fibrosarcomas. Multiple ulcerated nodules (courtesy H. Morvan, coll. J. Gourreau, AFSSA).

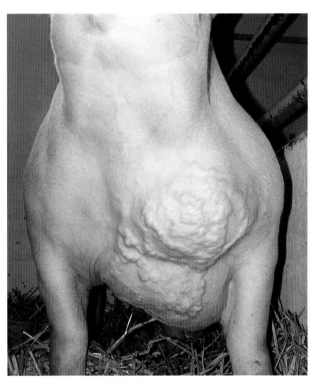

Figure 4.10-7 Neurofibroma. Large, multilobulated tumor on neck and sternum (courtesy J. Gourreau).

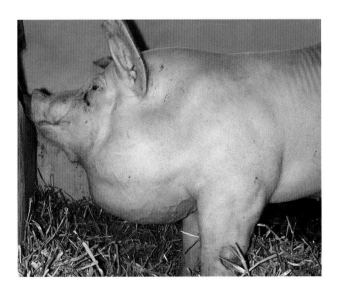

Figure 4.10-8 Neurofibroma. Huge tumor on neck (courtesy J. Gourreau).

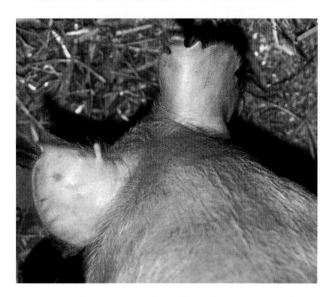

Figure 4.10-9 Organoid Nevus. Finger-like projection near base of left ear.

REFERENCES

Howard JO, Smith RL. 1999. Current Veterinary Therapy. Food Animal Practice. Ed 4. WB Saunders, Philadelphia, PA.

Jeong SM, et al. 2003. Subcutaneous Fibrosarcoma with Low Malignancy in a Pig. *Vet Rec* 152: 720.

Morvan H, et al. 2004. Neurofibromatose chez le Porc: un Nouveau Syndrome. *Bull Acad Vét France* 157: 31.

Nakamura T, et al. 1987. Fibroleiomyoma on a sow ear. *Jpn J Vet Sci* 49: 1177.

Scott DW. 1988. Large Animal Dermatology. WB Saunders, Philadelphia, PA.

Vítovec J, et al. 1999. Congenital Fibropapillomatosis in a Piglet. *Vet Pathol* 36: 83.

Zibrín M, et al. 2000. The Spontaneous Regression of Congenital Melanomas in Pigs: the Ultrastructure and Role of Macrophages, Mast Cells, and Plasma Cells. *Folia Vet* 44: 179.

INDEX

Italicized page locators indicate a figure; tables are noted with a *t* following the page locator.

A

A. israelii, actinomycosis and, 8

Abscess, 107*t*
 bacterial, 14*t*
 diagnosis of, porcine, 202
 features and differential diagnosis of, porcine, 201
 ovine, 155*t*
 subcutaneous, *14*
  on caudal aspect of udder, due to *Corynebacterium pseudotuberculosis, 108*
  on chest, due to *Corynebacterium pseudotuberculosis, 108*
  huge abscess involving face and neck due to *Arcanobacterium pyogenes, 203*
  multiple abscesses on left thoracic limb, *203*

Acral lick dermatitis, *89*

Actinic dermatitis, 77, 138, 182, 228

Actinic keratosis, 99*t,* 147*t*
 multiple crusts on lower eyelid, *99*
 ovine, 192*t*
 porcine, 239*t*

Actinobacillosis, 107*t,* 155*t*
 features and differential diagnosis/diagnosis of, bovine, 10
 firm, movable swelling over mandible, *155*
 multiple ulcerated nodules over back, *11*
 porcine, 205*t*
 ulcerated
  crusted mass subsequent to dehorning operation, *11*
  subcutaneous mass below ear, *11*

Actinobacillus lignieresii, 10
 actinomycosis and, 9
 Corynebacterium pseudotuberculosis granuloma and, 6

Actinomyces bovis, 10
 actinomycosis and, 8
 Corynebacterium pseudotuberculosis granuloma and, 6

Actinomycetic mycetoma, 107*t*

Actinomycosis, 8–10
 differential diagnosis/diagnosis of, bovine, 9–10
 features and differential diagnosis/diagnosis of, porcine, 202
 features of, bovine, 8
 firm, immovable, ulcerated nodule with draining tracts on mandible, *10*
 firm, immovable swelling over mandible, *9*
 firm, immovable swelling with alopecia and crusting over mandible, *9*

firm, ulcerated nodule with draining tracts on udder, *10*
 firm tumor in flank, *203*
 seropurulent exudate containing "sulfur granules" in a stainless steel bowl, *10, 203*

Actinomycosis ("lumpy jaw"), 107*t*

Acute erysipelas, 200
 widespread annular to angular papules and plaques, some of which have central necrosis, *201*

Acute exudative epidermitis, 197

Adenovirus infection, in swine, 218*t*

African swine fever *(Iridovirus),* 218*t*

Alcelaphine herpesvirus 1, *39*

"Allerton virus" (pseudolumpy skin disease), 48*t*

Alopecia areata, 55–56
 annular area of, with regrowth of fine, white hairs, *56*
 differential diagnosis/diagnosis of, bovine, 56
 features of, bovine, 55
 multiple annular to oval areas of, over cheek, neck, and shoulder, *55*
 multiple annular to oval areas of, over face and neck, *55*
 periocular alopecia with regrowth of fine, white hairs, *55*
 two annular areas of, on head, *55*

Amanita toxicosis, 79*t*

Anagen defluxion ("anagen effluvium"), 87–89, 189–190
 alopecia occurring seven days after onset of fever and diarrhea, *189*
 alopecia on leg beginning several days after onset of fever and pneumonia, *88*
 alopecic tail, *89*
 diagnosis of, bovine, 89
 differential diagnosis of, bovine, 87
 easy epilation of wool, *189*
 facial alopecia, *190*
 features and differential diagnosis/diagnosis of, ovine, 189
 features of, bovine, 87
 widespread alopecia associated with pneumonia, *88*
 widespread alopecia associated with severe systemic illness, *189*

Angora goats
 occurrence of papillomas in, 145
 squamous cell carcinoma in, 146

Angus cattle
 epidermolysis bullosa in, 62
 hereditary zinc deficiency in, 64

Anthrax, 14*t,* 155*t*
 porcine, 205*t*

"Aphthous fever," 42, 129*t,* 171, 216

Aphthovirus
 foot-and-mouth disease and seven principal serotypes of, 216–217
 foot-and-mouth disease caused by, 42

Aplasia cutis ("epitheliogenesis imperfecta"), 180*t,* 223
 congenital full thickness ulcer over carpus, *223*

Arcanobacterium pyogenes, 10
 abscess and, 201
 actinomycosis and, 9
 clostridial cellulitis and, 11
 Corynebacterium pseudotuberculosis granuloma and, 6
 huge subcutaneous abscess due to, *203*
 spirochetosis and, 199
 ulcerative lymphangitis and, 5

Arsenic toxicosis, 79*t*

Aspergillosis, 19*t,* 114*t*
 aborted fetus; multiple annular, brownish-black, felt-like lesions on skin, *19*
 porcine, 208*t*

Atopic dermatitis
 alopecia, hyperpigmentation, and lichenification of udder, ventral abdomen, ventral thorax, and axillae, *176*
 alopecia, hyperpigmentation, lichenification, and excoriation in perineum, *176*
 crust and alopecia on pinna, *176*
 ovine, 175
 periocular scale, crust, and hypotrichosis, *176*

Aujeszky's disease (pseudorabies), 48*t,* 129*t,* 174*t*

Aural hematomas, 225

Australian Border Leicester-Southdown crossbred lambs, cutaneous asthenia in, 177

Ayrshires
 epidermolysis bullosa in, 62
 semi-hairlessness in, 60
 viable hypotrichosis in, 60

B

Bacterial infections
 differential diagnosis for symmetrical cyanotic extremities, 204*t*
 differential diagnosis for symmetrical sloughing of extremities, 204*t*

Bacterial pseudomycetoma ("botryomycosis"), 14*t*

Bacterial skin diseases
 bovine, 3–16
 bovine, miscellaneous, 13, 14*t*
 caprine, 103–109
 caprine, miscellaneous, 107*t*
 ovine, 151–155